HIGH-YIELD
COGNITIVE-BEHAVIOR THERAPY
FOR BRIEF SESSIONS

AN ILLUSTRATED GUIDE

High-Yield
COGNITIVE-BEHAVIOR THERAPY
FOR **BRIEF SESSIONS**

An Illustrated Guide

Jesse H. Wright, M.D., Ph.D.
Professor and Vice Chair for Academic Affairs, Department of Psychiatry and Behavioral Sciences; Director, Depression Center, University of Louisville, Kentucky

Donna M. Sudak, M.D.
Professor of Psychiatry and Director of Psychotherapy Training, Drexel University College of Medicine, Philadelphia, Pennsylvania

Douglas Turkington, M.D.
Professor of Psychosocial Psychiatry, Institute of Neuroscience, Newcastle University, Royal Victoria Infirmary; Consultant Liaison Psychiatrist with Northumberland, Tyne and Wear NHS Trust, St. Nicholas Hospital, Gosforth, Newcastle-upon-Tyne, United Kingdom

Michael E. Thase, M.D.
Professor of Psychiatry and Director of the Mood and Anxiety Disorders Section, University of Pennsylvania School of Medicine, Philadelphia, Pennsylvania

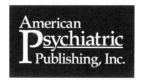

American Psychiatric Publishing, Inc.

Washington, DC
London, England

If you would like to buy between 25 and 99 copies of this or any other APPI title, you are eligible for a 20% discount; please contact APPI Customer Service at appi@psych.org or 800–368–5777. If you wish to buy 100 or more copies of the same title, please e-mail us at bulksales@psych.org for a price quote.

Copyright © 2010 American Psychiatric Publishing, Inc.
ALL RIGHTS RESERVED

Manufactured in the United States of America on acid-free paper
14 13 12 11 10   5 4 3 2 1
First Edition

Typeset in Adobe's Berling Roman and Frutiger.

American Psychiatric Publishing, Inc.
1000 Wilson Boulevard
Arlington, VA 22209–3901
www.appi.org

Library of Congress Cataloging-in-Publication Data
High-yield cognitive-behavior therapy for brief sessions : an illustrated guide / Jesse H. Wright ... [et al.].—1st ed.
      p. ; cm.
   Includes bibliographical references and index.
   ISBN 978-1-58562-362-4 (alk. paper)
  1. Cognitive therapy. 2. Brief psychotherapy. 3. Behavior therapy. I. Wright, Jesse H.
   [DNLM: 1. Cognitive Therapy—methods. 2. Mental Disorders—therapy. 3. Psychotherapy, Brief—methods. WM 425.5.C6 H638 2010]

   RC489.C63H54 2010
   616.89'1425—dc22
                                                                2010000569

British Library Cataloguing in Publication Data
A CIP record is available from the British Library.

Contents

List of Learning Exercises

LIST OF VIDEO ILLUSTRATIONS

Foreword

The authors begin this book with an important query: "Why should psychiatrists and other clinicians who prescribe medications consider using cognitive-behavior therapy (CBT) methods in brief sessions?" They answer with a powerful litany. CBT methods in brief sessions help produce better outcomes, promote adherence, help control co-occurring or co-existing components of major syndromes, aid in preventing recurrences, and accomplish these goals in briefer times. Perhaps that says enough. But to further encourage readers to learn more, I will substantiate the authors' rationale with additional perspectives. For brevity, I will focus on depression and bipolar disorders but fully recognize that the described CBT methods for brief sessions are applicable to other diagnoses as well.

We are in an exciting era of translational, personalized health care. One of this era's goals is to generate convincing new knowledge about really important clinical questions, such as the best and quickest ways to treat clinical depression and prevent recurrences. A second is to develop personalized treatments that work best for "me"—for *my* particular type of disorder, recognizing that my genes, my coping mechanisms, and my stresses may be different from yours. A third is to integrate knowledge from various fields by linking basic research advances with clinical acumen and experience; this goal intriguingly forces us to meld together what works best in clinical care rather than continually debating unhelpful questions that emphasize "versus," such as medications "versus" psychotherapy. A final goal is to more rapidly apply the knowledge that we are accumulating: "Knowledge heals"—but only when translated. This book provides a roadmap of the growing knowledge of CBT for brief sessions. It translates currently known best ways for clinicians to use front-line treatments in personalized, integrated approaches to help patients reach their desired destinations most effectively. In that sense, it is a vital part of our treatment roadmap.

What justifies this book being written now? We might start with the observation that pharmacotherapy and CBT are the best-documented pillars of treatment for major depressive disorder and related conditions and for most other major brain disorders. These two modalities are metaphorically the proud parents of most of the family of evidence-based tools in our treatment portfolio for mood disorders. Second, psychiatrists, psychologists, psychiatric social workers, and mental health workers of all disciplines work in an era when evidence of effectiveness must be presented, sometimes even to obtain reimbursement. Finally, while we may not like it, clinicians' time pressures are relentless. Integrating these observations explains why mental health professionals of all disciplines have little choice but to learn and incorporate CBT into their treatment armamentarium.

To further answer "why now?", using depression and bipolar disorder as illustrations, data repeatedly demonstrate that the 21% of Americans with meaningful clinical depressions and bipolar disorder almost always have better outcomes when pharmacotherapy and CBT—these two pillars—are combined, and this book guides the clinician in how to do it, providing illustrations to help show the way. The authors also address the often overlooked but arguably most important clinical challenge: once we get people better, how do we keep them better? Maintenance pharmacotherapy has been demonstrated to achieve this goal, among many. Maintenance CBT studies are fewer, so more research remains to be done—but already consistent with emerging trends, early evidence suggests that the combination of pharmacotherapy and CBT may provide the best approach to sustainability of wellness.

Drs. Wright, Sudak, Turkington, and Thase are icons in studying these two pillars—leaders in developing, refining, testing, teaching, and integrating CBT methods with the best of psychopharmacology. They study what they do, apply what they learn, continually challenge their assumptions, and always seek to integrate new advances. This iterative model has helped catalyze the progress that has occurred.

And the best may be yet to come. For psychiatry and other mental health professionals to achieve breakthroughs beyond the gains described in this text, we will need to evaluate treatment strategies among very large samples of individuals that are simultaneously assessed with standardized biomarkers, such as genetic/genomic, stress measures, neuroimaging, sleep, and immune responses. We have learned from colleagues studying cancer, cardiovascular, diabetes, and other diseases that we will only achieve true breakthroughs by developing large, integrated, standardized, and sustainable networks of centers of excellence. Happily, such a network has recently been established for depression, bipolar disorders, and related conditions: the National Network of Depression Centers (http://nndc.org). Drs. Wright and Thase are part of this network, and by working with NNDC colleagues, we might optimistically anticipate that future editions of this book will address advances that have occurred from studying tens of thousands of patients rather than being limited to the tens or hundreds that now tend to be our norm. The best is yet to come, and this text will help us achieve it.

John F. Greden, M.D.
Rachel Upjohn Professor of Psychiatry and Clinical Neurosciences; Founder and Executive Director, University of Michigan Comprehensive Depression Center; Founding Chair, National Network of Depression Centers; Research Professor, Molecular and Behavioral Neuroscience Institute, University of Michigan, Ann Arbor, Michigan

Preface

In the courses and workshops we teach on cognitive-behavior therapy (CBT), we have been hearing an increasing chorus of requests to help practicing clinicians learn how to use key CBT methods along with psychopharmacology in brief sessions. These requests are pertinent 1) because most psychiatrists and other clinicians who use psychopharmacology in treatment of mental disorders are devoting large portions of their practice to sessions that are briefer than the traditional "50-minute hour" and 2) because medications, while invaluable, frequently do not provide full relief from the symptoms of mental illness. If clinicians want to offer more than symptom assessment and medication management in these sessions, how can they pragmatically apply CBT methods to enhance the treatment process?

As psychiatrists who have been trained in both pharmacotherapy and CBT, we have been using a combined approach in brief sessions for a number of years and have learned ways of infusing these sessions with the collaborative-empirical style of CBT. We have also been working on methods of efficiently using "high yield" techniques to target specific symptoms or problems and have drawn on these experiences to write this guide to combining CBT and pharmacotherapy in brief sessions. The methods described here are offered as suggestions or clinical tips, not as a scientifically proven treatment approach. Randomized controlled trials of CBT have focused heavily on implementation in 45–60 minute sessions. Research on CBT in brief sessions is clearly needed, but we believe that there has been enough clinical experience in using CBT in shorter sessions with medication to present guidelines for practitioners who want to use this approach.

The book begins with chapters that 1) describe basic principles for combining CBT with pharmacotherapy in brief sessions, 2) explain the comprehensive cognitive-behavioral-biological-sociocultural model for treatment, and 3) describe indications and applications of the brief session format. Because CBT is formulation driven, even in shorter sessions, a chapter is included on how to perform a succinct case conceptualization, construct a "mini-formulation," and plan treatment interventions. Also, an early chapter discusses ways of promoting effective therapeutic relationships when brief sessions are being used. The first four chapters cover the core methods of combined CBT and pharmacotherapy that provide a solid platform for implementation of the specific procedures described in subsequent chapters.

Portions of the book devoted to targeted applications of CBT cover topics that we have found to be especially important in treatment of a broad range of clinical conditions, including mood and anxiety disorders and psychoses. One of the most important chapters is on medication adherence. Application of CBT in brief sessions might be justified by this indication alone because of the very high rate of nonadherence to psychotropic medications and the strong evidence for effectiveness of CBT in improving adherence. We think that CBT offers very practical methods for adherence that are easily adapted for use in medication management.

Other chapters focus on some of the key elements of CBT that we have found to be particularly helpful in brief sessions. These include behavioral methods for depression and anxiety, cognitive restructuring techniques, and interventions to reduce hopelessness and suicidality. Behavioral methods such as activity scheduling, graded task assignments, exposure and response prevention, and breathing retraining can be explained in brief sessions, assigned for homework, and followed up at subsequent visits. Simple, targeted cognitive restructuring can be performed either to reverse maladaptive patterns of thinking in mood disorders or to assist with other therapy tasks such as improving adherence. CBT methods can also be very helpful in working with patients who have hopelessness and suicidal thinking. Although longer sessions or hospitalization may be needed when suicide risk is high, we describe how CBT may have a place in shorter sessions for patients who are hopeless and despairing.

Insomnia is another very useful application for CBT in brief sessions. CBT has been shown to be at least as effective as sleeping medication for insomnia and does not have problems with side effects, tolerance, or rebound insomnia. In Chapter 10, "CBT Methods for Insomnia," we outline the CBT approach to insomnia including education on sleep hygiene, restructuring of cognitions about sleep, use of relaxation and imagery strategies, sleep logs, and other valuable techniques.

Chapter 11, "Modifying Delusions," and Chapter 12, "Coping With Hallucinations," deal with specialized CBT interventions for patients with delusions or hallucinations. Often, briefer sessions are preferentially selected for patients with psychotic disorders because problems with attention span, concentration, or agitation may decrease the value of longer interventions. After establishing a collaborative therapeutic relationship, clinicians can help normalize symptoms, perform effective psychoeducation, modify delusional thinking, and teach methods for coping with hallucinations. CBT methods for adherence described earlier in the book are especially helpful for working with patients with psychotic disorders.

CBT is gaining increasing acceptance in the treatment of substance abuse and can be delivered in some instances in short sessions in combination with other approaches, such as pharmacotherapy and 12-step involvement. For example, the authors have had positive outcomes of treatment of individuals with alcohol addiction who were seen for brief CBT-oriented sessions on a weekly basis, in addition to attending AA meetings and taking naltrexone. In Chapter 13, "CBT for Substance Misuse and Abuse," we detail a variety of methods of efficient adaptation of CBT techniques in treatment of substance abuse.

We discuss CBT methods for helping with problems of habits or lifestyle in Chapter 14, "Lifestyle Change: Building Healthy Habits." These techniques include helping patients stick with exercise or diet programs or break patterns of procrastination. In Chapter 15, "CBT in Medical Patients," we explain how to integrate a CBT approach into long-term medication management and how to use CBT to build the patient's strengths in preventing symptom return.

The final chapter covers one of the most useful applications of CBT in brief sessions—relapse prevention. In our clinical practices, we see many patients with conditions that require indefinite maintenance therapy with medications such as lithium carbonate, atypical antipsychotics, anticonvulsants, or antidepressants. For these patients, acquiring CBT skills for managing stress and spotting early signs of potential relapse can be a very useful addition to the treatment program.

As in two earlier books, we use video illustrations to convey key concepts and methods. Readers of these earlier books have told us that video illustrations help bring CBT alive and provide useful models for how to implement therapy. The video illustrations are integrated with specific content in the book so that you will find them to be most effective if viewed in sequence at the time recommended in the text. The videos were produced with the kind assistance of colleagues who role-played patients with various psychiatric problems. We used a naturalistic style of filming that attempted to show interventions much as they would appear in actual clinical practice. The videos were filmed in clinical offices at the University of Louisville in Kentucky and at Newcastle University in the United Kingdom with the help of video production departments from both of these institutions.

Case illustrations that appear in the videos or elsewhere in the text are either entirely fictitious or are amalgams of cases that we have treated in which identifiers have been removed or altered to protect confidentiality. We use the convention of writing about cases as if they have actually been treated by us in order to enhance the flow and appeal of the text. Instead of using the phrase he or she (or she or he), we alternate use of personal pronouns when not describing specific cases.

Throughout the book, we discuss various worksheets, forms, and resources that are useful tools for patients and clinicians to use in CBT. To aid our readers, we've collected these materials in Appendix 1, "Worksheets and Checklists," and Appendix 2, "CBT Resources for Patients and Families." We have included these appendixes online, available as free downloads and in larger format, on the American Psychiatric Publishing Web site: www.appi.org/pdf/62362. Permission is granted for readers to use these worksheets, handouts, and inventories in clinical practice. Please seek permission from the individual rights holder for any other use.

Two additional appendixes are provided to aid your use of this book and learning CBT methods. As a handy reference, Appendix 3, "CBT Educational Resources for Clinicians," lists courses and workshops, certification, fellowship opportunities, and a resource for computer-assisted CBT training. Appendix 4, "DVD Guide," contains a list of videos discussed in the text.

In writing this book on brief sessions of CBT and medication, we do not intend to recommend or advocate for this approach over the more conventional modes of treatment delivery for CBT. In fact, we typically perform CBT in 50-minute sessions with a portion of our patients and also frequently arrange for other therapists to provide this form of treatment. The purpose of the book is to help psychiatrists and other clinicians who perform pharmacotherapy to adapt CBT for use in their brief sessions, and thus add a cognitive-behavioral therapeutic dimension to routine clinical management. In Chapter 2, "Indications and Formats for Brief CBT Sessions," we explain clinical situations in which brief sessions may be indicated either as the sole treatment method or as an adjunct to longer sessions with another therapist.

Our own clinical practices have been enriched by the practical yet compelling methods of CBT, and we hope that you will also find that CBT helps your patients get the most from the time spent in treatment sessions.

Acknowledgments

Our ability to produce this book rested heavily on the skilled work of the volunteers who play the patients shown in the video illustrations. We thank these clinicians who developed engaging and realistic simulations of commonly experienced psychiatric problems. Leigh Ann Doerr, R.N., a psychiatric nurse who provides cognitive-behavior therapy (CBT) to hospitalized patients, created the character of Barbara, a recently discharged patient with bipolar disorder. Virginia Evans, L.C.S.W., a certified cognitive therapist and an invaluable member of the clinical team at the University of Louisville Depression Center, appears as Grace, a woman who is depressed following the death of her husband and is now facing the stress of a new job. Sara Tai, D.Clin.Psy., a psychologist at the University of Manchester and expert on recent developments in CBT theory and practice, depicts Helen, a woman with delusions and hallucinations. Alphonso Nichols, M.D., a child psychiatrist from Louisville, Kentucky, plays Darrell, a young man who has depression and alcohol abuse. Christopher Stewart, M.D., a cognitive-behavior therapist and specialist in addiction psychiatry, appears as Rick, a man with social anxiety. David Casey, M.D., a geropsychiatrist who is senior vice chairman of the department of psychiatry and behavioral sciences at the University of Louisville and who uses CBT in many of his brief therapy sessions, plays Allan, a man who has become depressed after experiencing a heart attack.

As for our other illustrated guides, the majority of the filming was done at the University of Louisville with the able assistance of Randy Cissell and Ron Harrison. Additional filming was completed by Stephen

Bradwel, Urwin Wood, and Kevin Dick at Newcastle University in the United Kingdom. Ann Schaap, Leslie Pancratz, and Deborah Dobiecz, librarians at Norton Healthcare in Louisville, were always ready to help us with literature searches and retrievals. Mary Hosey, L.C.S.W., and Christopher Stewart, M.D., provided valuable feedback on several chapters. We also want to give a special message of thanks to Carol Wahl and Christine Castle for their dedicated work in helping prepare the manuscript.

When we developed the concept for this book on using CBT in brief sessions, we wondered how clinicians might react. Would they be critical of the idea that psychiatrists and other prescribing clinicians could do meaningful therapeutic work with CBT in sessions shorter than the traditional 50-minute hour? Or, instead, would they welcome a book that is directed at the real-world clinical practice of many psychiatrists who want to integrate pharmacotherapy and psychotherapy? As it turned out, we received a great deal of encouragement from clinicians from all points of the compass—biological psychiatrists, practitioners of psychodynamic therapy, and of course those who have embraced CBT as a key therapeutic method. The support and encouragement of these colleagues meant a great deal to us as we readied this book for publication.

Finally, we want to thank the top-notch editorial staff at American Psychiatric Publishing, Inc. Robert Hales, M.D., John McDuffie, and Ann Eng have cheered us on to complete this practical book on CBT and have given us fine editorial guidance along the way.

Disclosures of Interest

The authors of this book have indicated a financial interest in or other affiliation with a commercial supporter, a manufacturer of a commercial product, a provider of a commercial service, a nongovernmental organization, and/or a government agency, as listed below:

Jesse H. Wright, M.D., Ph.D.
Dr. Wright may receive royalties or other compensation from MindStreet, publisher of software for computer-assisted cognitve-behavior therapy. He is on the speakers bureau for Pfizer and receives book royalties from Simon & Schuster, American Psychiatric Publishing, Inc., and Guilford Press.

Donna M. Sudak, M.D.
Dr. Sudak receives book royalties from Lippincott Williams & Wilkins and John Wiley & Sons, Inc. She receives honoraria from Elsevier.

Douglas Turkington, M.D.
Dr. Turkington has no disclosures to report.

Michael E. Thase, M.D.
Dr. Thase has provided scientific consultation to AstraZeneca, Bristol-Myers Squibb Company, Cephalon, Cyberonics, Eli Lilly & Company, Forest Pharmaceuticals, GlaxoSmithKline, Janssen Pharmaceutica, MedAvante, Neuronetics, Novartis, Organon International, Sepracor, Shire US, Supernus Pharmaceuticals, Transcept Pharmaceuticals, and Wyeth-Ayerst Laboratories. Dr. Thase has been a member of the speakers' bureaus for AstraZeneca, Bristol-Myers Squibb Company, Cyberonics, Eli Lilly & Company, GlaxoSmithKline, Schering-Plough (formerly Organon), Sanofi-Aventis, and Wyeth-Ayerst Laboratories. He receives grant funding from Eli Lilly & Company, GlaxoSmithKline, National Institute of Mental Health, and Sepracor. Dr. Thase has equity holdings in MedAvante, and receives royalty income from American Psychiatric Publishing, Inc., Guilford Publications, Herald House, Oxford University Press, and W. W. Norton & Company. He has provided expert testimony for Jones Day and Phillips Lyttle, L.L.P., and Pepper Hamilton, L.L.P. His wife is employed as the senior medical director for Advogent.

CHAPTER 1

Introduction

LEARNING MAP

Features of CBT that are useful in brief sessions

⇩

Combining CBT and pharmacotherapy

⇩

What clinicians need to know about CBT to use
it effectively in brief sessions

Why should psychiatrists and other clinicians who prescribe medications consider using cognitive-behavior therapy (CBT) methods in brief sessions? In what clinical situations could brief CBT interventions have a place? What CBT methods can be used effectively in sessions that are briefer than the traditional 50-minute hour? How can busy clinicians integrate targeted CBT methods with psychopharmacology? These are the types of questions that we attempt to answer in this book.

Because all the coauthors have practiced and taught CBT for many years and also do clinical work in which we see patients for brief sessions (ranging from 15 to 30 minutes depending on the setting and patient needs) and prescribe medications, we have developed methods for blending CBT into these shorter treatment interventions. We do not discard our knowledge and skills in CBT at the office door when a patient who is taking medication appears for a brief session. In a similar manner, when we have the opportunity to treat patients in more traditional 45- to 60-minute CBT sessions, we do not forget that we are psychiatrists who assess and manage the biological components of illnesses.

Even in brief, 15-minute medication checks or in medication groups, we have found that it is worthwhile to draw from the resources of CBT to augment standard clinical management and prescribing methods. If more time is available (e.g., 20–30 minutes), we are often able to implement CBT interventions such as thought records, behavioral activation, exposure and response prevention, or sleep enhancement strategies. In Chapter 2, "Indications and Formats for Brief CBT Sessions," we discuss a variety of options for providing treatment in brief sessions and detail clinical situations in which brief sessions may be an appropriate component of treatment.

Features of CBT That Are Useful in Brief Sessions

Collaborative Empiricism

Some of the general features of CBT that can be applied to advantage in brief sessions are listed in Table 1–1. The first item, collaborative empiricism, is perhaps the most important. The collaborative and empirical nature of the therapeutic relationship in CBT can be emphasized in even the shortest clinical encounters. Therapists can set a high priority on establishing a collaborative relationship in which the patient's attitudes and concerns are elicited and fully valued, a highly genuine and understanding approach is used, and the patient and therapist function as an investigative team (e.g., in checking out the usefulness of medications or CBT interventions, testing the validity of conclusions, being open to trying different approaches).

Instead of using a controlling style for medication management, the CBT-oriented clinician tries to forge a collaborative relationship in which the patient takes an active role in learning about the illness, making decisions, and implementing the treatment plan. We suspect that the collaborative-empirical relationship in CBT is one reason why this therapy has been shown to be helpful in promoting treatment adherence (Cochran 1984; Weiden 2007; Weiden et al. 2007). We discuss video illustrations of collaborative relationships in Chapter 2, "Indications and Formats for Brief CBT Sessions," and Chapter 3, "Enhancing the Impact of Brief Sessions," and provide further recommendations for developing effective treatment relationships and using other basic features of CBT in Chapter 3.

Table 1–1.	Features of cognitive-behavior therapy: advantages for brief sessions

Collaborative empiricism
Structuring techniques
Psychoeducational emphasis
Practical methods
Homework

Structuring

Structuring, another basic feature of CBT, is especially well suited to brief sessions. If only 20–25 minutes are available for the session, efficiency and organization would appear to be high on the list of desired traits. Clinicians can teach patients how to set agendas rapidly, focus their efforts on specific problems that can be addressed within the available time, pace sessions effectively, and give and receive feedback on treatment progress. Many of our patients who are seen in brief sessions come to each visit with a written agenda and have learned other ways of maximizing the time spent in the treatment encounter. For example, a patient might say that she wants to cover one specific agenda item in addition to discussing a possible increase in medication but that another agenda item can wait until the next visit.

Psychoeducation

CBT is well known for its psychoeducational emphasis. One of the important goals of CBT is to help patients learn enough about this approach that they can eventually become "self-therapists." Instead of relying on the therapist for solutions to their problems, they can reach the point where they can spot cognitive distortions or maladaptive behaviors and have the skills to reverse these patterns. When briefer sessions are used, the psychoeducational aspects of therapy may become somewhat more dominant. Thus, clinicians who use this form of CBT need to learn to tap educational resources that can be used outside of sessions (e.g., readings, Web sites, video recordings, audio recordings) to help patients build their knowledge.

A specialized form of brief CBT, computer-assisted CBT, has been shown to be particularly effective in educating patients and in providing opportunities to practice CBT methods. In a study performed by Wright et al. (2005), computer-assisted CBT delivered in 25-minute sessions was more effective than standard 50-minute sessions in helping patients acquire knowledge about CBT. Detailed suggestions on psychoeducation in brief sessions are provided in Chapter 4, "Case Formulation and Treatment Planning."

Practical Methods

One reason that CBT is often appealing to both clinicians and patients is that it is distinguished by a number of very practical methods that can provide good results by decreasing symptoms. In some cases, these methods can be learned fairly quickly and are suitable for applications in brief sessions. Table 1–2 contains a list of possible high-yield methods that could be considered for treatment plans with patients who are being seen in sessions shorter than 45–60 minutes. We have used these methods repeatedly and will illustrate them in clinical vignettes throughout the book and in video clips that appear in the accompanying DVD.

Homework

An additional feature of CBT that we find very helpful in brief sessions is the use of homework. This fundamental CBT procedure extends learning beyond the confines of the session and encourages self-help in the treatment process. An example from our clinical practice involves the treatment of Consuela, a 22-year-old woman with agoraphobia and fear of driving. After explaining the basic CBT model for anxiety disorders, the psychiatrist helped Consuela set up a hierarchy for graded exposure to her fear of driving and showed her how to use relaxation and breathing training to reduce anxiety levels. The exposure therapy was implemented by Consuela primarily in homework assignments. During each brief session, Consuela reported on her progress, did troubleshooting on ways to persevere with the exposure protocol, and set specific targets for homework to take on increasing steps in the hierarchy. Consuela's treatment is detailed further in Chapter 2, "Indications and Formats for Brief CBT Sessions," and Chapter 9, "Behavioral Methods for Anxiety."

Combining CBT and Pharmacotherapy

In many ways, CBT and pharmacotherapy are ideal partners in the treatment of mental disorders. Both have strong empirical bases, with a large number of randomized controlled trials supporting their effectiveness. They are pragmatic treatments that can give symptom relief in acute

Table 1–2.　High-yield cognitive-behavior therapy (CBT) methods for brief sessions

- Activity scheduling
- Breathing retraining
- CBT for insomnia
- CBT rehearsal
- Collaborative goal setting
- Computer-assisted CBT
- Coping cards
- Examining the evidence
- Exposure and response prevention
- Identifying cognitive errors
- Imagery
- Generating reasons for hope/living
- Graded task assignments
- Listing advantages and disadvantages
- Medication adherence interventions
- Mindfulness training
- Motivational interviewing
- Normalizing
- Problem solving
- Relapse prevention
- Socratic questioning
- Symptom diaries
- Thought recording
- Well-being logs

phase therapy, in addition to providing long-term relapse prevention effects. Also, each utilizes an active and direct treatment approach.

A Comprehensive, Integrated Treatment Model

We recommend that a comprehensive, integrated treatment model be used for combining CBT and pharmacotherapy in clinical practice (Wright 2004; Wright et al. 2008), as diagrammed in Figure 1–1. According to Wright (2004, p. 355), this model is based on the following assumptions:

1. Cognitive processes modulate the effects of the external environment (e.g., stressful life events, interpersonal relationships, social forces) on the central nervous system substrate (e.g., neurotransmitter function, activation of CNS [central nervous system] pathways, autonomic and neuroendocrine responses) for emotion and behavior.
2. Dysfunctional cognitions can be produced by both psychological and biological influences.
3. Biological treatments can alter cognitions.
4. Cognitive and behavioral interventions can change biological processes.
5. Environmental, cognitive, biological, emotional, and behavioral processes should be conceptualized as part of the same system.
6. It is valuable to search for ways of integrating or combining cognitive and biological interventions to enhance treatment outcome.

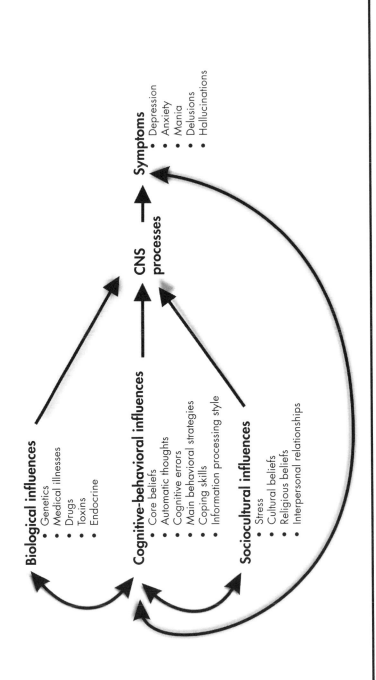

Figure 1–1.   A cognitive-behavioral-biological-sociocultural model for combined treatment.

CNS=central nervous system.

Assumption 1 is a key feature of the basic cognitive-behavioral model (Wright et al. 2008). Because humans are thinking beings, they attach meaning to the information signals in their environments, and these cognitions activate CNS biological processes involved in producing emotion and behavior. Assumptions 2–5 are based on a far-ranging research effort that has included neuroimaging and other biological investigations that have shown how CBT acts through CNS pathways and processes (Baxter et al. 1992; Furmark et al. 2002; Goldapple et al. 2004; Joffe et al. 1996; Thase et al. 1998); studies that have demonstrated that pharmacotherapy can reverse maladaptive cognitions (Blackburn and Bishop 1983; Simons et al. 1984); and the work of Kandel (2001, 2005), Kandel and Schwartz (1982), and others who have formulated an integrative approach to understanding the biology of psychotherapy. Assumption 6 is supported by outcome studies on combined treatment reviewed later in this chapter and by the accumulated experience of many psychiatrists and other mental health professionals who routinely use medications and psychotherapy together in clinical practice.

Core Elements of Combined CBT and Pharmacotherapy

If an integrated model is used for combined therapy (as shown in Figure 1–1), debates on the merits of biological versus psychological approaches can be dropped in favor of a unified approach. Clinicians can then strive to find the best ways to combine treatments to achieve desired results. In some respects, an ideal method may be to have a psychiatrist, other physician, or nurse practitioner who has expertise in both CBT and pharmacotherapy provide the entire course of therapy. When a single clinician practices both CBT and pharmacotherapy, a very cohesive and fully integrated approach can be presented to the patient; also, possible conflicts between treatment methods or miscommunications that may occur when a physician or nurse practitioner prescribes medication and a nonphysician therapist performs CBT are avoided. However, the most common method of delivering combined therapy involves a "team" of a pharmacotherapist and a nonphysician cognitive-behavior therapist. Table 1–3 lists the core elements of an integrated approach to combined treatment.

When more than one clinician is involved in treatment, we highly recommend that the clinicians work together regularly, agree on an integrated model for therapy, and express a shared, favorable attitude about combined treatment to the patient. For some patients, all of the CBT and pharmacotherapy is provided by the psychiatrist, often using brief sessions for a part or all of the treatment. For other patients, the nonphysician cognitive-behavior therapist delivers a series of traditional-length 50-minute sessions (the term *50-minute session* is used throughout the book to describe traditional-length sessions that may range from 45 minutes to 1 hour). In Chapter 2, "Indications and Formats for Brief CBT Sessions," we explain some of the criteria that may be helpful in choosing the format and intensity of the treatment plan.

In either a single- or dual-therapist mode, combined treatment can be facilitated by using a flexible approach that is tailored to each patient's unique blend of problems and strengths. In the research studies described in the following section, medication was typically prescribed with limited opportunity for the clinician to vary doses or types of treatment. Similarly, CBT was usually delivered according to a manualized protocol. We value the information gleaned from controlled studies, but in our clinical practices we make efforts to adjust both the pharmacotherapy and CBT components of treatment to match the patient's needs and to take advantage of therapeutic opportunities. The formulation-based method of treatment planning described in Chapter 3, "Enhancing the Impact of Brief Sessions," underlies this flexible strategy for performing combined CBT and pharmacotherapy.

Research on Combined CBT and Pharmacotherapy

Investigations of combined therapy compared with either CBT or pharmacotherapy alone have been highly influential in establishing the efficacy of treatments for depression and anxiety disorders (e.g., see meta-analyses and reviews by Friedman et al. 2006; Hollon et al. 2005; Wright et al. 2008). However, many features of these studies limit generalization of results to the real-world practice of combining CBT and medication in clinical settings (Hollon et al. 2005; Wright et al. 2005). Designed as efficacy investigations, these comparisons have typically screened out many of the complex cases that are typically seen in clinical practice. Also, these studies were primarily focused on pitting CBT against pharmacotherapy, usually employing different clinicians to provide the psychotherapy and pharmacotherapy components of treatment. Thus, the studies were not geared toward developing or investigating an integrated, flexible model for combined therapy.

One of the principal criticisms of research on combined treatment is that studies have been underpowered to detect advantages of combined treatment (Friedman et al. 2006; Hollon et al. 2005). In a meta-analysis of studies of combined treatment for depression, Friedman et al. (2006) found that some individual studies of CBT for depression demonstrated only a trend for superiority for using CBT and pharmacotherapy together.

Table 1–3. Core elements of an integrated approach to combined treatment

Therapy is guided by a comprehensive, cognitive-behavioral-biological-sociocultural model.

Treatment is delivered by either a physician or a nurse practitioner alone who is trained in both psychopharmacology and cognitive-behavior therapy or by a collaborative team of a physician and nonphysician cognitive-behavior therapist.

Treatment methods are flexible and are customized to fit the diagnosis and the specific needs of each patient.

However, when results of all investigations were taken together, the combined approach gave the best results.

Investigations of pharmacotherapy, CBT, and combined treatment for anxiety disorders have been reviewed by several groups, including Bakker et al. (2000), Hollifield et al. (2006), Westra and Stewart (1998), and Wright (2004). All of the above reviews and a meta-analysis (van Balkom et al. 1997) concluded that combined treatment with CBT plus antidepressants appeared to offer benefits beyond those achieved with monotherapy. However, when alprazolam was combined with CBT, the long-term results were worse than if CBT was used with a placebo (Marks et al. 1993). This finding is a rare example of a potential negative interaction between medication and CBT. Although benzodiazepines with longer half-lives, such as diazepam, do not appear to have this deleterious effect on CBT (Westra and Stewart 1998), the work of Marks et al. (1993) suggests caution in using some benzodiazepines with CBT for anxiety disorders.

Randomized controlled trials of CBT and antidepressant medication for bulimia nervosa have usually found advantages for combined treatment. Based on a meta-analysis of seven studies, Bacaltchuck et al. (2000) reported that the remission rate for combined treatment was almost double the rate achieved with medication alone. The benefits of combined treatment for bulimia nervosa may be somewhat dependent on the length of treatment. For example, Agras et al. (1994) found that after 16 weeks of treatment, both combined treatment and CBT were superior to imipramine alone. However, after 32 weeks of treatment, only combined treatment gave better results than medication.

For conditions such as bipolar disorder and schizophrenia, for which pharmacotherapy is the principal treatment approach, no studies have compared a combined approach with CBT alone. However, a large number of investigations have demonstrated a positive additive effect for adjunctive CBT (e.g., see Drury et al. 1996; Lam et al. 2003; Miklowitz et al. 2007; Naeem et al. 2005; Rector and Beck 2001; Sensky et al. 2000; Tarrier et al. 1993; Turkington et al. 2006). Although not all studies have shown advantages for adding CBT to pharmacotherapy for schizophrenia and bipolar disorder, the overall pattern suggests that CBT can make a valuable contribution in the treatment of many patients with these disorders. Readers who are interested in reading further on studies of combined treatment can consult publications by Friedman et al. (2006), Hollifield et al. (2006), Hollon et al. (2005), Wright (2004), and Wright et al. (2008).

What Clinicians Need to Know About CBT to Use It Effectively in Brief Sessions

The old saying "don't put the cart before the horse" fits well for understanding the learning sequence that we recommend for building expertise in using CBT in brief sessions. Because CBT in brief sessions requires an ability to rapidly and skillfully implement techniques and to effectively weave together the pharmacotherapy and psychotherapy components of treatment, clinicians need to have a solid grounding in basic CBT theories and methods. In Table 1–4, we give suggestions for recommended basic knowledge and skills in CBT.

Before attempting to use CBT in brief sessions, we believe that clinicians should have significant experience in performing CBT in standard 45- to 50-minute sessions as described in texts such as *Cognitive Therapy: Basics and Beyond* (Beck 1995), *Cognitive Behavioral Therapy for Clinicians* (Sudak 2006), or *Learning Cognitive-Behavior Therapy: An Illustrated Guide* (Wright et al. 2006). In doing this work, clinicians need to become adept at performing CBT case conceptualizations and planning treatment based on these formulations (for methods of developing CBT case conceptualizations, see Wright et al. 2006; Wright et al. 2009; and Chapter 4, "Case Formulation and Treatment Planning"). When sessions are brief, clinicians must be able to generate succinct and targeted formulations that include the key pieces of information that allow for full understanding of the patient, while honing in on specific problems or issues that are likely to yield positive results. All of the attributes of good CBT in standard-length sessions, such as forming highly collaborative relationships, showing genuineness and accurate empathy, structuring and pacing sessions to promote efficiency and learning, and providing effective psychoeducation, need to be refined even further when sessions are brief.

Some of the specific CBT skills that need to be acquired are as follows: identifying and changing automatic thoughts; modifying schemas; com-

---

Table 1–4. Recommended basic knowledge and skills in cognitive-behavior therapy (CBT)

Understand the basic CBT model for treatment.

Obtain experience in conducting standard 45- to 50-minute sessions.

Perform case conceptualizations and plan treatment based on CBT principles.

Structure and pace treatment to enhance learning.

Elicit and modify automatic thoughts and schemas.

Use standard behavioral methods such as behavioral activation, activity scheduling, exposure and response prevention, breathing retraining, and relaxation training.

Identify and implement CBT strategies for specific disorders.

---

monly used behavioral methods for depression (e.g., behavioral activation, activity scheduling, and graded task assignments); and behavioral techniques for anxiety disorders (e.g., exposure and response prevention, breathing training, relaxation training). Because different disorders (e.g., depression, anxiety disorders, psychoses) may respond best if techniques are tailored to match the unique characteristics of the disorder, the platform of skills for effective use of brief sessions should also include an understanding of the CBT approach to major forms of psychiatric illnesses. Books listed in Appendix 3, "CBT Educational Resources for Clinicians," such as *Learning Cognitive-Behavior Therapy: An Illustrated Guide* (Wright et al. 2006), *Psychological Treatment of Panic* (Barlow and Cherney 1988), *Cognitive-Behavioral Therapy for Bipolar Disorder* (Basco and Rush 2005), *Cognitive Therapy of Schizophrenia* (Kingdon and Turkington 2005), and *Cognitive-Behavior Therapy for Severe Mental Illness: An Illustrated Guide* (Wright et al. 2009), can help readers better understand how to apply CBT for commonly encountered psychiatric conditions.

Many training opportunities exist for learning CBT (see Table 1–5). Because psychiatry residents in the United States are now required to attain competency in this approach, most residency training programs offer basic courses and supervision in CBT. The typical curricula at residency programs at universities where we teach include an extensive series of didactic sessions; many video, role-play, and/or live demonstrations of CBT; case write-ups to gain formulation skills; experiences in treating a variety of patients with CBT; and individual and/or group supervision. Many CBT training programs and CBT centers also offer continuing medical education for practicing clinicians and ongoing seminars for learning advanced CBT techniques. Courses in CBT are also offered at annual meetings of the

American Psychiatric Association, the American Psychological Association, the Association for Behavioral and Cognitive Therapies, and other regional, national, and international scientific organizations.

In addition to basic texts in CBT, engaging training materials are available in video and computerized formats. For example, books by Wright et al. (2006, 2009) contain DVDs with a number of illustrations of core CBT methods. Also, a novel computer-based training program, Praxis, has been developed in the United Kingdom by Turkington and others (www.praxiscbtonline.co.uk). Praxis teaches CBT for depression, anxiety, and psychosis using interactive computer exercises, video demonstrations, and case vignettes. Supervision via telephone and Internet is included in the basic cost of the computer-assisted training. Other training materials and opportunities are available at several Web sites, including the Academy of Cognitive Therapy (www.academyofct.org), the Beck Institute (www.beckinstitute.org), and the University of Louisville Depression Center (www.louisville.edu/depression). Appendix 3, "CBT Educational Resources for Clinicians," contains lists of organizations that provide training in CBT, plus books, a computer program, and Web sites that may be useful in building CBT skills.

This book, with its video illustrations and learning exercises, has been designed to help readers sharpen their basic CBT techniques and to effectively apply this knowledge in the stimulating and rewarding domain of brief sessions.

Summary

Key Points for Clinicians

- Some of the key features of CBT that may be especially useful in brief sessions are collaborative empiricism, structuring techniques, a psychoeducational emphasis, pragmatic methods, and homework.
- CBT and pharmacotherapy can be effective partners in treatment of patients with psychiatric disorders.
- A comprehensive cognitive-behavioral-biological-sociocultural model is used for combining CBT and medication in psychiatric treatment.
- Research on combined therapy has not directly tested the flexible, fully integrated method suggested in this book. However, the overall results of investigations on short-term CBT generally support the use of combined treatment in clinical practice.
- A basic grounding in CBT concepts and methods is recommended for clinicians who want to adopt CBT methods for use in brief sessions.

Table 1–5. Training opportunities in cognitive-behavior therapy (CBT)

Psychiatry residency or other graduate education programs for CBT

Continuing medical education courses offered by universities or other training programs

Courses and workshops at scientific meetings

Workshops at regional conferences

Basic texts on CBT

Videos that demonstrate CBT

DVD-ROMs and Internet-delivered educational programs

Fellowships in CBT

Concepts and Skills for Patients to Learn

- CBT offers practical help for managing many of the symptoms of psychiatric disorders.
- CBT methods and skills can be learned in brief sessions.
- Excellent collaboration or "teamwork" with a clinician is an important ingredient of effective treatment.
- A combined approach of medication and CBT can offer advantages to some people in getting well and staying well.

References

Agras WS, Rossiter EM, Arnow B, et al: One-year follow-up of psychosocial and pharmacologic treatments for bulimia nervosa. J Clin Psychiatry 55:179–183, 1994

Bacaltchuk J, Trefiglio RP, Oliveira IR, et al: Combination of antidepressants and psychological treatments for bulimia nervosa: a systematic review. Acta Psychiatr Scand 101:256–264, 2000

Bakker A, van Balkolm AJ, van Dyck R: Selective serotonin reuptake inhibitors in the treatment of panic disorder and agoraphobia. Int Clin Psychopharmacol 15 (suppl 2):25–30, 2000

Barlow DH, Cherney JA: Psychological Treatment of Panic. New York, Guilford, 1988

Basco MR, Rush AJ: Cognitive-Behavioral Therapy for Bipolar Disorder, 2nd Edition. New York, Guilford, 2005

Baxter LR Jr, Schwartz JM, Bergman KS, et al: Caudate glucose metabolic rate changes with both drug and behavior therapy for obsessive-compulsive disorder. Arch Gen Psychiatry 49:681–689, 1992

Beck J: Cognitive Therapy: Basics and Beyond. New York, Guilford, 1995

Blackburn IM, Bishop S: Changes in cognition with pharmacotherapy and cognitive therapy. Br J Psychiatry 143:609–617, 1983

Cochran SD: Preventing medical noncompliance in the outpatient treatment of bipolar affective disorders. J Consult Clin Psychol 52:873–878, 1984

Drury V, Birchwood M, Cochrane R, et al: Cognitive therapy and recovery from acute psychosis: a controlled trial, I: impact on psychotic symptoms. Br J Psychiatry 169:593–601, 1996

Friedman ES, Wright JH, Jarrett RB, et al: Combining cognitive therapy and medication for mood disorders. Psychiatr Ann 36:320–328, 2006

Furmark T, Tillfors M, Marteinsdottir I, et al: Common changes in cerebral blood flow in patients with social phobia treated with citalopram or cognitive-behavioral therapy. Arch Gen Psychiatry 59:425–433, 2002

Goldapple K, Segal Z, Garson C, et al: Modulation of cortical-limbic pathways in major depression: treatment-specific effects of cognitive behavior therapy. Arch Gen Psychiatry 61:34–41, 2004

Hollifield M, Mackey A, Davidson J: Integrating therapies for anxiety disorders. Psychiatr Ann 36:329–338, 2006

Hollon SD, Jarrett RB, Nierenberg AA, et al: Psychotherapy and medication in the treatment of adult and geriatric depression: which monotherapy or combined treatment? J Clin Psychiatry 66:455–468, 2005

Joffe R, Segal Z, Singer W: Change in thyroid hormone levels following response to cognitive therapy for major depression. Am J Psychiatry 153:411–413, 1996

Kandel ER: Psychotherapy and the single synapse: the impact of psychiatric thought on neurobiological research. N Engl J Med 301:1028–1037, 2001

Kandel ER: Psychiatry, Psychoanalysis, and the New Biology of the Mind. Washington, DC, American Psychiatric Publishing, 2005

Kandel ER, Schwartz JH: Molecular biology of learning: modulation of transmitter release. Science 218:433–443, 1982

Kingdon DG, Turkington D: Cognitive Therapy of Schizophrenia. New York, Guilford, 2005

Lam DH, Watkins ER, Hayward P, et al: A randomized controlled study of cognitive therapy for relapse prevention for bipolar affective disorder: outcome of the first year. Arch Gen Psychiatry 60:145–152, 2003

Marks IM, Swinson RP, Basoglu M, et al: Alprazolam and exposure alone and combined in panic disorder with agoraphobia: a controlled study in London and Toronto. Br J Psychiatry 162:776–787, 1993

Miklowitz DJ, Otto MW, Frank E, et al: Psychosocial treatments for bipolar depression: a 1-year randomized trial from the Systematic Treatment Enhancement Program. Arch Gen Psychiatry 64:419–426, 2007

Naeem F, Kingdon D, Turkington D: Cognitive behavior therapy for schizophrenia in patients with mild to moderate substance misuse problems. Cogn Behav Ther 34:207–215, 2005

Rector NA, Beck AT: Cognitive behavioral therapy for schizophrenia: an empirical review. J Nerv Ment Dis 189:278–287, 2001

Sensky T, Turkington D, Kingdon D, et al: A randomized controlled trial of cognitive-behavioral therapy for persistent symptoms in schizophrenia resistant to medication. Arch Gen Psychiatry 57:165–172, 2000

Simons AD, Garfield SL, Murphy GE: The process of change in cognitive therapy and pharmacotherapy for depression. Arch Gen Psychiatry 41:45–51, 1984

Sudak D: Cognitive Behavioral Therapy for Clinicians. Philadelphia, PA, Lippincott Williams & Wilkins, 2006

Tarrier N, Beckett R, Harwood S, et al: A trial of two cognitive-behavioural methods of treating drug-resistant residual psychotic symptoms in schizophrenic patients: I. outcome. Br J Psychiatry 162:524–532, 1993

Thase ME, Fasiczka AL, Berman SR, et al: Electroencephalographic sleep profiles before and after cognitive behavior therapy of depression. Arch Gen Psychiatry 55:138–144, 1998

Turkington D, Kingdon D, Weiden PJ: Cognitive behavior therapy for schizophrenia. Am J Psychiatry 163:365–373, 2006

van Balkom, AJ, Bakker A, Spinhoven P, et al: A meta-analysis of the treatment of panic disorder with or without agoraphobia: a comparison of psychopharmacological, cognitive-behavioral, and combination treatments. J Nerv Ment Dis 185:510–516, 1997

Weiden PJ: Understanding and addressing adherence issues in schizophrenia: from theory to practice. J Clin Psychiatry 68 (suppl 14):14–19, 2007

Weiden PJ, Burkholder P, Schooler NR, et al: Improving antipsychotic adherence in schizophrenia: a randomized pilot study of a brief CBT intervention, in 2007 New Research Program and Abstracts, American Psychiatric Association 160th Annual Meeting, San Diego, CA, May 19–24, 2007. Washington, DC, American Psychiatric Association, 2007, p 346

Westra HA, Stewart SH: Cognitive behavioral therapy and pharmacotherapy: complementary or contradictory approaches to the treatment of anxiety? Clin Psychol Rev 18:307–340, 1998

Wright JH: Integrating cognitive-behavioral therapy and pharmacotherapy, in Contemporary Cognitive Therapy: Theory, Research, and Practice. Edited by Leahy RL. New York, Guilford, 2004, pp 341–366

Wright JH, Wright AS, Albano AM, et al: Computer-assisted cognitive therapy for depression: maintaining efficacy while reducing therapist time. Am J Psychiatry 162:1158–1164, 2005

Wright JH, Basco MR, Thase ME: Learning Cognitive-Behavior Therapy: An Illustrated Guide. Washington, DC, American Psychiatric Publishing, 2006

Wright JH, Beck AT, Thase ME: Cognitive therapy, in The American Psychiatric Publishing Textbook of Clinical Psychiatry, 5th Edition. Edited by Hales RE, Yudofsky SC, Gabbard GO. Washington, DC, American Psychiatric Publishing, 2008, pp 1211–1256

Wright JH, Turkington D, Kingdon DG, et al: Cognitive-Behavior Therapy for Severe Mental Illness: An Illustrated Guide. Washington, DC, American Psychiatric Publishing, 2009

CHAPTER 2

Indications and Formats for Brief CBT Sessions

LEARNING MAP

Brief CBT sessions: a practice survey

Indications for combining CBT and pharmacotherapy in brief sessions

Formats for brief sessions of combined CBT and pharmacotherapy

Examples of brief sessions of combined CBT and pharmacotherapy

---

In this chapter, we discuss possible clinical situations in which brief sessions of combined cognitive-behavior therapy (CBT) and pharmacotherapy might be used and detail several ways to deliver combined treatment. These recommendations and suggestions are derived from our clinical experiences in providing combined treatment in a variety of settings and from our work with multidisciplinary teams. Two general implementation strategies are explained: 1) use of brief sessions when a psychiatrist, other physician, or nurse practitioner[†] is the sole provider, and 2) use of brief sessions along with 50-minute sessions when there are two providers (a prescribing clinician and a nonphysician cognitive-behavior therapist).

Brief CBT Sessions: A Practice Survey

We begin this chapter's exploration of indications and formats by sharing the results of a survey from our own practices. This survey was designed to answer questions such as these: How frequently do we use the brief session format? What are the diagnoses of patients seen for brief visits of combined CBT and pharmacotherapy? What are some of the clinical reasons for treating patients in brief sessions?

We completed a log of 265 sequential patient visits in our practices to provide a snapshot of the frequency of brief visits compared with longer sessions and to provide information on some of the indications for selecting the brief session format. We provided CBT in all but 39 of these sessions; therefore, we focused on the 226 sessions that included therapy (Table 2–1). For the purpose of this survey, we defined a brief visit as lasting less than 30 minutes. The percentage of brief sessions in our clinical practices was 51% (116/226); the modal length of brief sessions was 20 minutes (range: 15–30 minutes). The vast majority of brief visits (92%; 107/116) were with patients who were taking psychotropic medications. In 86% (100/116) of the brief visits, we were the only provider. The intervals between brief sessions ranged from 1 week to 6 months, with the majority (64%; 74/116) of the sessions occurring at least monthly. When these data are considered together, it is clear that we commonly use brief visits and almost always provide CBT, that we most commonly use CBT techniques in combination with medication, and that we apply brief CBT sessions across all stages of treatment (i.e., from acute visits to maintenance sessions).

Our scheduling system is simple: we arrange appointments in blocks of one patient per hour (for initial evaluations or traditional 50-minute

---

[†] To simplify the writing style, we primarily use the term *psychiatrist* or *prescribing clinician* throughout the rest of this book instead of repetitively noting that clinicians who can deliver both CBT and pharmacotherapy include psychiatrists, other physicians trained in CBT, and nurse practitioners.

Table 2–1. Principal diagnoses of patients seen for brief visits compared with 50-minute sessions[a]

Diagnoses	Brief visits (*n*=116)	Longer sessions (*n*=110)
Major depression, single episode	19 (16%)	22 (20%)
Major depression, recurrent or chronic	31 (27%)	28 (25%)
Bipolar disorder	12 (10%)	9 (8%)
Schizophrenia or schizoaffective disorder	20 (17%)	14 (13%)
Anxiety disorders	18 (16%)	19 (17%)
Other	16 (14%)	18 (16%)

[a]From survey of 226 sequential visits in each of four authors' practices. Initial evaluations are excluded from this analysis.

psychotherapy plus pharmacotherapy sessions) or in blocks of three patients per hour. When three patients are scheduled per hour, the average is about one patient per hour who can be seen for 15 minutes or less for a medication check and two patients who can benefit from longer sessions of 22–25 minutes. Over the course of several hours of work, we can usually blend these types of visits into our schedules in a smooth and efficient way while providing meaningful sessions to a variety of patients.

The principal diagnoses of patients in our practice survey are shown in Table 2–1. As is the case in most ambulatory practices, the largest proportion of patients has mood disorders, followed by anxiety disorders. However, the proportion of patients with schizophrenia (15%; 34/226) is not small. The "other" category is quite heterogeneous and includes small numbers of patients with substance abuse, adjustment disorder, attention-deficit/hyperactivity disorder, and somatization disorder, along with a handful of patients with emotional and behavioral problems related to severe or chronic medical illnesses. There were no notable differences in the diagnostic composition of the groups receiving shorter and longer sessions.

Because our practice survey was performed with only four psychiatrists, each of whom is highly experienced in CBT and is clearly committed to an integrated cognitive-behavioral and biological treatment model, a survey of a larger and more varied sample would be unlikely to have the same results. Nevertheless, we believe these data provide a valuable glimpse into a practice style that includes a significant proportion of brief CBT sessions along with initial evaluations, traditional 50-minute sessions, and visits for medication management without specific CBT interventions.

Indications for Combining CBT and Pharmacotherapy in Brief Sessions

The indications for CBT and pharmacotherapy in the dual-therapist mode are rather straightforward. Because standard 50-minute sessions of CBT are being delivered plus brief sessions with a prescribing physician, any of the classic indications for CBT (e.g., major depression and anxiety disorders, eating disorders, substance abuse disorders, personality disorders, and adjunctive treatment for psychoses, bipolar disorder, and medical disorders; Wright et al. 2009) are reasonable targets for treatment. Indications for using brief sessions of combined CBT and pharmacotherapy in the sole-clinician mode have not been studied in randomized controlled trials. However, the general indications for this form of treatment would appear to be the same as for pharmacotherapy because medication is used in all cases.

Traditional 50-minute sessions remain the standard method of delivering a full course of CBT. The majority of outcome studies have used 50-minute sessions, and most cognitive-behavior therapists who are not licensed to prescribe medication devote all or most of their efforts in individual therapy to sessions of this length. In certain situations, we do *not* consider using briefer sessions in the single-therapist mode. Table 2–2 lists some of these situations. The first item listed—"patient has not had a full course of standard CBT, and diagnosis and symptoms suggest this approach is needed"—is the most important.

In performing an assessment, psychiatrists trained in both CBT and pharmacotherapy should ask themselves this question: Would this patient's needs be best met with a full course of 50-minute sessions, or at least a combination of longer and briefer sessions? If the answer is that 50-minute sessions would be the preferred approach, and if the patient wants and has the resources for this type of treatment, we try to arrange for a course of longer sessions. In some cases, we provide all of this treatment ourselves. However, as noted in the next section of this chapter, "Formats for Brief Sessions of Combined CBT and Pharmacotherapy," we often organize a teamwork approach to having 50-minute sessions with a nonphysician therapist and brief sessions with a psychiatrist.

The complexity and chronicity of each patient's problems should also play a role in determining the type of sessions used for combined CBT and pharmacotherapy. Patients who have been traumatized or who have long-

---

Table 2–2. Possible reasons not to use brief sessions alone for combined cognitive-behavior therapy (CBT) and pharmacotherapy

---

Patient has not had full course of standard CBT, and diagnosis and symptoms suggest this approach is needed.

Patient wants standard, full-length sessions and has resources to enter this form of treatment.

Condition is complicated by serious interpersonal problems that are not amenable to brief sessions.

Patient has significant history of trauma or abuse and needs extensive help in coping with these influences.

Axis II pathology is present and requires intensive treatment.

Brief sessions have been tried but do not appear to be meeting patient's needs.

---

standing problems with low self-esteem, self-efficacy, and interpersonal conflicts may require full sessions over a significant period of time. Also, those with personality disorders usually need more intensive treatment. In contrast, a person with rather circumscribed panic or depressive symptoms, obsessive-compulsive disorder, or social phobia who has a good basic self-concept and who is functioning fairly well in everyday life might do well with brief sessions coupled with medication and self-help exercises.

When brief sessions are chosen but the results are not ideal (e.g., symptoms worsen or a patient reaches a plateau and is making no further progress), a change of treatment plan may be needed. In addition to formulating changes in the pharmacotherapy regimen, clinicians should also consider intensifying the CBT component of treatment—by scheduling either longer sessions or more frequent brief sessions. Some of the formats for accomplishing this are explored in the next section of this chapter.

Learning Exercise 2–1 Choosing Brief Sessions for Combined CBT and Pharmacotherapy

1. Identify at least three patients in your practice whom you believe could be treated appropriately with brief sessions of combined CBT and pharmacotherapy in the single-therapist mode.

2. Identify at least three patients in your practice whom you think should be treated with 50-minute CBT sessions.

Formats for Brief Sessions of Combined CBT and Pharmacotherapy

We use several different formats that we can recommend to psychiatrists or other licensed prescribers who perform CBT in brief sessions (Table 2–3). The case formulation (see Chapter 4, "Case Formulation and Treatment Planning") and the considerations noted in Tables 2–2 and 2–3 should be used to guide the selection of a format.

When a Psychiatrist or Other Medication Prescriber Is the Sole Provider

Following the initial evaluation, some patients immediately begin having brief sessions with a sole provider. Another single-provider scenario is to schedule a few 50-minute sessions for initial treatment intensity and then transition to briefer sessions. Still another format for a sole provider who can prescribe medications is to mix 50-minute and briefer sessions together depending on the clinical status of the patient and the severity or complexity of issues that might need discussion.

Dual-Clinician Combined CBT and Pharmacotherapy

The term *split treatment* has sometimes been used to describe a form of the dual-therapist mode for delivering combined pharmacotherapy and psychotherapy (Riba and Balon 2005). The word *split* emphasizes the potential problems of having two therapists who may not agree on a theoretical approach or a treatment plan, who may not understand or support the work of the other, who may have professional or turf rivalries, and who do not communicate effectively in joining their efforts on behalf of the patient. In our clinical practices, we try hard to avoid any splits between clinicians. Instead, we emphasize close collaboration and teamwork wherever possible.

An illustration of a team approach to combined therapy can be found in the first author's (Wright's) clinical setting at the University of Louisville. The staff at this center includes several psychiatrists who are trained in CBT, in addition to nonphysician therapists who are experts in providing CBT with individuals, families, and groups. Some of the therapists have special interests and skills in areas such as mood and anxiety disorders, women's mental health, substance abuse, eating disorders, and psychoses. When patients are seen in a dual-therapist mode, format 4 in Table 2–3 is used (i.e., brief sessions with a psychiatrist are coordinated

Table 2–3. Formats for brief sessions of combined cognitive-behavior therapy (CBT) and pharmacotherapy

Format type	Provider(s)	Description
1	Psychiatrist[a]	Initial evaluation followed by brief sessions only
2	Psychiatrist[a]	Several 50-minute sessions to begin therapy and then transition to briefer sessions
3	Psychiatrist[a]	A mixture of 50-minute and briefer sessions depending on patient need and phase of therapy
4	Team of psychiatrist[a] and nonphysician cognitive-behavior therapist	Brief sessions with psychiatrist are coordinated with 50-minute sessions with nonphysician cognitive-behavior therapist
5	Psychiatrist[a] and nonphysician cognitive-behavior therapist who work largely in parallel	Brief sessions with psychiatrist and 50-minute sessions with nonphysician cognitive-behavior therapist, but clinicians do not work together or communicate regularly
6	Psychiatrist[a] and nonphysician therapist not trained in CBT	Brief sessions with psychiatrist and longer sessions with nonphysician therapist (e.g., pastoral counselor, psychodynamic therapist, family therapist) who provides therapy from a different orientation

[a]A psychiatrist, other licensed physician, or nurse practitioner who is trained to deliver both CBT and pharmacotherapy.

with 50-minute sessions with a nonphysician cognitive-behavior therapist). A joint treatment plan is formulated that draws on the strengths and experiences of the various clinicians, an overall cognitive-behavioral-biological-sociocultural model is used, a unified approach is presented to the patient, and communication is facilitated in a number of ways.

An obvious advantage of providing combined therapy in the same practice is the use of a single medical record. An electronic medical record with the capacity to send internal e-mail messages regarding patient care can be especially helpful. Another plus of working together in the same office is the opportunity to talk together on a daily basis about treatment issues. At the University of Louisville, a peer supervision group, held weekly to help clinicians build and maintain their abilities to perform CBT, provides additional help in forging an effective clinical team. The other authors of this book have very similar practice settings that place a high priority on delivering combined CBT and pharmacotherapy in a highly collaborative and tightly integrated manner.

Many psychiatrists and other prescribing clinicians may have work environments that are quite different from the one described above. They may work in solo practices or may not have nonphysician cognitive-behavior therapists in their groups. Therefore, they may be more likely to use formats 5 and 6 in Table 2–3. We also use these formats when working with patients who have a cognitive-behavior therapist from outside our groups or who are seeing a therapist who uses a different theoretical approach. Even in situations such as these, we think it is important for the physician and nonmedical therapist to communicate about the treatment plan and to attempt to coordinate efforts.

Examples of Brief Sessions of Combined CBT and Pharmacotherapy

In the first case example below, a detailed description of some of the interventions used in the treatment of Barbara, a 46-year-old woman with bipolar disorder, is provided to demonstrate how CBT can be delivered productively in brief sessions. The second and third case examples give shorter illustrations of different formats for brief visits of combined CBT and pharmacotherapy.

Barbara

The DVD that accompanies this book presents a wide variety of demonstrations of CBT in brief sessions. We recommend viewing these videos in sequence as we discuss them throughout the volume. The first video demonstrates a variation on the use of treatment format 1 (see Table 2–3).

> Barbara was first seen by Dr. Wright during a short hospital stay for a manic episode about 3 weeks before the session shown in Video Illustration 1 (we recommend viewing this video later in this section). She was admitted after not sleeping at all for 4 days, going on an extensive spending spree that led to overdrafts on her checking accounts, and being told by her boss that she

had to get help because she was acting erratically and was "all over the place." During the hospitalization, Barbara was treated with a combination of lithium carbonate and an atypical antipsychotic. Adjunctive treatment with CBT was also initiated (see Wright et al. 2009 for a description of CBT methods for bipolar disorder). The initial evaluation of about 50 minutes was followed by four briefer visits ranging from 15 to 25 minutes each. Barbara also met with nurses who assisted Dr. Wright in teaching basic principles of CBT. After a 6-day stay in the hospital, the manic episode was largely resolved, and Barbara was discharged to outpatient treatment.

The session shown in Video Illustration 1 was the second of a planned series of many brief outpatient sessions. This plan included the scheduling of brief sessions every 1–2 weeks for about 2–3 months, with a tapering to monthly and then quarterly visits depending on Barbara's response to treatment, adherence pattern, and ability to learn CBT skills. If this pattern of sessions helped Barbara to achieve a remission and avoid relapse, a brief quarterly session format could continue. However, if significant exacerbations occurred or other problems emerged, the frequency of brief sessions could be increased, some longer sessions could be added, or Barbara could be referred for more intensive CBT with a nonphysician therapist (formats 3 and 5 in Table 2–3). Also, the pharmacotherapy component of the regimen would be monitored closely and modified if needed.

Barbara reported a history of three previous episodes of depression but no suicidal ideation or attempts. Her first mania did not occur until her late 30s. She had not been hospitalized until the current episode—her second experience with mania. She had no history of substance abuse. Barbara's father had depression for much of his life and was eventually diagnosed with bipolar disorder. He was treated with lithium, which apparently worked well. Although her parents divorced when she was age 15 years, Barbara noted that she had a "good childhood" and has remained close to both parents. Her own marital relationships have been marked by much conflict. She has been divorced twice and is currently single. Her last marriage failed after she had an affair with a married man while she was manic. Barbara has three children, ages 13, 15, and 17. Her oldest child has been giving her "trouble"; although he is doing well in school, he sometimes cuts class and comes home later than expected. Barbara has had a successful career developing displays for department stores and other commercial businesses. She enjoys hobbies of quilting and making porcelain dolls.

Barbara's previous treatment was primarily with antidepressant medication. She took lithium briefly after the previous episode of mania, but she stopped after about a year because she concluded that she did not really have bipolar disorder. She had not had CBT before her recent hospitalization.

In the beginning of the session shown in Video Illustration 1, Barbara shows Dr. Wright her written agenda for the visit and a symptom summary worksheet. As we detail in Chapter 3, "Enhancing the Impact of Brief Sessions," techniques such as preparing an agenda in advance and using checklists or scales for symptom reviews can be used to make sessions more efficient. Symptom summary worksheets are used in CBT with patients who have bipolar disorder (Wright et al. 2009) for several purposes: to help patients log and record their symptoms, to encourage them to become more aware of early warning signs of shifts into hypomania or depression, and to work on plans to manage symptoms before they escalate into full episodes of illness.

Barbara's agenda had two items: 1) "Help me to stop 'losing it' when I get into arguments with my son" and 2) "Doing something about the tremor." Her symptom summary worksheet had been started when she was hospitalized. Barbara's homework before the session shown in Video Illustration 1 had been to review the worksheet and to circle any symptoms that she observed in herself. Figure 2–1 shows her worksheet for hypomanic and manic symptoms. The only symptom that she had experienced was irritability. As shown in the video illustration, recognizing this symptom provided an excellent opportunity for a brief CBT intervention.

We recommend viewing Video Illustration 1 now and then reading some of our observations on the highlights of this demonstration of CBT using a brief format. The first section of Barbara's session (a CBT intervention for her first agenda item, "Help me to stop 'losing it' when I get into arguments with my son") is shown in Video Illustration 1. The last part of her session (work on her second agenda item, "Doing something about the tremor") is discussed in Chapter 5, "Promoting Adherence."

▶ **Video Illustration 1.** A Brief CBT Session: Dr. Wright and Barbara

The first video demonstrates several CBT methods that can be delivered successfully in brief sessions. An agenda is set, and the session is structured to help Barbara stay on track to perform significant CBT work in a brief time frame. Dr. Wright reminds Barbara of her previous efforts to learn about automatic thoughts while she was hospitalized and then employs a very brief "mini-lesson" to review the definition. He then asks her to go back over the scene of the argument with her son to recognize some of her automatic thoughts.

Dr. Wright: Can you try to think back to it? Try to put yourself back in that scene in your mind.
Barbara: It probably started before he walked in the front door after school.
Dr. Wright: What was going through your mind then?
Barbara: I had just felt like I had had it. You know, I've been a single

Symptom	Mild	Moderate	Severe
Irritability	Edgy, quick to criticize others, voice may have a sharp tone.	May throw dishes or other things, yell at kids, show little concern for others' problems.	Scream and rant and rave. Have trouble sitting still —others better stay out of my way. Always on edge—work, home, everywhere.
Thinking I can do more than is realistic—not paying attention to real concerns.	Minimize real problems in my life—pay less attention to genuine worries like bills or work responsibilities.	Starting to get pumped up about special projects—taking on way more than I can actually handle. I push my way into positions where I am overcommitted.	Grandiosity out of control. I think I am the best in everything I do. I push others out of the way, don't listen to them—do it my way.
Sleeping too little	Stay up about 1 hour extra most nights because I am really enjoying myself or am involved in a special project.	Staying up 2 or more hours extra most nights. I am on a roll. I have lots of trouble shutting off my mind to go to sleep. Don't really want to sleep.	I am going a mile a minute—don't want to sleep at all. I could stay up for 3 or 4 nights before crashing.
Mind racing	Thoughts begin to pick up speed. This is subtle, but I start to feel more creative and full of life.	Thoughts definitely are speeding along. I don't pay much attention to what others are saying.	Thoughts are jumping around so fast that sometimes I don't make a lot of sense.
Getting into trouble	A bit of extra risk taking. I might drive 5–10 miles faster, and I might flirt more with men.	I say things that I shouldn't —off-color jokes. I wear more provocative clothes. I'm spending more than I should.	I am really in trouble now—spending more money than I have, racking up credit card debt, getting involved with the wrong kind of men.

Figure 2–1. Symptom summary worksheet for hypomanic and manic symptoms: Barbara's example.

> mom…I've worked hard. I don't get any respect. I don't get any help from him…I'd just had it!
>
> Dr. Wright: …And as this thing evolved, were there any more intense thoughts that went through your head…more extreme than that?
>
> Barbara: Yeah. I did have a few thoughts that he's going to be like his dad…He's going to be a loser and a bum.
>
> Dr. Wright: And as you got closer to the time that you actually had the blowup, were those the kinds of thoughts that were going through your head? Like he is a loser…He's going to be a bum?
>
> Barbara: Yes, exactly.
>
> Dr. Wright: So, I have a hunch this was really building up the strength of your anger.
>
> Barbara: Yes.
>
> Dr. Wright: And once you did get angry like that, how did you behave?
>
> Barbara: …I just get so angry, I throw things. Whatever is around, I reach for it and throw it…I just have no control. I scream, yell, and throw things.

After eliciting automatic thoughts, Dr. Wright then suggests that Barbara might get a better handle on these types of situations by recognizing that her thinking is quite extreme and absolute. He notes that these types of thoughts (e.g., "I don't get any respect…He's going to be a loser and a bum") can be inflammatory—"They can set you on fire…set your emotions on fire because they are so extreme."

The next step in this intervention was working on developing a more rational perspective. Although Barbara admits that she believes her automatic thoughts "100%" when she is in the middle of the situation, her belief is only "30%" when she is thinking "in the cool light of day." Dr. Wright then asks her to break through the absolutistic thinking by recognizing some of her son's positives.

> Dr. Wright: Does he do anything to help around the house? Or does he do anything you really like?
>
> Barbara: He mows the lawn sometimes. He's helped me out with the dishes before. And he's been on the honor roll before…made the basketball team.
>
> Dr. Wright: It sounds like you're proud of him to some extent. Is that true?
>
> Barbara: Yes, that's true…I love him.

After Barbara and Dr. Wright agree that her extreme reactions get in the way of showing her love, they use another valuable CBT method for brief sessions—a coping card—to capture the ideas they have generated for managing irritability and anger (Figure 2–2). This vignette ends with a suggestion that they will continue to work on the problem with irritability in future sessions and that the principles Barbara has learned from the example of a "blowup" with her son can be applied to many other sit-

---

Problem: Anger and irritability with son

1. *When I start to get angry or irritable, stop to spot my automatic thoughts and check them out to see how accurate they are.*
2. *Try to take a balanced look at the situation.*
3. *Do something to step away from the situation...like take a walk or a "timeout."*
4. *Try talking with my son and work out a solution for the problem.*

Figure 2–2. Barbara's coping card.

uations where she becomes irritable and angry. We think that this video illustration gives a good example of how key elements of CBT can be delivered in brief sessions when a psychiatrist is the sole therapist and how interventions from a series of sessions can be linked together in an overall plan for combined CBT and pharmacotherapy.

Wayne

The second case briefly illustrates how the dual-therapist format can be used effectively in combined therapy.

> Wayne was a 52-year-old manufacturing supervisor who had treatment-resistant depression. He was referred from another psychiatrist who had tried a wide variety of medications, none of which had led to a full or sustained remission. Although Wayne was still able to work, he had ongoing depressive symptoms that limited his effectiveness and interfered with his psychosocial functioning. After work, he became a "couch potato"—spending virtually all of his time staring at the TV or doing "nothing." He had dropped out of all his social activities (e.g., bowling, church groups, fishing) and spent little time in family activities. His self-esteem was very low. Although he had hopeless thoughts about not being able to recover, he did not consider suicide an option.

Because Wayne had never had CBT, had very long-standing symptoms, and appeared to be stuck in depression, a concentrated treatment plan of brief sessions with Dr. Thase and 50-minute CBT visits with a social worker was developed (format 4 in Table 2–3). Dr. Thase scheduled brief sessions every 2–4 weeks in which he initiated a series of augmentation strategies for pharmacotherapy of treatment-resistant depression but also used CBT methods that were coordinated with the efforts of the social worker. Some of the CBT influences and techniques used by Dr. Thase in these sessions were 1) case formulation based on the comprehensive cognitive-behavioral-biological-sociocultural model; 2) collaborative empiricism; 3) structuring the session with overall goals, an agenda, and feedback; 4) inquiring about the CBT work done by the social worker and supporting the value of this therapy; 5) asking Wayne to briefly explain his homework assignments from the 50-minute sessions; 6) suggesting and/or reinforcing behavioral activation assignments that were consistent with the overall treatment plan; 7) spotting obvious maladaptive cognitions, asking the patient to try to revise his thinking, and recommending that he discuss the cognitions at more length in his next visit with the social worker; and 8) writing a coping card for a problem discussed in the session and asking Wayne to show the card at his next 50-minute CBT session.

Just as Dr. Thase made a clear effort to promote the value of the 50-minute CBT sessions, the social worker who was providing more intensive CBT also worked to support Wayne's sessions with Dr. Thase. For example, at each session, she asked Wayne for a brief summary of the previous brief visit with Dr. Thase, a report on the strategies they were using for pharmacotherapy, and feedback on any suggestions that Dr. Thase had made. In this manner, the two clinicians implemented a cohesive and integrated treatment strategy that steered away from the potential pitfalls of split therapy.

Consuela

A case from Dr. Sudak's practice demonstrates a method of using brief sessions along with 50-minute visits with a therapist who is using a different model for treatment (format 6 in Table 2–3).

> Consuela was a 22-year-old-woman who was referred by her primary care doctor to Dr. Sudak for treatment of agoraphobia. During the initial evaluation, Dr. Sudak learned that Consuela had been seeing a pastoral counselor about twice a month for almost a year because of grief after the death of a close friend in a car accident. Consuela and her friend had been passengers in a car that was hit by a drunk driver. The accident had also led to spiritual questions and issues—Consuela had been questioning how a "loving God" could let such a tragedy occur. Although Consuela valued the sessions with the pastoral counselor very much, she realized that they were not helping her with her agoraphobic symptoms that had been present to some extent since about age 16 or 17. The principal symptoms were fear and avoidance of driving (now worse after the accident) and crowded places such as malls or grocery stores. Dr. Sudak also diagnosed Consuela with posttraumatic

stress disorder. Although fear of driving was present to some extent before the tragic death of her friend, the avoidance problem was much worse now, and Consuela was having "flashbacks." She had been unable to drive alone, or with assistance, in any areas that reminded her of the accident (e.g., four-lane highways, congested spots, roads close to malls).

Because Consuela was already in therapy with a pastoral counselor, Dr. Sudak 1) explained a combined CBT and pharmacotherapy approach to anxiety disorders to Consuela; 2) asked Consuela for permission to discuss treatment with her pastoral counselor; 3) determined Consuela's preferences about therapy and found that she wished to continue pastoral counseling while participating in CBT; 4) discussed a joint treatment plan with the pastoral counselor and decided on a series of 8–12 brief sessions plus use of a selective serotonin reuptake inhibitor; and 5) agreed with the pastoral counselor and Consuela to communicate with updates about progress in both CBT and pastoral counseling. The choice of brief sessions seemed appropriate because Consuela was participating in full-length sessions in pastoral counseling, was strongly motivated for CBT, and appeared willing and able to engage in a self-help exposure protocol with homework outside therapy sessions. More details on Consuela's treatment are provided in Chapter 9, "Behavioral Methods for Anxiety."

> **Learning Exercise 2–2**   Selecting Formats for Combined CBT and Pharmacotherapy
>
> 1. Review the six formats for brief sessions of combined CBT and pharmacotherapy listed in Table 2–3. Try to identify patients from your practice who could be (or are) treated with each of the six formats.
>
> 2. List at least three problems or barriers you have encountered in using any of the formats for brief combined sessions. Write out some possible solutions that you could implement for each of these problems or barriers.

Summary

Key Points for Clinicians

- There are many possible indications for using brief sessions for delivery of all or part of the treatment plan in combined CBT and pharmacotherapy.
- Examples of indications for brief visits in which a psychiatrist or other prescribing clinician is the sole provider include the following situa-

tions: 1) CBT is being used as an adjunct to pharmacotherapy for a major mental disorder, 2) brief CBT visits appear to be a reasonable approach for a circumscribed problem, and 3) patient and psychiatrist agree on this preference.

- Indications for dual-therapist delivery of combined CBT and pharmacotherapy include the following situations: 1) patient's diagnosis and symptoms suggest that full course of CBT is needed; 2) patient's condition is complicated by trauma, abuse, serious interpersonal problems, or significant Axis II pathology; and 3) patient and psychiatrist agree on this preference.
- Brief visits of combined CBT and pharmacotherapy can be delivered in several different formats. The choice of the format for therapy should be based on a thorough assessment and case formulation.
- In the single-clinician mode, the psychiatrist or other prescribing physician should select session length and intensity that match the patient's needs and capacities.
- In the dual-clinician mode, the clinicians should use a cognitive-behavioral-biological-sociocultural model for treatment, present a unified approach to the patient, and communicate regularly.
- Even when full 50-minute CBT sessions are being conducted by a nonmedical therapist, psychiatrists and other prescribers can use CBT principles in brief sessions to enhance the overall treatment plan.

Concepts and Skills for Patients to Learn

- Much can be accomplished in brief sessions of combined CBT and pharmacotherapy.
- In developing a treatment plan, patients and clinicians should discuss the possible benefits of brief sessions, 50-minute sessions, or a mixture of different visit lengths and make a collaborative decision on the form of therapy that will be used.
- If one form of therapy does not appear to be working well, a discussion should be held about options for modifying the treatment plan.
- If 50-minute sessions have been conducted but no longer appear to be needed, the patient and clinician can consider transitioning to briefer sessions.

References

Riba MB, Balon R: Competence in Combining Pharmacotherapy and Psychotherapy: Integrated and Split Treatment. Washington, DC, American Psychiatric Publishing, 2005

Wright JH, Turkington D, Kingdon DG, et al: Cognitive-Behavior Therapy for Severe Mental Illness: An Illustrated Guide. Washington, DC, American Psychiatric Publishing, 2009

CHAPTER 3

Enhancing the Impact of Brief Sessions

LEARNING MAP

Maximizing the therapeutic relationship

⇩

Symptom checks

⇩

Structuring and pacing: keys to high-yield sessions

⇩

Psychoeducation

⇩

Using technology to improve efficiency

⇩

Homework and self-help as therapy extenders

⇩

Capitalizing on positive interactions between pharmacotherapy and CBT

When brief sessions are being used for combined cognitive-behavior therapy (CBT) and pharmacotherapy, clinicians need to find ways to get the most from the available time. Both clinician and patient should leave the session with a sense that they have had excellent communication, have done productive work, and have a reasonable treatment plan to carry forward. In this chapter, we describe some methods that can be used to enhance the impact of brief sessions.

Maximizing the Therapeutic Relationship

The collaborative-empirical therapeutic relationship in CBT (Beck et al. 1979; Sudak 2006; Wright et al. 2006) is especially well suited to brief sessions because it emphasizes teamwork and an action-oriented approach to therapy. Although during brief visits clinicians may feel somewhat pressured to compact a considerable amount of work into a short time, attention still needs to be paid to the fundamental attributes of all effective therapeutic relationships—genuineness, positive regard, warmth, and accurate empathy (Beck et al. 1979; Wright et al. 2006). Striking a balance between these essential therapist activities and the business of structuring and providing specific CBT and pharmacotherapy interventions is a critically important challenge for clinicians who are providing treatment in brief sessions.

In writing about brief CBT sessions conducted in Japan, Ono and Berger (1995) observed that clinicians might model their behavior on the undivided attention of the server to the recipient in the traditional Japanese tea ceremony. The authors highlight the term *ichigo ichie*, which is often used to describe the relationship between the host and the guest: *ichigo* means a whole life, and *ichie* means one meeting. Although CBT is certainly a more collaborative process, the authors' point is well taken. Clinicians need to show patients their deepest concern and concentrated thoughtfulness in brief sessions.

As demonstrated in Video Illustration 2, the therapeutic relationship can make a strong contribution to the outcome of brief sessions. This video shows Dr. Sudak working with Grace, a woman who has depression after the loss of her husband from cancer and who is now trying to take on a new job. While demonstrating genuine concern and empathy, the clinician moves the session along with a plan to assist Grace in revising some negative automatic thoughts. The video also illustrates the use of effective Socratic questions to help Grace gain a healthier perspective on her problems. The Socratic questioning method is a primary element of the collaborative-empirical relationship in CBT. We describe more about Grace's treatment in Chapter 7, "Targeting Maladaptive Thinking."

▶ **Video Illustration 2.** Modifying Automatic Thoughts I: Dr. Sudak and Grace

In the following excerpt from Video Illustration 2, Dr. Sudak demonstrates how to weave empathic comments into a therapeutic effort to change distressing cognitions.

> Dr. Sudak: When you said, "I might get fired again…," what actually happened with the old job?
> Grace: Well, I didn't get fired. They were downsizing, and a few of us got laid off…I know it wasn't directed at me, but I still lost my job.
> Dr. Sudak: Right…It's really a big stressor to lose your job…There's a lot going on here.
> Grace: Yeah.
> Dr. Sudak: But by the same token, you said you knew that it wasn't about you.
> Grace: Yeah…It wasn't…I did OK.
> Dr. Sudak: It wasn't about your work performance?
> Grace: No, it wasn't. But I did lose it…I've lost a lot of things. And I'm scared about that happening again.
> Dr. Sudak: …You've got a lot on your shoulders, I know.

Some suggestions for building strong therapeutic relationships in brief sessions are listed in Table 3–1. In addition to the collaborative, empathic, and highly attentive therapy style we discussed above, the relationship in brief sessions can be enhanced by selecting targets that yield rapid and/or especially welcome results. If patients are getting relief from symptoms or are finding solutions to problems, their confidence and trust in the clinician are likely to grow. Thus, we recommend that a mini-formulation (see Chapter 4, "Case Formulation and Treatment Planning") be constructed as quickly as possible and that clinicians choose targets and interventions that 1) are clearly important to the patient, 2) are suitable for treatment in brief sessions, and 3) have a good chance of leading to positive outcomes.

A focus on clear communication is another feature of good therapeutic relationships in brief sessions. Because time is limited, therapists need to make special efforts to listen very carefully to patients and to be effective communicators. Some of the techniques that we like to use to improve communication are 1) working to pare down our explanations and comments to "nuggets" of information that patients can easily understand and use, 2) providing brief but incisive summaries of key points, and 3) asking for feedback to check for understanding.

Humor can also be an appropriate tool for promoting good relationships in brief sessions. Some of our video illustrations demonstrate how

---

Table 3–1. Ways to enhance collaborative empiricism in brief sessions

---

Emphasize a team approach in which there is shared responsibility for the work of therapy.

Stay tuned to the patient's emotions and respond with accurate empathy when appropriate.

Give the patient your full attention; try to avoid digressions.

Use Socratic questions to show more rational perspectives and to build rapport.

Choose targets for change that have both high relevance and good opportunities for success in a brief session format.

Burnish your communication skills: listen carefully, give clear and succinct explanations, summarize key points, and ask for and give feedback.

Do not forget that humor can sometimes be a very effective method of enhancing the relationship and promoting learning.

---

use of a judicious sense of humor can be a genuine and effective way of normalizing the relationship and helping patients gain fresh perspectives. Another possible benefit of humor is that it can be used as a coping skill in responding to stress or in managing life problems. Taking a few moments to laugh together or to encourage use of humor as a coping strategy can often be time well spent in brief sessions.

Symptom Checks

An important component of every session is symptom assessment, which can be performed in brief visits through several time-saving ways. A patient can be educated to give a succinct report on progress or setbacks at the beginning of each session, and the clinician can follow up on this report by asking several incisive questions about key symptoms. For example, if sleep problems have been a focus of treatment, the clinician can ask a few brief questions about any recent changes in the patient's sleep pattern. Another commonly used method is to ask the patient to rate the overall degree of symptoms (e.g., depression, anxiety, the interference of obsessive-compulsive disorder [OCD] with daily life) on 0- to 10-point scales, with 10 representing the most extreme distress and 0 representing no symptoms. If this technique is used over a series of sessions, the clinician and patient will have a simple but useful method of measuring the impact of treatment.

Routine use of self-report rating scales can provide a more systematic way of assessing symptoms and checking on progress. Although most clinicians do not use rating scales in their clinical work, this practice has the potential for significantly improving the quality of care (Zimmerman and McGlinchey 2008). A reasonable plan for integrating rating scales into brief sessions might be to ask patients to arrive 15 minutes before the scheduled start time of the visit with the clinician and to use this time to complete one or two brief rating scales. If an electronic medical record is being used, patients can do the rating on a computer in the waiting room so that the scale is available at the start of the session. If a paper chart is being used, the rating scale can be scored by office staff and attached to the medical record before the visit with the clinician begins.

In Table 3–2, we list brief self-report rating scales that are suitable for routine use in clinical settings. Except the Beck Depression Inventory and Beck Anxiety Inventory, the scales are in the public domain and can be used without charge. We list the Beck scales because they have been employed extensively in research studies and clinical practice and are considered standard measures. However, the cost of these copyrighted instruments is a consideration when they are used for each patient visit. Readers who are interested in learning more about brief self-report rating scales can consult reviews by Lam et al. (2005) or Goodwin and Jamison (2007).

Structuring and Pacing: Keys to High-Yield Sessions

Set Goals

Goal setting—one of the standard structuring methods for CBT sessions of all lengths—can be a powerful tool for getting the most from brief visits. Therapy goals provide a direction for the entire course of treatment and, if made explicit between clinician and patient, can help them stay on focus and use time wisely. In our experience, specific achievable goals usually work best (e.g., reduce OCD rituals to less than 10% of baseline; sustain a remission from depression; be able to drive at least daily with little or no fear; minimize the risk of relapse from bipolar disorder; be able to cope with hallucinations so that they are only like "background noise" and don't upset me; return to and be able to stay at my job). In contrast, vague or poorly thought out goals may lead clinicians and patients to wander through unproductive discussions and miss good opportunities to apply high-impact methods in brief sessions.

Table 3–2. Brief self-report rating scales

Application	Rating scale and source	Reference
Anxiety	Beck Anxiety Inventory (www.pearsonassessments.com/pai)	Beck et al. 1988
	Penn State Worry Questionnaire (Meyer et al. 1990)	Meyer et al. 1990
Delusions and hallucinations	Psychotic Symptom Rating Scales (Haddock et al. 1999)	Haddock et al. 1999
Depression	Beck Depression Inventory (www.pearsonassessments.com/pai)	Beck et al. 1961
	Patient Health Questionnaire–9 (www.mapi-trust.org/test/129-phq)	Kroenke et al. 2001
	Quick Inventory of Depressive Symptomatology Self-Report Version–16 (www.ids-qids.org)	Rush et al. 2003

Note. These scales are listed in Appendix 1, "Worksheets and Checklists."

The following are some useful questions for clinicians to ask themselves:

1. Have we set specific, meaningful, and achievable goals for treatment?
2. Are these goals appropriate for brief sessions?
3. Can the patient articulate the goals? Does the patient have a clear idea of what we are trying to accomplish? If not, what questions should I ask to better define the goals?
4. Have I asked for feedback often enough to see if we are staying on course to achieve the goals?
5. Do the goals need to be reconsidered or revised?
6. Do the patient and I agree on the goals? If we disagree on the goals for treatment, can we collaborate on modifying the goals to help us use brief sessions more productively?

Sharply Focus the Therapy Effort

When effective goals are chosen and therapy is guided by an accurate formulation (see Chapter 4, "Case Formulation and Treatment Planning"), clinicians and patients can narrow their attention to central problems, themes, or processes that can offer excellent opportunities for making solid progress. Some of the possible advantages of maintaining a sharp focus in brief sessions are listed in Table 3–3. The first two benefits are

---

Table 3–3. Advantages of having a clear focus for brief sessions

Can reduce a sense of being overwhelmed

Can stimulate hope when progress is made on a specific problem

Can enhance learning

If cognitive-behavior therapy methods for one problem can be learned well, these skills can be transferred to other situations and problems

Helps to avoid digressions and inefficiencies

Can improve the productivity of brief sessions

---

demonstrated in Video Illustration 2. Grace was initially overwhelmed with the various problems that she was confronting in starting a new job and coping with the loss of her husband. However, when Dr. Sudak narrowed the focus of the session to a specific component of the problem (coping with negative predictions about her work situation), Grace felt a substantial degree of relief and became more optimistic about her future.

In supervising trainees in CBT, we often find that they try to do too much in a single session. They may not stick with one problem or idea long enough for the patient to understand key points or to thoroughly learn a CBT concept or skill. We think that doing one or two things well in a therapy session is preferable to trying to "cover the waterfront." If patients can fully grasp a basic CBT principle as it applies to a circumscribed situation, then they can apply what they have learned to many other problems in their lives. A template of understanding can be developed that can have wide-ranging effects. As Arieti (1985) noted, the study of "cognition teaches us that the human being is *Homo symbolicus* for which a small part becomes a symbol which stands for the whole" (p. 240).

Use a Session Agenda

In CBT, agendas are used to keep individual sessions on track and to relate the work in the individual session to the overall goals of treatment. In *Learning Cognitive-Behavior Therapy: An Illustrated Guide*, Wright et al. (2006) explained agenda setting in detail and gave a video example of agenda setting in a 50-minute session. This example, from very early in therapy, lasts almost 8 minutes—an amount of time that may be needed in the opening phase of treatment when patients are being socialized to the nature and structure of 50-minute sessions. However, time spent in agenda setting is typically reduced considerably as patients enter the middle and later stages of CBT in 50-minute sessions, and also is shortened a great deal in sessions of 25 minutes or less.

Table 3–4.   Agenda-setting techniques for brief sessions

Educate patients on methods for making effective agendas.

Instruct patients on the value of preparing an agenda in advance.

Ask patients to take primary responsibility for constructing the agenda.

If the patient has not prepared an agenda in advance, useful targets for a brief session often can be chosen quickly by asking questions such as these:

- What do you want to put on the agenda for today?
- What could we work on today that would help us stay focused on our goal (list goal)?
- Would it be OK to work on _____ (list a key target that the clinician believes to be important)?
- What could we follow up on from the last session? (Clinician looks at medical record.)
- Can we put the homework assignment from last time on the agenda?

In brief sessions, we try to use abbreviated agenda-setting techniques that provide needed structure for therapy but may only require a few moments to implement (Table 3–4). Perhaps the most important strategy is to educate patients on the benefits and methods of preparing, setting, and following agendas. We do this in two major ways: through mini-lessons (see "Psychoeducation" section later in this chapter) and by modeling the use of agendas in sessions.

We try to convey to our patients the following key points about effective agenda setting for brief sessions: 1) agenda items should be linked to the overall goals of therapy; 2) specific agenda items (e.g., develop a coping strategy for problem at work, resolve questions about medication dose and side effects, decide on next steps in following the exposure therapy plan for fear of driving, review homework) usually work better than general discussion topics; 3) a beneficial practice is to state agenda items in a way that will allow the patient and clinician to know if progress is being made and/or the item has been satisfactorily addressed; and 4) agenda items can lead to useful homework assignments and also can be carried over from visit to visit, thus linking sessions together to reach the overall objectives of treatment (Wright et al. 2006).

As part of the educational effort, we often encourage patients to prepare a written agenda in advance of the therapy appointment. A written agenda can help patients bring their concerns to the immediate attention of the clinician, ensure that important items are not forgotten, and

> 1. Help me stop "losing it" when I get into arguments with my son.
> 2. Do something about the tremor.

Figure 3–1. An agenda prepared in advance for a brief session: Barbara's example.

prompt the patient and clinician to get to work rapidly to solve problems. Because agenda setting is a collaborative process in CBT, clinicians always need to retain the option of suggesting other items that might be covered productively during the current visit or considered for future sessions.

Video Illustration 1, discussed in Chapter 2, "Indications and Formats for Brief CBT Sessions," shows the beginning of a brief session to which Barbara, a woman with bipolar disorder, brought a written agenda. Barbara's agenda is shown in Figure 3–1. Most of the video illustrations in this book (e.g., see Video Illustration 2 with Dr. Sudak and Grace in this chapter) do not show the beginning of the visit when an agenda is set but instead pick up at a point in the session where a specific method or technique is demonstrated. However, in all of the cases, an agenda of some type was negotiated very early in the visit.

Many of our patients like to prepare written agendas in advance. Others may think of agenda items before the session but, instead of writing out a list, prefer to spend a short time at the beginning of the visit outlining the agenda with the clinician. Examples of efficient and effective questions that can be used to help shape agendas are listed at the end of Table 3–4. The examples include open-ended queries that give the patient the chance to outline the agenda and others that are more directive or targeted. These questions can be used with patients who have given the agenda some forethought but have not yet solidified their plans for the session. The questions also can be used with patients who come to sessions without a clear idea of what they want to accomplish. In the latter situation, the clinician may need to take the lead in constructing an agenda and suggesting topics, while continuing to teach the patient about the value of structuring brief sessions with agendas.

The agenda-setting methods described above are recommended for routine use in treatment of patients with nonpsychotic Axis I disorders. In CBT for patients with schizophrenia or other psychoses, a specific agenda may not be discussed at the beginning of the session (for detailed descriptions of CBT methods for these conditions, see Chapter 11, "Modifying Delusions"; Chapter 12, "Coping with Hallucinations"; Wright et al. 2009). However, the clinician still keeps an implicit agenda in mind while guiding and structuring the flow of the session.

Learning Exercise 3–1   Agenda Setting

1. Practice agenda-setting methods for brief sessions with at least one of your patients.

2. Educate the patient on the value of having an agenda for each session.

3. Ask the patient to prepare an agenda in advance for the next session.

4. Use the agenda to structure the session.

Pace Interventions

Throughout brief sessions, we make a concentrated effort to pace interventions in a manner that uses time well, while not giving patients a sense that we are rushing or not giving full attention to their concerns. In a way, a well-paced brief CBT visit requires the clinician to think like an accomplished chess player who plots several moves ahead and conceptualizes a variety of options in advance. Although an overall collaborative stance needs to be maintained, guiding the session on a constructive and efficient path from its beginning to its conclusion is the clinician's responsibility.

Table 3–5.   Pacing goals for brief sessions

Session phase	Pacing goals
Opening phase	Set agenda.
	Perform symptom check.
Middle phase	Review pharmacotherapy regimen and modify if needed.
	Review homework, if any, from previous session.
	Focus on one or more agenda items with cognitive-behavior therapy methods.
	Check for understanding, and ask for feedback and/or questions from patient.
	Assign homework if appropriate.
Closing phase	Review and wrap-up.
	Check for understanding, and ask for feedback and/or questions from patient.
	Assign homework if appropriate.

Pacing goals for the opening, middle, and closing phases of brief sessions are summarized in Table 3–5. A great deal can be accomplished in a well-paced brief session. In the opening phase, the clinician greets the patient, does a symptom check, and sets an agenda. Although the time needed to accomplish these tasks can vary widely, we typically can move to the middle phase of a brief session in less than 5 minutes. In the middle phase, medication issues are discussed if needed, homework is reviewed, and CBT work is done on one or more specific agenda items. New homework can be developed in the middle or the closing phase of the session. In the closing phase, the clinician should offer a review and a wrap-up of the session. In both these middle and closing phases, the clinician should ask for and give feedback and should check to see if the patient has any questions or comments about the work that is being done in the session.

If these pacing goals are to be accomplished, clinicians may need to use a variety of artful comments and directions to shape the session. Although many communication styles can work effectively in pacing brief sessions, we think that the methods in Table 3–6 will work well for most clinicians.

Psychoeducation

The psychoeducational emphasis of CBT is one of the primary reasons that we think this treatment approach has great potential for use in brief sessions. Although the clinician's role as teacher/coach is highly important in CBT, educational efforts do not typically require large amounts of time. In fact, psychoeducation in longer sessions of 45–50 minutes is usually delivered in "mini-lessons" (short explanations or demonstrations) or by suggesting readings or other homework to be completed between visits with the clinician (Basco and Rush 2005; Beck 1995; Sudak 2006; Wright et al. 2006).

The following are some of our recommendations for providing psychoeducation in brief CBT sessions:

1. **Try to directly relate teaching points to situations or problems in the patient's own life.** If educational moments are highly relevant to the patient's current dilemma or way of thinking, the patient may be more likely to recall and use them.
2. **Use Socratic questioning to stimulate the patient's involvement in the learning process.** Questions that prime patients to be curious and to "think about their thinking" may be more effective than lecturing or the use of an overly didactic teaching style.

Table 3–6. Tips for pacing brief sessions

Use a conversational, collaborative style of asking questions and guiding the course of therapy so patients do not feel that they are being pushed or prodded through the session.

If patients digress, make judicious comments that bring them back to the task.

If needed, remind patients of overall goals of treatment or make suggestions that help them attend to main themes.

Use therapy notes to keep patients centered on useful discussions (e.g., if session seems to be drifting, say "Let's check our notes to see if we are staying on track…What is the main thing we have been working on?").

Plan ahead. Use a formulation to chart a course through the session.

Emphasize the use of questions and comments that have a direct link to the goals and purposes of the treatment; minimize questions and comments that fill time with unfocused conversation. A bit of social communication (e.g., comments about the weather, a holiday, a trip the patient just had or is planning to take) at the beginning and end of the session is fine, but if the session is weighted heavily with this type of commentary, the tenets of pacing brief cognitive-behavior therapy sessions have been breached.

Give and ask for feedback to be sure that the pace of the session is not too fast or too slow (e.g., "Can you recap the main points that we have covered so far today?" "Are we covering the things you wanted to do today?" "How does the session seem to be going?" "Is there anything you suggest I do differently?").

---

3. **If a didactic lesson seems to be needed (e.g., to explain the concept of exposure therapy or to teach the value of a coping card), keep it short and focused on a specific problem or issue.** Mini-lessons can often be delivered in a very succinct manner. Watch the video illustrations that accompany this book for examples of didactic explanations that are made within very brief time frames.

4. **Use a friendly touch.** Research on the therapeutic relationship has found that the most productive interpersonal processes are observed when clinicians are "friendly teachers" (Muran 1993; Wright and Davis 1994). Thus, we suggest that clinicians teach in a conversational, kind, and empathic manner while maintaining appropriate professional boundaries.

5. **Be a good coach or mentor.** While teaching patients in brief sessions, think of the attributes that are valuable in an effective coach. We

have had the good fortune of having superb coaches and mentors who have exhibited some of the following traits: 1) a stimulating and motivating approach, 2) a genuine interest in teaching, 3) use of empowering methods, 4) clear evidence of expertise, 5) patience and persistence, and 6) respect for the student/mentee.

6. **Use written diagrams, instructions, or logs as learning tools.** A written exercise in a session can be very useful for helping patients understand a key concept. Examples include diagramming the basic CBT model, working on a thought change record, or starting an activity schedule. We also typically encourage patients to keep therapy notebooks for storing and reviewing their work. Logs, diaries, or other written self-monitoring efforts (e.g., sleep logs, mood graphs, exposure and response prevention logs, medication adherence diaries) are valuable for encouraging learning.

7. **Prepare a "library" of educational handouts to give to patients.** To maximize the time available for psychoeducation, we use a variety of printed materials (e.g., worksheets, thought records, definitions of cognitive errors, pamphlets) that we keep easily accessible at our desks. A number of different worksheets, checklists, and other educational exercises are detailed throughout this book. We provide copies of some useful handouts in Appendix 1, "Worksheets and Checklists," and some of these items may be copied from the appendix or downloaded in larger format from the publisher's Web site (www.appi.org/pdf/62362).

8. **Organize a reading list of books that can help educate patients on psychiatric illnesses, CBT, and pharmacotherapy.** Many patients are eager to read about their condition or to spend time outside sessions learning more about CBT concepts and skills. A short list of some books that we often recommend is contained in Table 3–7. In assigning readings, be careful to not overload the patient. If the patient is quite symptomatic or is having trouble concentrating, he may have a better learning experience with assignment of only one chapter or a portion of a chapter instead of being asked to tackle an entire book.

9. **Learn about Internet resources for psychoeducation. Prepare a list of Web sites, and/or develop a Web site that has useful links.** Patients wishing to learn about psychiatric illnesses and treatments have been increasingly using the Internet (Fox 2008; Schwartz et al. 2006). Clinicians can have a positive influence by steering patients to Web sites that provide accurate and solid information. We discuss use of technology as an adjunct to brief sessions and provide a list of useful Web sites in the next section of this chapter.

Table 3–7. Psychoeducational readings for patients and families

---

Books for patients and families

Antony MM, Norton PJ: The Anti-Anxiety Workbook: Proven Strategies to Overcome Worry, Phobias, Panic, and Obsessions. New York, Guilford, 2009

Basco MR: Never Good Enough. New York, Free Press, 1999

Basco MR: The Bipolar Workbook. New York, Guilford, 2006

Burns DD: Feeling Good. New York, Morrow, 1999

Craske MG, Barlow DH: Mastery of Your Anxiety and Panic, 3rd Edition. San Antonio, TX, Psychological Corporation, 2000

Foa EB, Wilson R: Stop Obsessing! How to Overcome Your Obsessions and Compulsions. New York, Bantam Books, 1991

Greenberger D, Padesky CA: Mind Over Mood. New York, Guilford, 1995

Jamison KR: Touched With Fire: Manic-Depressive Illness and the Artistic Temperament. New York, Simon & Schuster, 1996

Miklowitz DJ: The Bipolar Survival Guide: What You and Your Family Need to Know. New York, Guilford, 2002

Mueser KT, Gingerich S: The Complete Family Guide to Schizophrenia. New York, Guilford, 2006

Romme M, Escher S: Understanding Voices: Coping With Auditory Hallucinations and Confusing Realities. London, Handsell, 1996

Turkington D, Kingdon D, Rathod S, et al: Back to Life, Back to Normality: Cognitive Therapy, Recovery and Psychosis. Cambridge, UK, Cambridge University Press, 2009

Wright JH, Basco MR: Getting Your Life Back: The Complete Guide to Recovery From Depression. New York, Touchstone, 2002

Personal accounts of mental illness

Duke P: Brilliant Madness: Living With Manic Depressive Illness. New York, Bantam Books, 1992

Jamison KR: An Unquiet Mind. New York, Knopf, 1995

Nasar SA: A Beautiful Mind: The Life of Mathematical Genius and Nobel Laureate John Nash. New York, Touchstone, 1998

Shields B: Down Came the Rain. New York, Hyperion, 2005

Styron W: Darkness Visible: A Memoir of Madness. New York, Random House, 1990

Note.   This list is also included in Appendix 2, "CBT Resources for Patients and Families."

> **Learning Exercise 3–2**   Starting a Library of Educational Handouts
>
> 1. A suggested reading list is provided in Table 3–7. These books are also listed in Appendix 2, "CBT Resources for Patients and Families." Either copy the list from the appendix or construct your own list to give as a handout to patients.
>
> 2. Organize other handouts that you may already be using or could use to help patients learn about psychiatric treatment and CBT. Our earlier books—*Learning Cognitive-Behavior Therapy: An Illustrated Guide* (Wright et al. 2006) and *Cognitive-Behavior Therapy for Severe Mental Illness: An Illustrated Guide* (Wright et al. 2009)—have a number of worksheets, checklists, and self-help exercises that could become a part of your library of handouts.
>
> 3. Add to the library as you work through this book and find handouts that might be useful to your patients.

Using Technology to Improve Efficiency

The most obvious way to use technology in improving the efficiency of brief visits is the electronic medical record. Time can be saved and the quality of care can be enhanced if this medical record has drop-down menus and other point-and-click methods to record symptoms, construct and modify treatment plans, select medications and write prescriptions, note use of CBT methods, check for medication interactions, and document other critical clinical functions (Lawlor 2008; Luo 2006; Tsai and Bond 2008). However, technology can be used in a number of other ways to assist clinicians and patients in using brief sessions effectively.

Although a detailed review of the use of technology in psychiatric practice is beyond the scope of this book, we believe that the items listed in Table 3–8 can provide significant opportunities for enhancing clinical practice in brief visits of combined CBT and pharmacotherapy. Readers who are interested in learning more about this topic are referred to *Using Technology to Support Evidence-Based Behavioral Health Practices: A Clinician's Guide* (Cucciare and Weingardt 2009).

A number of excellent educational Web sites can give patients general information about psychiatric illnesses and treatment, and several sites specialize in providing education and, in some cases, self-help exercises on CBT. Web sites that clinicians might consider recommending to patients are listed in Table 3–9. Other sites offer online self-help groups (e.g., the Depression and Bipolar Support Alliance, Walkers in the Darkness) or assistance in managing symptoms of psychosis.

Table 3–8.   Opportunities for using technology to enhance brief sessions

---

Electronic medical records

Patient and/or clinician Internet searches

Computer-assisted cognitive-behavior therapy

Use of Web sites that provide self-help and/or support

E-mail

Telepsychiatry

Computer-assisted CBT is a particularly interesting and potentially useful adjunct for brief sessions (see Table 3–9). Studies of two multimedia computer programs for depression—*Beating the Blues* (Proudfoot et al. 2004) and *Good Days Ahead: The Multimedia Program for Cognitive Therapy* (Wright et al. 2002, 2005)—have demonstrated that substantial reductions in symptoms can be achieved even if clinician time is reduced to 4 hours or less for the entire course of treatment. In a study of drug-free patients with major depression, Wright et al. (2005) found no significant differences in the effects of computer-assisted CBT when patients were seen for 25-minute sessions or for standard 50-minute sessions. Kenwright et al. (2001) have also shown that clinician time can be lowered considerably in the treatment of anxiety disorders with the use of a multimedia computer program. Other studies of computer-assisted CBT for anxiety disorders (Carlbring et al. 2006; Litz et al. 2007; Spek et al. 2007) have explored models of providing CBT by Internet-delivered programs along with brief therapist sessions conducted either in person, by telephone, or through e-mail.

Reviews of computer-assisted CBT have found that significant clinician involvement is a key element in effectiveness (Spek et al. 2007; Wright 2008). Low levels of completion of program content and symptom reduction are typically observed when patients use a Web site on their own. For example, a study of the MoodGYM self-help Web site (www.moodgym.anu.edu.au) found that a large majority of users were browsers and "one-hit wonders" (Christensen et al. 2006). However, programs that include clinician screening, supervision, and guidance—for example, *Beating the Blues* (www.beatingtheblues.co.uk), *Good Days Ahead* (www.mindstreet.com), and virtual reality programs supplied by Virtually Better (www.virtuallybetter.com)—have fared much better in outcome studies.

Virtual reality therapy is another computer-assisted therapy tool that can be quite useful in implementing CBT (Difede et al. 2007; Rothbaum et al. 1995, 2000, 2001). However, because virtual reality requires a cli-

Table 3–9. Computer resources

Web sites with general information on psychiatric treatment and/or cognitive-behavior therapy (CBT)

Academy of Cognitive Therapy
  www.academyofct.org

Depression and Bipolar Support Alliance
  www.dbsalliance.org

Depression and Related Affective Disorders Association
  www.drada.org

Massachusetts General Hospital Mood and Anxiety Disorders Institute
  www2.massgeneral.org/madiresourcecenter/index.asp

National Alliance on Mental Illness
  www.nami.org

National Institute of Mental Health
  www.nimh.nih.gov

University of Louisville Depression Center
  www.louisville.edu/depression

University of Michigan Depression Center
  www.depressioncenter.org

Computer-assisted CBT programs

Beating the Blues
  www.beatingtheblues.co.uk

FearFighter: Panic and Phobia Treatment
  www.fearfighter.com

Good Days Ahead: The Multimedia Program for Cognitive Therapy
  www.mindstreet.com

Virtual reality programs by Rothbaum and associates
  www.virtuallybetter.com

Psychoeducational Web site for CBT

MoodGYM Training Program
  www.moodgym.anu.edu.au

Web sites for online support groups

Depression and Bipolar Support Alliance
  www.dbsalliance.org

Walkers in Darkness (for people with mood disorders)
  www.walkers.org

Table 3–9.   Computer resources *(continued)*

Web sites for helping persons with psychosis

Hearing Voices Network
  www.hearing-voices.org
  (Provides practical advice for understanding voice hearing)

Gloucestershire Hearing Voices & Recovery Groups
  www.hearingvoices.org.uk/info_resources11.htm
  (Gives examples of coping skills for voice hearing)

Paranoid Thoughts
  www.paranoidthoughts.com
  (Gives advice on coping with paranoia)

Note.   This list is also included in Appendix 2, "CBT Resources for Patients and Families."

---

nician to administer the exposure therapy for time periods that typically extend beyond 30 minutes, it is usually not employed in treatments where only brief sessions are used. Virtual reality could be a helpful component of formats for brief visits in which a nonphysician therapist is providing this part of the treatment plan or a psychiatrist schedules several longer sessions along with brief visits (see Chapter 2, "Indications and Formats for Brief CBT Sessions"). The primary application of virtual reality is in exposure-based therapies for anxiety disorders (Difede et al. 2007; Rothbaum et al. 1995, 2000, 2001).

E-mail and teleconferencing are other technologies that might be considered for the brief session format of combined CBT and pharmacotherapy. Although e-mail can have certain advantages (e.g., reminders to perform homework, access to clinicians to ask questions, having a hard copy of communications outside sessions), many clinicians are hesitant to use this method (Callan and Wright 2010; Mehta and Chalhoub 2006). Some of the concerns about using e-mail as a therapy extender are confidentiality issues, excessive demands on clinician time, lack of reimbursement for time spent on e-mail communications, potential for miscommunication (e.g., with patients who have concentration problems related to Axis I disorders), and medicolegal vulnerability.

Teleconferencing has been shown to be an effective method of delivering CBT in sessions of standard length (Bouchard et al. 2004; De Las Cuevas et al. 2006; Simpson et al. 2006) and may also be useful for brief sessions. This technology could allow psychiatrists and other prescribing clinicians to deliver combined CBT and pharmacotherapy in sessions of varied length to persons who are in remote sites where such treatment is not available.

Homework and Self-Help as Therapy Extenders

Homework can provide abundant opportunities for leveraging the work of clinicians in brief visits. Patients can be engaged in highly productive work outside sessions to build their knowledge of CBT and their ability to apply these principles in daily life. For example, in Video Illustration 2, Dr. Sudak reviewed homework from the previous session (a thought record), drew from this homework to target an important and successful intervention (modified maladaptive cognitions about starting a new job), and then worked with Grace to design a useful new assignment (listing rational cognitions, deciding they should be posted on Grace's bathroom mirror, and completing additional thought records) that reinforced the material learned in the session and strengthened Grace's skills for coping with the new job situation.

The degree to which homework and self-help can be used to extend the therapist's activities in CBT varies widely from patient to patient. Some patients with anxiety disorders can have successful outcomes of treatment with CBT when the majority of the work is performed through self-help, either with printed materials or with computer-assisted CBT (Carr et al. 1988; Ghosh et al. 1984; Kenright et al. 2001). We have had many patients with conditions such as agoraphobia, panic disorder, and OCD who have readily taken to the brief session format and have completed large amounts of homework (e.g., exposure and response prevention protocols, breathing retraining exercises, relaxation training) outside sessions that appeared to play a fundamental role in achieving positive results. Illustrations of such cases are provided in Chapter 9, "Behavioral Methods for Anxiety." Also, many patients with major depression, bipolar disorder, addictions, psychoses, and other conditions have also appeared to benefit greatly from doing homework assigned in brief sessions. However, other patients with a variety of diagnoses have not routinely completed homework or have had significant difficulties in making this part of CBT a productive experience.

We discussed methods of troubleshooting lack of homework completion in an earlier book (Wright et al. 2006). The following are some of the methods we use to prevent problems with homework:

1. Develop homework assignments collaboratively.
2. Rehearse homework assignments in advance (especially if they are complicated or challenging).
3. Be sure to always follow up on homework from the previous session. (Otherwise, the patient may assume that homework is not important.)

4. Normalize difficulties with completing homework (explain that lots of people may have problems doing assignments—the clinician will help if the assignment does not work out as planned).

If the patient comes to the session without completing any homework or other difficulties are encountered, then the clinician can do the following (Wright et al. 2006):

1. Evaluate the acceptability and appropriateness of the assignment. (Was the assignment too difficult or too easy? Was it explained clearly enough? Was the assignment directed at a target that was relevant to the patient?)
2. Have the patient complete the assignment in the session (e.g., educate the patient further on how to carry out the assignment, model ways of using CBT in homework activities).
3. Check for any negative thoughts about the homework task. (Did the homework trigger any self-condemning cognitions or other automatic thoughts?)
4. Identify barriers to homework completion and try to find ways to overcome these roadblocks.

A large number of potential homework assignments can be used to promote learning outside therapy sessions. Many of these are detailed and illustrated in other chapters of this book. A short list of some of our favorite types of assignments is displayed in Table 3–10.

Capitalizing on Positive Interactions Between Pharmacotherapy and CBT

Our focus to this point in the chapter has been on cognitive and behavioral methods for enhancing the impact of brief sessions. Before closing, we want to suggest a few general psychopharmacological strategies that also may have a place in making brief visits more productive. As reviewed in Chapter 1, "Introduction," the overall results of research on combined pharmacotherapy and CBT suggest that the two treatments can have positive interactions that can have a favorable effect on outcome. In Table 3–11, we list some possible influences of pharmacotherapy on CBT that could be used to advantage in clinical practice (Wright 2004).

A way to help patients get more out of brief sessions of CBT is to effectively use pharmacotherapy to reduce symptoms that interfere with attention or concentration. We have seen patients who presented with severe

Table 3–10. Examples of homework assignments for brief sessions

Activity schedules

Breathing retraining rehearsal

Coping cards

Educational readings

Examining-the-evidence exercises

Exposure logs (hierarchical exposure)

Generating a list of reasons for hope

Positive imagery rehearsal

Practicing coping skills for hallucinations

Problem-solving activities

Simple behavioral activation exercises

Sleep logs

Spotting cognitive errors in thought patterns

Thought change records

Table 3–11. Possible positive effects of pharmacotherapy on cognitive-behavior therapy (CBT)

Medications can improve attention and concentration and thus facilitate CBT.

Medications can reduce painful emotions or excessive physiological arousal, thereby increasing accessibility to CBT.

Medications can be used appropriately for sleep disruption in acute episodes of Axis I disorders. Improved sleep allows the patient to make better use of CBT interventions.

Medications can decrease distorted or irrational thinking, thus adding to the effect of CBT.

Source. Reprinted from Wright JH: Integrating cognitive-behavior therapy and pharmacotherapy, in *Contemporary Cognitive Therapy: Theory, Research, and Practice*. Edited by Leahy RL. New York, Guilford, 2004, p. 343. Copyright © 2004 The Guilford Press. Reprinted with permission of The Guilford Press.

depression, manic symptoms, or psychotic disorganization that made psychotherapy of any length a difficult if not impossible proposition. Extreme examples of this problem are frequently encountered in hospitalized patients who have such florid symptoms of psychosis or mania, or who have such profound psychomotor retardation from depression, that psycho-pharmacological interventions must come before attempts to engage in CBT. A more common situation in outpatient practice is a patient who is struggling with learning concepts in CBT, with practicing them at home, or with doing self-help assignments because an Axis I disorder is interfering with attention or concentration.

Clinicians who are providing effective psychopharmacology for these types of problems need to consider the potential alerting or cognitive-enhancing actions of medications (e.g., antidepressants for major depression or anxiety disorders, mood stabilizers and atypical antipsychotics for bipolar disorder, antipsychotics for schizophrenia, stimulants for attention-deficit/hyperactivity disorder) while being cautious to avoid or limit potential negative effects of certain medications on cognition. In addition to the possibility of sedative effects of antipsychotics, mood stabilizers, and some antidepressants (e.g., mirtazapine, trazodone), special concern needs to be paid to the possible adverse effects of benzodiazepines on a patient's concentration and learning and memory functioning. As demonstrated by Marks et al. (1993), alprazolam can interfere in some cases with the effectiveness of CBT for anxiety, presumably because it interferes with learning.

The choice of type and dose of the psychopharmacological agent can also influence psychotherapy when patients are having intense emotional and physiological arousal, insomnia, or other symptoms that may be impeding their ability to benefit from CBT. For example, a depressed patient with intense anxiety and agitation who is having trouble focusing on simple behavioral interventions (see Chapter 6, "Behavioral Methods for Depression") might require the addition of a benzodiazepine to the antidepressant regimen on a short-term basis, or a switch to another antidepressant might be considered as a way to reduce the anxiety and help the patient gain more from the CBT component of therapy.

Although CBT techniques can be very effective for insomnia (see Chapter 10, "CBT Methods for Insomnia"), in some situations psychopharmacological management of sleep disruption is clearly required. Appropriate use of sleeping medication and/or antidepressants, mood stabilizers, or antipsychotic drugs for Axis I disorders (e.g., major depression, bipolar disorder, schizophrenia) not only can reverse a destructive sleep pattern and contribute to overall recovery but also can make CBT interventions more successful. A patient who is rested will probably be better able to understand and follow through with CBT assignments than a patient who is exhausted from sleep deprivation.

Psychopharmacology can also benefit patients participating in CBT by targeting negatively distorted thoughts, delusions, hallucinations, or other cognitive symptoms of Axis I disorders. Relief from these symptoms—a key goal of medication treatment—gives a bonus to patients who are receiving CBT. For example, Samantha, a depressed patient being treated with combined pharmacotherapy and CBT, reported that she had finally been able to use CBT skills to discount intrusive, negative automatic thoughts after the addition of an augmenting agent (an atypical antipsychotic medication); Roberto, a man being treated with OCD, was able to complete more challenging exposure and response prevention assignments after the dose of a selective serotonin reuptake inhibitor was increased to a high level; and Gail, a woman with chronic paranoid schizophrenia, began to effectively use CBT coping strategies for hallucinations after she began treatment with clozapine. These are just a few examples of how effective use of psychotropic medications not only can reduce core symptoms of Axis I disorders but also can have a positive influence on the implementation of CBT.

> **Learning Exercise 3–3**   Using Psychopharmacology to Enhance CBT
>
> 1. In the next 10 patients that you see in your practice, carefully examine the possible positive or negative influences of medication on capacity to participate in psychotherapy.
>
> 2. From these 10 cases, identify any in which you believe a medication has already helped and/or is currently helping the patient better use psychotherapy methods.
>
> 3. Identify any patients in which a medication adjustment or change might assist in reducing symptoms and improving ability to participate in CBT.

Summary

Key Points for Clinicians

- The collaborative-empirical therapeutic relationship in CBT can work well in brief sessions. In short visits, clinicians need to redouble their efforts to be fully attentive and to be excellent communicators.
- Symptom checks can be done efficiently and effectively with targeted questions, use of 0- to 10-point global ratings, and standardized self-report scales.
- The productivity of brief visits can be enhanced greatly with structuring methods. The primary techniques are 1) developing specific goals

for treatment, 2) finding a clear focus for CBT interventions, 3) setting agendas, and 4) carefully pacing the flow of the session.

- Some especially useful psychoeducational tools for brief sessions include Socratic questions; mini-lessons; written diagrams, instructions, or logs; libraries of educational handouts; and reading assignments. Clinicians can improve the efficiency of their teaching by preparing educational materials in advance.

- Computer tools can serve as useful adjuncts to the efforts of clinicians in brief sessions. Fully developed computer-assisted therapy programs have been shown to be effective in clinical trials. Also, educational and self-help Web sites can offer helpful suggestions and advice.

- Homework can multiply the impact of the clinician's efforts in brief visits.

- An advantage of combining pharmacotherapy and CBT is the use of medications to enhance potential benefits from psychotherapy. The prescribing clinician can use medication regimens that decrease symptoms (e.g., poor concentration, low energy, negatively biased thinking, sleep disorder, delusional thinking, severe mood swings) that may interfere with participation in CBT.

Concepts and Skills for Patients to Learn

- People can get the most out of brief treatment sessions if they practice good teamwork in their relationship with their clinician. Effective collaboration is very important to the success of CBT.

- A beneficial practice is to come to the appointment prepared to report on progress and to have a clear agenda in mind for what you want to accomplish in the session.

- Staying focused on a specific topic often leads to good results. If you can understand one problem or strategy well, you can apply this knowledge in many other areas of your life.

- CBT is geared toward teaching people effective coping skills. The more you work on learning principles of CBT, the more likely you are to benefit from the treatment.

- Homework—an essential part of CBT—is not like the homework you had in school. It should be something that makes you feel better because you are learning ways to overcome your problems. Usually, people who put effort into CBT homework get a lot of help from these activities. If you have questions about the homework or have difficulties with assignments, be sure to discuss these with your doctor or therapist.

- When medication is used along with CBT, your doctor will try to prescribe drugs that reduce symptoms and help you use the CBT more effectively. Medication questions or issues are usually routine agenda items when you are receiving both pharmacotherapy and CBT.

References

Arieti S: Cognition in psychoanalysis, in Cognition and Psychotherapy. Edited by Mahoney MJ, Freeman A. New York, Plenum Press, 1985, pp 223–241

Basco MR, Rush AJ: Cognitive-Behavioral Therapy for Bipolar Disorder, 2nd Edition. New York, Guilford, 2005

Beck AT, Ward CH, Mendelson M, et al: An inventory for measuring depression. Arch Gen Psychiatry 4:561–571, 1961

Beck AT, Rush AJ, Shaw BF, et al: Cognitive Therapy of Depression. New York, Guilford, 1979

Beck AT, Epstein N, Brown G, et al: An inventory for measuring clinical anxiety: psychometric properties. J Consult Clin Psychol 56:893–897, 1988

Beck J: Cognitive Therapy: Basics and Beyond. New York, Guilford, 1995

Bouchard S, Paquin B, Payeur R, et al: Delivering cognitive-behavior therapy for panic disorder with agoraphobia in videoconference. Telemed J E Health 10:13–25, 2004

Callan JA, Wright JH: Mood disorders, in Using Technology to Support Evidence-Based Behavioral Health Practices: A Clinician's Guide. Edited by Cucciare MA, Weingardt KR. New York, Routledge, 2010, pp 3–26

Carlbring P, Bohman S, Brunt S, et al: Remote treatment of panic disorder: a randomized trial of Internet-based cognitive behavior therapy supplemented with telephone calls. Am J Psychiatry 163:2119–2125, 2006

Carr AC, Ghosh A, Marks IM: Computer-supervised exposure treatment for phobias. Can J Psychiatry 33:112–117, 1988

Christensen H, Griffiths K, Groves C, et al: Free range users and one hit wonders: community users of an Internet-based cognitive behaviour therapy program. Aust N Z J Psychiatry 40:59–62, 2006

Cucciare MA, Weingardt K (eds): Using Technology to Support Evidence-Based Behavioral Health Practices: A Clinician's Guide. New York, Routledge, 2009

De Las Cuevas C, Arredondo MT, Cabrera MF, et al: Randomized clinical trial of telepsychiatry through videoconference versus face-to-face conventional psychiatric treatment. Telemed J E Health 12:341–350, 2006

Difede J, Cukor J, Jayasinge N, et al: Virtual reality exposure therapy for the treatment of posttraumatic stress disorder following September 11, 2001. J Clin Psychiatry 68:1639–1647, 2007

Fox S: The engaged e-patient population: people turn to the Internet for health information when the stakes are high and the connection fast. Pew Internet and American Life Project, August 26, 2008. Available at: www.pewinternet. org/~/media//Files/Reports/2008/PIP_Health_Aug08.pdf.pdf. Accessed August 21, 2009.

Ghosh A, Marks IM, Carr AC: Controlled study of self-exposure treatment for phobics: preliminary communication. J R Soc Med 77:483–487, 1984

Goodwin FK, Jamison KR: Manic-Depressive Illness: Bipolar Disorders and Recurrent Depression. New York: Oxford University Press, 2007

Haddock G, McCarron J, Tarrier N, et al: Scales to measure dimensions of hallucinations and delusions: the Psychotic Symptom Rating Scales (PSYRATS). Psychol Med 29:879–889, 1999

Kenwright M, Liness S, Marks I: Reducing demands on clinicians by offering computer-aided self-help for phobia/panic: feasibility study. Br J Psychiatry 179: 456–459, 2001

Kroenke K, Spitzer RL, Williams JB: The PHQ-9: validity of a brief depression severity measure. J Gen Intern Med 16:606–613, 2001

Lam RW, Michalak EE, Swinson RP: Assessment Scales in Depression, Mania, and Anxiety. London, Taylor & Francis, 2005

Lawlor T: Behavioral health electronic medical record. Psychiatr Clin North Am 31:95–103, 2008

Litz BT, Engel CG, Bryant RA, et al: A randomized, controlled proof of concept trial of an Internet-based, therapist-assisted self-management treatment for post-traumatic stress disorder. Am J Psychiatry 164:1676–1683, 2007

Luo JS: Electronic medical records. Prim Psychiatry 13(2):20–23, 2006

Marks IM, Swinson RP, Basoglu M, et al: Alprazolam and exposure alone and combined in panic disorder with agoraphobia: a controlled study in London and Toronto. Br J Psychiatry 162:776–787, 1993

Mehta S, Chalhoub N: An e-mail for your thoughts. Child Adolesc Ment Health 11:168–170, 2006

Meyer TJ, Miller ML, Metzger RL, et al: Development and validation of the Penn State Worry Questionnaire. Behav Res Ther 28:487–495, 1990

Muran JC: The self in cognitive-behavioral research: an interpersonal perspective. The Behavior Therapist 16:69–73, 1993

Ono Y, Berger D: Zen and the art of psychotherapy. Journal of Practical Psychiatry and Behavioral Health 1:203–210, 1995

Proudfoot J, Ryden C, Everitt B, et al: Clinical efficacy of computerized cognitive-behavioral therapy for anxiety and depression in primary care: randomised controlled trial. Br J Psychiatry 185:46–54, 2004

Rothbaum BO, Hodges LF, Kooper R, et al: Effectiveness of virtual reality graded exposure in the treatment of acrophobia. Am J Psychiatry 152:626–628, 1995

Rothbaum BO, Hodges L, Smith S, et al: A controlled study of virtual reality exposure therapy for the fear of flying. J Consult Clin Psychol 60:1020–1026, 2000

Rothbaum BO, Hodges LF, Ready D, et al: Virtual reality exposure therapy for Vietnam veterans with posttraumatic stress disorder. J Clin Psychiatry 62: 617–622, 2001

Rush AJ, Trivedi MH, Ibrahim HM, et al: The 16-item Quick Inventory of Depressive Symptomatology (QIDS) Clinician Rating (QIDS-C) and Self-Report (QIDS-SR): a psychometric evaluation in patients with chronic major depression. Biol Psychiatry 54:573–583, 2003

Schwartz KL, Roe T, Northrup J, et al: Family medicine patients' use of the Internet for health information: a MetroNet study. J Am Board Fam Med 19: 39–45, 2006

Simpson S, Bell L, Britton P, et al: Does video therapy work? A single case series of bulimic disorders. Eur Eat Disord Rev 14:226–241, 2006

Spek V, Cuijpers P, Nyklicek I, et al: Internet-based cognitive-behavior therapy for symptoms of depression and anxiety: a meta-analysis. Psychol Med 37: 319–328, 2007

Sudak D: Cognitive Behavioral Therapy for Clinicians. Philadelphia, PA, Lippincott Williams & Wilkins, 2006

Tsai J, Bond G: A comparison of electronic medical records to paper records in mental health centers. Int J Qual Health Care 20:136–143, 2008

Wright JH: Integrating cognitive-behavioral therapy and pharmacotherapy, in Contemporary Cognitive Therapy: Theory, Research, and Practice. Edited by Leahy RL. New York, Guilford, 2004, pp 341–366

Wright JH: Computer-assisted psychotherapy. Psychiatr Times 25:14–15, 2008

Wright JH, Davis DD: The therapeutic relationship in cognitive-behavioral therapy: patient perceptions and therapist responses. Cogn Behav Pract 1:25–45, 1994

Wright JH, Wright AS, Salmon P, et al: Development and initial testing of a multimedia program for computer-assisted cognitive therapy. Am J Psychother 56:76–86, 2002

Wright JH, Wright AS, Albano AM, et al: Computer-assisted cognitive therapy for depression: maintaining efficacy while reducing therapist time. Am J Psychiatry 162:1158–1164, 2005

Wright JH, Basco MR, Thase ME: Learning Cognitive-Behavior Therapy: An Illustrated Guide. Washington, DC, American Psychiatric Publishing, 2006

Wright JH, Turkington D, Kingdon DG, et al: Cognitive-Behavior Therapy for Severe Mental Illness: An Illustrated Guide. Washington, DC, American Psychiatric Publishing, 2009

Zimmerman M, McGlinchey JB: Why don't psychiatrists use scales to measure outcome when treating depressed patients? J Clin Psychiatry 69:1916–1919, 2008

CHAPTER 4

Case Formulation and Treatment Planning

LEARNING MAP

Comprehensive formulations

Case example: developing a comprehensive
formulation for Grace

Efficient methods for using formulations in
brief sessions

Practice case: constructing a mini-formulation

Even in the briefest sessions, a solid formulation is needed to guide treatment choices in cognitive-behavior therapy (CBT). The fundamentals of CBT formulation strategies are explained in basic texts, such as those by Beck (1995), Sudak (2006), and Wright et al. (2006), and are also detailed on the Academy of Cognitive Therapy Web site

(www.academyofct.org). In this chapter, we briefly review essential features of the methods recommended by the Academy of Cognitive Therapy and then explain how formulations can be used as efficient and
practical treatment tools in brief sessions.

Comprehensive Formulations

We recommend that a comprehensive biopsychosocial formulation be developed for all patients who receive CBT. In the initial evaluation, the clinician can start to build the formulation by taking a full history that assesses all
the domains shown in boxes in Figure 4–1. As treatment evolves, more detail
can be added to the formulation until the clinician has a deep understanding
of the patient, and treatment is guided by a clear and well-considered plan.

The Academy of Cognitive Therapy guidelines for case conceptualization suggest that both cross-sectional and longitudinal perspectives be considered in constructing the formulation (www.academyofct.org [click on
the following menu options: Professionals > Certificate in CT > Application Process > Candidate Handbook]; Wright et al. 2006). In the *cross-sectional* part of the formulation, clinicians identify characteristic examples,
from the present or the recent past, of how events trigger automatic
thoughts that influence emotions and shape behavioral responses. Coupled
with knowledge of basic CBT theories for the major types of psychiatric
disorders, these examples help in planning treatment interventions that
target specific cognitive and behavioral dysfunctions that may be amenable
to change. To illustrate, we introduce Rick, a man with social phobia whose
case is described in detail in Chapter 9, "Behavioral Methods for Anxiety."

Rick had classic social anxiety. Whenever he was confronted with having to attend a social event, he had automatic thoughts that were consistent with the characteristics of cognitive pathology in anxiety disorders:
1) excessive fears of danger, harm, and/or vulnerability; 2) increased estimate of risk in these situations; 3) decreased estimate of ability to manage these situations; and 4) heightened attention and vigilance about
potential threats (see Chapter 9 for more information about the CBT
model for anxiety disorders). The cross-sectional component of the case
formulation for Rick might include this example:

Event: Driving to a fund-raising event
Automatic thoughts: "I won't know what to say…I'll want to leave right
    away…I'll freeze and look stupid."
Emotion: Anxiety, tension
Behavior: Try to avoid event altogether, or make an excuse and leave very
    early.

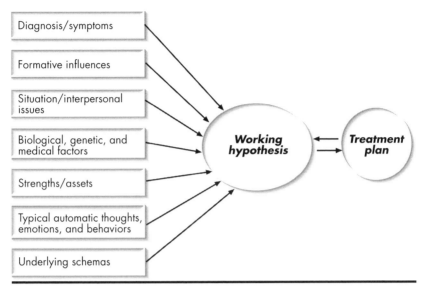

Figure 4–1. Case conceptualization flowchart.

Source. Reprinted from Wright JH, Basco MR, Thase ME: *Learning Cognitive-Behavior Therapy: An Illustrated Guide.* Washington, DC, American Psychiatric Publishing, 2006, p. 51. Used with permission. Copyright © 2006 American Psychiatric Publishing.

Because Rick had maladaptive automatic thoughts about social cues, excessive anxiety and tension that appeared to be driven by the dysfunctional cognitions, and a pattern of avoidance, the treatment plan was directed at modifying all three of these components of his problem with social anxiety disorder. Thought records and examining the evidence, among other cognitive techniques, were used to change his maladaptive automatic thoughts; relaxation training was used to reduce his anxiety and tension; and hierarchical exposure was used to modify his pattern of avoidance.

The *longitudinal* part of the formulation adds a developmental perspective for understanding the patient's symptoms and planning treatment. Formative influences, such as early childhood experiences, peer relationships and school activities, marital and work history, and important events in adult life, are considered. Both negative and positive influences are taken into account. In CBT, the developmental part of the conceptualization usually centers on the evolution of core beliefs (schemas) and long-standing behavioral patterns that accompany these beliefs.

The amount of attention given to the longitudinal elements of the conceptualization in patients being seen for brief sessions can vary depending on the type of disorder, the degree of childhood pathology, and the chronicity and severity of symptoms. In patients with chronic low self-esteem rooted in negative experiences from earlier phases of their lives, or in those who report significant traumas or abuse, the longitudinal conceptualization may be critical to developing understanding and planning effective treatment. However, in patients with circumscribed symptoms who do not have firmly entrenched or dominating maladaptive schemas, a primary focus on the cross-sectional elements of the formulation may be sufficient to plan useful and productive treatment interventions.

For patients being seen in brief sessions, clinicians should first construct a comprehensive formulation that includes cross-sectional and longitudinal elements, in addition to observations on the impact of other components of the cognitive-behavioral-biological-sociocultural model (see Chapter 1, "Introduction," and Figure 4–1). Then, decisions can be made to sharpen the focus of treatment with the types of mini-formulations that are described later in the chapter.

Case Example: Developing a Comprehensive Formulation for Grace

The following case example shows the work that Dr. Sudak did in developing a comprehensive conceptualization for the treatment of Grace, a woman with depression. Video Illustration 2, discussed in Chapter 3, "Enhancing the Impact of Brief Sessions," showed a section of one of Dr. Sudak's brief sessions with Grace.

Background Information

> Grace is a 41-year-old woman who has been experiencing grief and major depression after the death of her husband from brain cancer 10 months ago. His illness was rapid and progressive and resulted in a substantial change in his personality. Grace cared for him at home throughout his illness and managed to keep the children's lives reasonably normal. She assumed responsibility for the entire household and was the major support during all of her husband's medical appointments.
>
> Grace was referred to a pastoral counselor by her minister 3 months after her husband's death. The referral was initially for grief work with her children. Grace's primary care doctor referred her to Dr. Sudak about 6 months ago because of depressive symptoms. The pastoral counselor continued to see Grace and her children for 3 months after the referral, and Dr. Sudak communicated with the counselor to coordinate their efforts. After Dr. Sudak started treatment with a selective serotonin reuptake inhibitor (SSRI), Grace improved significantly and was able to return to work as an office manager. However, her company downsized 2 months ago, and she became unemployed.

Grace quickly obtained a better job as an administrative assistant to a chief executive officer of a trucking company; however, she has been much more symptomatic since accepting the new job. She has been ruminating about her capabilities and the possibility of failure in this position, particularly now that she sees herself as the only source of support for her children and the sole parent in the household. She thinks, "I might get fired again…My boss won't like me…I'll make a mistake and get fired." Grace has especially intense worries at night when she is trying to sleep (e.g., being overwhelmed by thoughts of not waking up on time if she has slept insufficiently, having to get lunches made, getting to work on time, taking care of her kids, doing her housework, balancing her checkbook). Because the new job is a "jump" in responsibility, she has many questions about her own competence and is highly concerned about the catastrophe she believes failure would bring to her life. She has returned to Dr. Sudak because she is aware that she needs to be less anxious before she begins the new job.

Grace has been avoiding simple tasks, such as paying the bills on time and balancing the checkbook. Her friends want her to date, but she is not ready. She is isolating herself from family and friends—she does not visit with her deceased husband's family and she avoids her girlfriends. Thus, they are not calling her as often. She describes herself as feeling "lonely and alone." Her three children are doing better. Grace was involved in her children's school and taught Sunday school prior to her husband's illness. Although she previously enjoyed outdoor recreational exercise with her husband and kids, she has stopped this, because she feels guilty when she takes any time for herself. She does not spend as much time on personal grooming as she did in the past.

Family/Social History

Grace is the second of two children born to married, religious, lower-middle-class parents. Her brother, 4 years her senior, was an athletic and gregarious boy who was highly successful in school and the favored child. Grace's parents seemed to expect little from her except to marry and have a family. She was always a good student and a diligent and careful person. She married Jim, her high school sweetheart, after she finished 2 years at a community college. By all accounts, they had a loving and supportive relationship. They had three children, who were 14, 11, and 8 at the time of Jim's death. Grace has always been active at church and in her children's schools. She returned to work as an office manager when her youngest child started preschool. Before her husband's illness and the onset of Grace's depression, she maintained an active social life with friends and family.

Treatment History

Grace has completed grief-oriented therapy with the pastoral counselor and has been on an SSRI with good results since starting treatment with Dr. Sudak 6 months ago. Monthly sessions of about 20 minutes with Dr.

Sudak were increased to every 2 weeks when Grace relapsed after the stress from losing her job and the anticipation of her new job responsibilities. Grace had no prior psychiatric history before her husband's death.

Case Formulation

Dr. Sudak's conceptualization is shown on the CBT case formulation worksheet in Figure 4–2. As experienced cognitive-behavioral therapists, we do not typically *take* the time to formally write out a full conceptualization such as the one shown in Figure 4–2, but we do routinely assess and consider all of the elements in the formulation worksheet while planning treatment. Also, we highly recommend that trainees or others who are familiarizing themselves with CBT case conceptualizations write out several of these to build their skills in this approach. (A blank CBT case formulation worksheet is provided in Appendix 1 and can be downloaded in larger format from www.appi.org/pdf/62362.)

> **Learning Exercise 4–1**   Constructing a Comprehensive Case Formulation
>
> 1. Review the case history of a patient you are seeing in brief sessions or might consider treating in a brief session format.
>
> 2. Download the CBT case formulation worksheet from www.appi.org/pdf/62362.
>
> 3. Write out a comprehensive case formulation.
>
> 4. Review and update your treatment plan based on the formulation.
>
> 5. If you are currently treating this patient, add detail to the case conceptualization as it becomes available.

Efficient Methods for Using Formulations in Brief Sessions

In brief visits, as in CBT sessions of all lengths, clinicians need to keep in mind all of the valuable information from the comprehensive conceptualization while they help patients select a productive focus for their work. A strategy that may have special merit for brief sessions is to engage patients in constructing an abbreviated, emotionally relevant summary of key elements of the formulation. If patients help write out an easily understood construction of the CBT model and can see how it di-

Patient Name: Grace

Diagnoses/Symptoms: Major depression, single episode with predominant symptoms of sadness, lack of interest, insomnia, anxiety, social isolation, and withdrawal

Formative Influences: Temperamentally cautious, lots of input about "being careful" from her parents; family expected little from her—saw brother as the competent and successful child; acculturated to see herself as wife and mother and not take much credit for her accomplishments

Situational Issues: Death of husband 10 months ago; single parent now; downsized at workplace 2 months ago—laid off; social isolation; demands of new job

Biological, Genetic, and Medical Factors: No family history of depression. No medical illnesses.

Strengths/Assets: Hardworking; healthy; smart; engaging; religious faith; support from family and friends; has new, better job

Treatment Goals: 1) Reduce anxiety and worry to appropriate levels for starting a new job; 2) sleep 7–8 hours per night; 3) build coping skills for recent stresses; 4) develop more realistic standards of performance and build self-esteem; 5) resume predepression level of social involvement and participation in pleasurable activities.

Event 1	Event 2	Event 3
Thinking about new job	Asked to join friends for dinner	Making kids' lunches at night
Automatic Thoughts	**Automatic Thoughts**	**Automatic Thoughts**
"I will make a mistake and get fired." "The boss might not like me."	"I'm not any fun anymore. I would be a drag on them." "It would be too much for me."	"How will I ever manage at my new job?" "I will never be able to stay organized." "Everything is on my shoulders."

Figure 4–2. Cognitive-behavior therapy case formulation worksheet: Grace's example .

Emotions	Emotions	Emotions
Anxiety Tension	Sadness Anxiety	Sadness Anxiety
Behaviors	**Behaviors**	**Behaviors**

Ruminate about job
Stay awake
	Turn down invitation
	Spend time alone
		Watch TV late into
		  the night
		Restless, can't settle
		  down

Schemas: "I am incapable." "If something is not perfect, I will fail." "I must always put other people first."

Working Hypothesis: Grace has always been a careful and deliberate person, modeling herself after her parents. Her world changed abruptly with the illness and death of her husband. This extraordinary stress left her without her main source of interpersonal support. She has been socially isolated since his death and has struggled to resume pleasurable activities with friends and to participate in physical exercise. Her symptoms had improved, and she was beginning to be more involved with others before she lost her job. The new job that Grace found is more demanding. Because of her developmental influences, she has never considered herself very capable or credited her accomplishments. This cognitive vulnerability, in combination with the very real demands on her as a single parent and breadwinner, has precipitated an increase in her anxiety and dysphoria, more intense self-deprecating thoughts, insomnia, and a heightened pattern of social isolation.

Treatment Plan: 1) Antidepressant pharmacotherapy; 2) modify dysfunctional automatic thoughts and core beliefs about competency and realistic standards with Socratic questioning, thought change records, examining the evidence, and other core CBT methods; 3) use activity scheduling to help with time management and to increase pleasurable events and exercise; 4) sleep habit management and relaxation exercises; 5) self-credit logs; 6) coping cards to record and encourage implementation of strategies.

Figure 4–2. Cognitive-behavior therapy case formulation worksheet: Grace's example *(continued)*.

rectly applies to their life, they can be more fully engaged as clinicians proceed to implement specific CBT techniques. They also become well educated on basic CBT concepts, and thus can become active partners in performing treatment in brief, efficient sessions.

Because formulations that are only communicated verbally with patients may be forgotten easily, a useful practice is to sketch out the core concepts on paper or to use a whiteboard or flipchart with colored pens to enhance the impact of the collaborative work in building the formulation. Written diagrams or mini-formulations can then be taken home by the patient or can be copied into a homework diary. Such formulations do not include all of the detail shown in Grace's comprehensive conceptualization (Figure 4–2), but they give a shorthand version of the concepts that will give direction to the patient-therapist team in using CBT to tackle symptoms. These written shorthand formulations can also greatly enhance communications with other professionals and should be considered for placement in the patient's medical record. In the following subsections, we describe mini-formulations and timelines, which are both useful methods of diagramming key elements of the formulation.

Mini-Formulations

Mini-formulations are succinct illustrations of how the basic CBT model can be employed to understand and treat symptoms. One of the common methods for constructing a mini-formulation is based on the cross-sectional part of the case conceptualization described earlier in this chapter. An example of the relationship between events, automatic thoughts, emotions, and behaviors is used to help patients develop a constructive plan for using cognitive and behavioral techniques. Mini-formulations can help patients to zero in on especially salient components of the comprehensive conceptualization and to use time productively in brief sessions.

Our first example of a mini-formulation comes from the treatment of Grace, whose comprehensive conceptualization is shown in Figure 4–2. A mini-formulation drawn out by Dr. Sudak and Grace is displayed in Figure 4–3.

Our second example of a mini-formulation, shown in Figure 4–4, is drawn from the treatment of Terrell, a man with agoraphobia. This slightly more detailed mini-formulation also describes safety behaviors and includes plans to reduce this impediment to making progress in treatment. We explain safety behaviors—attempts to cope that perpetuate avoidance—in Chapter 9, "Behavioral Methods for Anxiety." Terrell and his therapist identified typical automatic thoughts that drove his anxiety

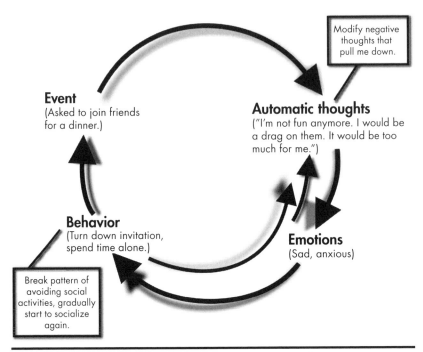

Figure 4–3.   A mini-formulation: Grace's example.

and avoidance, and they sketched out the general outlines of a plan to interrupt this vicious cycle of dysfunctional cognitions and behavior.

A related way of diagramming mini-formulations is to use the ABC
model first described by Ellis (1962). Patients often find this simple way
of constructing a formulation quite easy to comprehend. In the case of
Helen, a patient with schizophrenia featured in several chapters later in
this book (Chapter 5, "Promoting Adherence"; Chapter 11, "Modifying
Delusions"; and Chapter 12, "Coping With Hallucinations"), the ABC
explanation worked in the following manner:

   A=Activating event
      John (boyfriend) looked at me strangely.
   B=Belief
      "He must be possessed. His eyes turn pale when he is possessed."
   C=Consequence
      Emotion: anxiety.
      Behavior: Don't look in his eyes.

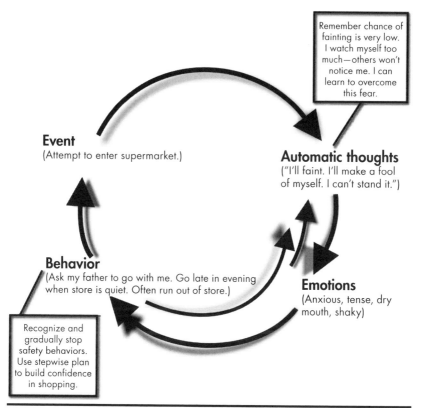

Figure 4–4. A mini-formulation: Terrell's example.

When patients begin to realize that they are continually appraising events from their environment (the A's), they can understand that the beliefs they have about these events (the B's) have consequences (the C's) for their emotions and behaviors. Also, they can start to see how attempts to target distorted interpretations can have benefits.

In the following example, the psychiatrist diagrammed the ABC mini-formulation on a piece of paper and asked Jerry, a patient with chronic low self-esteem, to review it for homework.

Jerry: I feel really bad. My neighbor completely ignored me when he passed me in the street…I'm worthless.
Psychiatrist: Can you sketch out the ABCs of the situation?
Jerry: Well, the A is he walked straight past me and didn't even look at me. I suppose the B is…no wonder he ignored me; I am useless. And the C is a deep sadness.
Psychiatrist: It might help to look at the A and the B here. Are you sure he ignored you on purpose? Could anything be distracting him?

Jerry: I heard he has been having problems with getting in debt.

Psychiatrist: So maybe your neighbor has been distracted with money problems, and perhaps you are not as useless as you think.

Jerry: You have a point there.

Psychiatrist: Also, I wonder if everyone you know ignores you when they see you. Do you ever feel like people pay attention to you?

Jerry: Sure, people at work talk with me a lot, and my friends don't ignore me.

Psychiatrist: Can you take this diagram of the ABCs home and review it so you will remember to check out the B's if you are feeling upset? We can use this same strategy to help you cope with many of your other problems.

Jerry: OK, I think I get it.

Timelines

With some patients, constructing a timeline of critical events in their life history can be useful. This longitudinal method of diagramming some of the important formative influences has been used successfully by Dr. Turkington and others in helping patients with psychotic disorders to understand how stressors may have played a role in the development of symptoms and how attempts to cope with stressors can play a role in reducing symptoms (Wright et al. 2009). Working on timelines can have the following benefits:

1. Allow patients to consider the positive as well as the negative events in their lives that led up to the development of a psychiatric disorder
2. Help patients answer questions that often perplex them, such as "Why me?" or "Why now?"
3. Allow patients to understand their illnesses in terms of a stress-vulnerability conceptualization, which thus may help in normalizing and destigmatizing symptoms
4. Allow patients to access critical life event relationships that have not previously been acknowledged
5. Help patients gain a healthier perspective on negative events and negatively biased interpretations of events
6. Improve rapport between patients and clinicians as they develop a shared model for the development of symptoms

In working with patients to construct timelines, clinicians can use Socratic questions and guided discovery to help discuss the occurrences that may have played a role in beginning and maintaining a psychiatric disorder. Clinicians should ask patients about key memories and achievements, as well as crucial relationships. Figure 4–5 shows an example of a timeline for Grace, the woman who became depressed after the death of

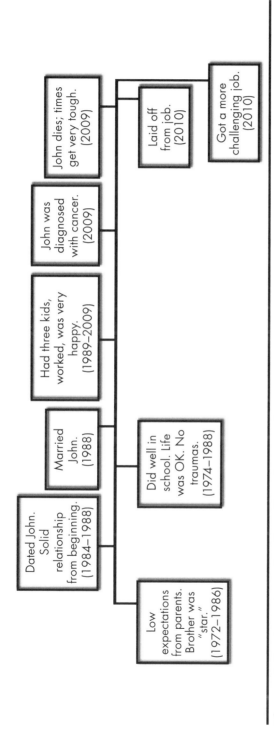

Figure 4–5. Long-term timeline: Grace's example.

her husband and later had to deal with the stresses of starting a new job. The timeline includes notes on early experiences but focuses primarily on more recent influences on symptom development. In this example, the timeline underscores all of the difficult challenges that have so recently come into Grace's life. Dr. Sudak was able to use the timeline to help Grace appreciate some of her long-standing positives, such as successes in school, work, marriage, and raising children. Also, targets for therapy were identified (e.g., enhancing self-esteem, building her capacities to manage life as a single mother, improving coping with recent stresses).

Practice Case: Constructing a Mini-Formulation

Samuel is a 19-year-old African American man who has developed auditory hallucinations. In the following learning exercise, you will be asked to construct a mini-formulation for Samuel.

> **Learning Exercise 4–2**   Developing a Mini-Formulation
>
> 1. Samuel has just recently been diagnosed with schizophrenia. He began hearing voices about 2 years ago, but until very recently he has kept them hidden from everyone, including his close family members. After he attempted to attend a technology training program at a vocational school, his hallucinations intensified, he became paranoid toward other students, and he began to act strangely (e.g., pacing outside his classroom and often being unable to actually sit in the class, wearing a heavy stocking cap that mostly covered his face even in the heat of summer). Fortunately, Samuel wants help and has been coming to see you for brief visits for the past 2 months.
>
>   In the first mini-formulation that you develop with Samuel, you use the CBT model to help him understand and cope with the stigma that he feels for having hallucinations and other symptoms of psychosis. Fill in the blank spots in the diagram shown in the first mini-formulation. Use terms that would be understood by Samuel. Imagine you are writing out this diagram with him in a brief therapy session.
>
> 2. Your mini-formulation directed at destigmatizing was fairly successful. Samuel is blaming himself much less for his symptoms and is now more engaged in working on coping with hallucinations. In the next mini-formulation, you help him understand the role of safety behaviors in maintaining symptoms and sketch out the beginnings of a plan to reduce

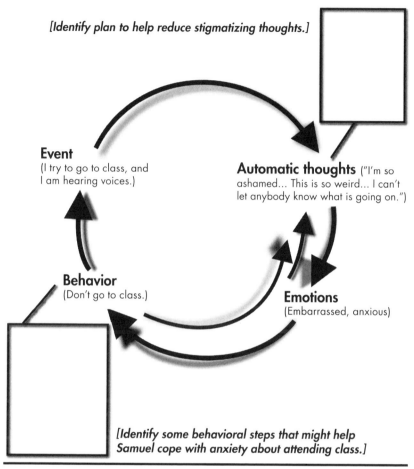

[Identify plan to help reduce stigmatizing thoughts.]

Event
(I try to go to class, and I am hearing voices.)

Automatic thoughts ("I'm so ashamed... This is so weird... I can't let anybody know what is going on.")

Behavior
(Don't go to class.)

Emotions
(Embarrassed, anxious)

[Identify some behavioral steps that might help Samuel cope with anxiety about attending class.]

Mini-formulation 1: Samuel's example.

these behaviors. Fill in the blanks in the second mini-formulation. If you are not familiar with CBT methods for psychosis, try to think of a strategy that may work. You will learn more about CBT for psychosis in Chapter 11, "Modifying Delusions," and Chapter 12, "Coping With Hallucinations."

Summary

Key Points for Clinicians

- A comprehensive case formulation is used in CBT to synthesize information from biological, cognitive-behavioral, and sociocultural domains in planning effective treatment.

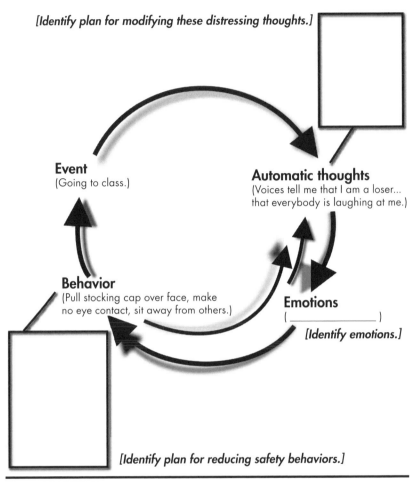

[Identify plan for modifying these distressing thoughts.]

Event
(Going to class.)

Automatic thoughts
(Voices tell me that I am a loser...
that everybody is laughing at me.)

Behavior
(Pull stocking cap over face, make
no eye contact, sit away from others.)

Emotions
(_____)

[Identify emotions.]

[Identify plan for reducing safety behaviors.]

Mini-formulation 2: Samuel's example.

- The CBT case formulation worksheet can provide a useful template for performing comprehensive conceptualizations.
- Both cross-sectional and longitudinal perspectives on symptom development are included in comprehensive case formulations.
- Mini-formulations, timelines, and other shorthand methods are used to help patients understand and use the CBT model.
- These shorthand methods are ideally suited for brief sessions because they sharpen the focus of interventions and give clinicians and patients a clear roadmap for collaborative therapeutic work.

Concepts and Skills for Patients to Learn

- Many different influences can contribute to the development of symptoms. These influences can include genetics, medical and physical problems, early life experiences, family and other close relationships, and the style of thinking and behaving that people develop over their lifetimes.
- In planning treatment, it can help to consider all of the major influences that may have played a role in symptom development. Your doctor or therapist will help you describe these influences and better understand how they may have led to problems.
- It is also very important to identify the positive experiences that have shaped you and to recognize your strengths and capacities. Your doctor or therapist will help you use these strengths in fighting symptoms.
- Your doctor or therapist may work with you to diagram or write out some of the key concepts from CBT. These diagrams or explanations will help you learn more about how this approach can be used to overcome problems.

References

Beck J: Cognitive Therapy: Basics and Beyond. New York, Guilford, 1995

Ellis A: Reason and Emotion in Psychotherapy. New York, Lyle Stuart, 1962

Sudak D: Cognitive Behavioral Therapy for Clinicians. Philadelphia, PA, Lippincott Williams & Wilkins, 2006

Wright JH, Basco MR, Thase ME: Learning Cognitive-Behavior Therapy: An Illustrated Guide. Washington, DC, American Psychiatric Publishing, 2006

Wright JH, Turkington D, Kingdon DG, et al: Cognitive-Behavior Therapy for Severe Mental Illness: An Illustrated Guide. Washington, DC, American Psychiatric Publishing, 2009

CHAPTER 5

Promoting Adherence

LEARNING MAP

General treatment strategies for adherence problems

⇩

Twelve CBT methods for promoting adherence

⇩

Examples of using CBT methods to promote adherence

⇩

Practice case: using CBT to promote adherence

Most patients know that it is a good idea to take medication regularly, but many have problems following prescription instructions. Research studies have typically found rather high rates of nonadherence. For example, significant problems with adherence were found in 48% of patients with schizophrenia (Rosa et al. 2005), 51% of patients with bipolar disorder (Keck et al. 1997), and 49% of patients with depression (Akincigil et al. 2007). In this chapter, we describe cognitive-behavior therapy

(CBT) methods that can be used to promote adherence and give illustrations of how to implement these procedures in clinical practice.

General Treatment Strategies for Adherence Problems

Before describing techniques for helping patients take medications reliably, we want to take a moment to explain our use of the terms *adherence* and *compliance*. Some clinicians object to the term *compliance*. They accurately point out that the power balance in the doctor-patient relationship can become dysfunctional when it is skewed toward physicians forcing their agenda for taking medication on patients who are expected to dutifully "comply" with the doctor's wishes. Because CBT employs a highly collaborative therapeutic relationship with a great deal of cooperation and teamwork, we are much less concerned about negative consequences from using the term *compliance* to describe medication-taking behavior. We prefer the term *adherence*, but we use both words interchangeably here to provide some variety in our writing about medication use.

Some basic treatment strategies that can encourage adherence to pharmacotherapy are listed in Table 5–1. These methods are so universal and obvious that they almost could go without mentioning; however, we suspect that prescribing clinicians do not always maximize the use of these strategies. Like many other physicians, we have sometimes strayed from some of these basic principles and have later discovered that adherence problems were occurring.

Although an excellent therapeutic relationship does not ensure that patients will take medications reliably, many studies have found a strong association between the quality of the doctor-patient relationship and adherence (Kikkert et al. 2006; Sajatovic et al. 2005; Zeber et al. 2008). The collaborative-empirical relationship in CBT (see Chapter 3, "Enhancing the Impact of Brief Sessions") emphasizes respect for patients' opinions and involves them as active partners in the therapeutic process. The teamwork approach includes asking for patient input and feedback on a regular basis. Thus, a CBT-influenced treatment session would typically include open discussions with the patient about how the medication is working; what problems, if any, have been encountered; and what strategies should be pursued to manage problems or improve the outcome. The video illustrations discussed later in this chapter demonstrate the collaborative-empirical style of CBT that we recommend for promoting adherence to pharmacotherapy.

One of the traps that doctors can fall into is to assume that patients are taking the medication as prescribed when the therapeutic relation-

---

Table 5–1. General treatment strategies for enhancing adherence

---

Establish and maintain a collaborative-empirical therapeutic relationship.

Routinely inquire about adherence to pharmacotherapy.

Devise uncomplicated dosing schedules.

Assess and effectively manage side effects.

Address practical concerns such as cost and availability of medication.

---

ship seems to be in excellent shape and the patient's symptoms are in good control. Sometimes the doctor can conclude that patients who have been seen for long periods of time and are very well known to the doctor must be taking medications reliably. At other times, a doctor might get busy with other concerns during treatment sessions and forget to check for adherence. These types of problems have happened to us more often than we would like to admit. We get overconfident in our estimate of how well the patient is adhering to the pharmacotherapy regimen and do not ask about medication-taking habits. At times, we become consumed with other issues and simply do not ask needed questions about compliance. Then we find out later, when symptoms return, that the patient has not being taking medications as planned. To avoid these problems, whenever there is any suspicion that adherence could be wavering, the clinician can routinely ask questions such as these:

"How are you doing with following the schedule for taking medication?"

"How often do you miss a dose or forget to take the pills?"

"Over a month's period of time, what percentage of the medication do you actually take?"

Overly complicated dosing schedules can be another reason for nonadherence. It is well known that patients are more likely to take all doses if a medication can be administered once a day than if it must be taken multiple times during the day (Fincham 2007; Julius et al. 2009). One of us takes four prescribed medications each day. Fortunately, all of these medications can be consumed in the morning after shaving, which facilitates remembering to take the medications routinely. In contrast, we have seen many patients who have multiple doctors and who have been prescribed large numbers of medications that are scheduled to be taken three or even four times a day. When complex medication regimens are reported, we suggest that clinicians attempt to contact other prescribing physicians and work together to simplify the medication plan. If the psychiatrist is the only prescribing clinician, efforts should be made to devise practical, clear, and uncomplicated dosing schedules for the psychotropic medications.

One of the most frequent reasons that patients decline to take or decide to stop their medications is side effects (Julius et al. 2009; van Geffen et al. 2008). Thus, clinicians need to prepare patients in advance for common side effects, discuss what might be done if side effects appear, and keep an open line of communication so that patients feel comfortable in reporting side effects and asking for advice on how to manage these problems. The video illustrations discussed later in this chapter give two examples of nonadherence related to side effects: One woman skipped or "forgot" many doses of lithium after experiencing a tremor that interfered with her favorite hobby, quilting. Another woman had a long history of stopping antipsychotic medications because of weight gain. In each case, the psychiatrist was able to work together with the patient to design an acceptable medication regimen that accounted for and managed the patient's concern about side effects.

Practical concerns—such as the affordability of medication, need for prior authorization for certain medications, changes in insurance plans, arrangements for lab tests (e.g., complete blood counts for patients taking clozapine; lithium levels and thyroid and renal monitoring in patients taking lithium), and ready access to refills—can also play a significant role in medication adherence. Thus, it may not be enough for the clinician to simply prescribe a medication and explain how to use it. If there are practical obstacles to adherence, a plan will need to be devised to surmount these problems, or a change in the medication regimen may be required so that the patient can secure the medication and take it on a regular basis.

Twelve CBT Methods for Promoting Adherence

A number of more specific CBT methods for improving adherence can be added to the general approach described above. The following 12 methods are well suited for brief sessions:

1. **Normalize problems with taking medication.** Patients may be more likely to discuss their adherence problems freely if the doctor normalizes problems with not taking medications as prescribed. The clinician can make comments such as, "Almost everybody has problems at one time or another in forgetting to take medication or not following the prescription exactly" or "Missing medication doses is a really

common problem, so you are not alone in having this difficulty." Another normalizing strategy is to use self-revelation: "I can understand the problem you have been having with taking medications routinely. When I was first prescribed medicine for hypertension, I missed a fair number of doses until I finally figured out a routine that worked for me." The normalizing strategy does not excuse or condone nonadherence but rather opens this topic for discussion and sets the stage for productive work on finding ways to improve consistency in medication taking.

2. **Educate the patient about the illness and its treatment.** The psychoeducational emphasis of CBT is well suited to helping patients better understand and accept their illnesses. Socratic questions, mini-lessons, handouts, recommended readings, and Internet searches can be used to promote learning. Lists of recommended books and Web sites are provided in Appendix 2, "CBT Resources for Patients and Families," and can also be downloaded from www.appi.org/pdf/62362.

3. **Inquire about the patient's daily routine.** In asking patients about their medication-taking behavior, we have found that people who have a fairly consistent routine may be more likely to take their medications regularly. On the other hand, people who have disorganized, chaotic daily schedules may have more difficulty adhering to a medication regimen. If the patient has an irregular schedule, efforts can be made to help him better organize the day. An activity schedule could be employed to plan key daily events, such as sleep and wake times, mealtimes, and medication taking. Alternatively, a simple behavioral plan could be devised that improves reliability by targeting a certain time of day for taking pills (e.g., morning awakening, preparing for bedtime).

4. **Suggest that medications be stored in a consistent and memorable place.** One of the highly useful questions that can be asked about adherence is, "Where do you store your medications?" Opportunities to improve adherence are indicated if you hear answers such as, "It varies"; "In my purse, but sometimes I forget that I have switched purses so the medicine is left at my mother's house"; or "I usually stick it away under some clothes in a drawer, but other times it can be in my desk or on top of the refrigerator." A behavioral plan to place the medication in the same place all the time where it can be seen easily every day without fail can often be a helpful component of the overall strategy to enhance compliance.

5. **Pair medication taking with a routine activity.** Another valuable behavioral intervention that we frequently use is pairing—that is, coupling medication taking with a behavior that the patient completes every

day. If the patient already has a behavioral routine that is consistently accomplished each day, this pattern can be linked to medication taking as a memory prompt and to help make the pharmacotherapy an "automatic" part of the daily routine. We previously noted that one of us takes four medications at one time each day. He uses pairing with his morning ritual of shaving as a principal reminder strategy. His medication is placed beside the shaving cream so that he sees it every day.

Some other examples of behaviors that our patients have used for pairing include taking medication during mealtimes, after putting on pajamas each evening, and after pouring a first cup of coffee each day. In using pairing, it is important to find an activity that is accomplished every day. For some patients with severe mental illness or for others who have highly irregular schedules, it may be hard to find a consistent behavior to associate with medication taking. In such cases, a behavioral plan to perform an activity daily (e.g., teeth brushing, having breakfast, eating an evening meal reliably) could be practiced for homework. The patient could log her efforts to carry out the plan and to take medication at the same time.

6. **Use a pill box or other reminder system.** Many patients find that pill boxes or other reminder systems can help them stick with a medication regimen. Although such reminder systems are recommended widely in medical practice and are thus not unique to CBT, they can be conceptualized as behavioral interventions within the CBT framework for treatment.

    Seven-day pill containers can be loaded once weekly on the same day at the same time (e.g., after the last pills for the week are taken on Sunday evening), and the boxes can be checked regularly to make sure that all pills have been taken as scheduled. Pill boxes may be especially useful when complex regimens (e.g., multiple medications and multiple times for dosing during the day) are required or for elderly persons or others who may have problems with forgetting. Other reminder systems that might be considered are 1) low-tech solutions such as logs, calendars, and Post-it notes, and 2) electronic aids such as setting cell phone alarms or using commercially available pill boxes with computerized beeps or voice alerts that tell users when it is time to take the medication.

7. **Assess barriers to adherence.** When patients report problems with adherence, an analysis can be conducted of barriers or obstacles to taking medications reliably, and then a plan can be devised for overcoming these problems. Sometimes the obstacles are practical ones that can be remedied by straightforward behavioral plans. Table 5–2 lists some examples of such plans.

Table 5–2. Practical plans to overcome barriers to adherence

Barrier	Behavioral plan
"I don't have insurance for medication, and I run out of samples before my next doctor visit."	Write note on daily calendar to call at least 10 days in advance to ask doctor to set aside samples.
"I forget to pack medication when I am rushing to leave town for business trips."	Get extra prescription or samples and place in laptop case so that medication is available during travel.
"I always take meds in the morning after I take a shower. But if my wife has put the bathroom drinking glass in the dishwasher, I tell myself I will take the meds later—then I forget to do it."	Buy paper cups and keep supply in bathroom at all times.
"I often wake up too late in the morning, skip most of my morning routine, and head off to work without taking my medication."	Set alarm every evening, and place alarm clock away from bed as incentive to get out of bed to turn it off. Allow time every morning to shower and take medications.

If barriers are more complex or challenging (e.g., the family is adamantly opposed to taking medication for psychiatric illness and believes that the patient just needs to try harder, or the patient fears that her boyfriend will be scared off if he finds out she is taking medication), the clinician can try to develop strategies for managing these obstacles. For example, the clinician might 1) schedule family visits to help break through any negative attitudes about psychiatric treatment and pharmacotherapy or 2) recommend readings and Web sites to educate family members.

8. **Ask patients about the meaning of symptoms.** The meanings that patients attach to their symptoms can have a large impact on adherence. Patients who have a disease explanation for their malady and who fully accept the illness may be more likely to embrace the need for medication than those who have dysfunctional attributions about experiencing symptoms. Some of the meanings that can lead patients away from routine medication taking are denying explanations (e.g., "It is just because I was stressed—I really don't have an illness that needs treatment"), psychotic explanations (e.g., "It is the devil that is talking to me"), or alternative explanations that may have a partial

ring of truth but still interfere with commitment to regular medication taking (e.g., "I am an artist, and my up times are when I am really creative and get a lot done—this isn't bipolar disorder, it's just the way I am wired"). When the meaning of the illness is undercutting compliance, clinicians can use Socratic questioning, examining the evidence, and other standard CBT methods to help patients develop more adaptive explanations. The video illustration of Dr. Wright and a woman with bipolar disorder, which is discussed later in this chapter, demonstrates a cognitive-behavioral approach to working with maladaptive explanations for psychiatric symptoms.

9. **Identify automatic thoughts and core beliefs about taking medication.** Clinicians need to determine whether patients are having negative automatic thoughts that are influencing medication nonadherence and whether underlying schemas are playing a role in medication-taking behavior. Common CBT methods such as guided discovery, thought records, and using the downward arrow technique to uncover core beliefs (see Wright et al. 2006) can help in answering these questions and readying the patient for modifying these dysfunctional cognitions.

10. **Modify automatic thoughts and core beliefs about taking medication.** Table 5–3 displays some typical automatic thoughts that we have observed in patients who have been having difficulties taking medications regularly. Many CBT techniques can be used in brief sessions to generate rational alternatives. These methods, such as examining the evidence, identifying cognitive errors, and using thought change records, are explained in detail in Chapter 7, "Targeting Maladaptive Thinking."

    The last example in Table 5–3 is from the treatment of Glenn, an inpatient with schizophrenia, who was rejecting a recommendation to take clozapine because he believed that Dr. Wright was trying to get him to take an "experimental drug." Figure 5–1 outlines an exercise in examining the evidence that was conducted with this patient, who had not responded to many other antipsychotic medications. During his hospital stay, he was seen almost daily for a total of eight brief sessions of about 15–20 minutes each. By gradually building trust, strengthening the therapeutic relationship, and exploring the evidence for Glenn's dysfunctional belief, Dr. Wright was able to eventually help this patient accept and comply with a needed medication.

    Part of the work on revising Glenn's dysfunctional thinking involved looking at illogical conclusions in the "evidence" for his belief. Although a research study was being conducted at the hospital, it had nothing to do with clozapine. Also, Glenn's assumption that penicil-

Table 5–3. Automatic thoughts and rational thoughts about pharmacotherapy

Automatic thoughts	Rational thoughts
"Taking an antidepressant means I am weak."	"Depression is an illness just like diabetes or high blood pressure. Antidepressants are helpful treatments that are taken by a large number of people—even those who are very successful and very strong willed."
"I am always the one to get the side effects. If a side effect is possible, I will get it."	"I may have had more side effects than the average person, but I am using extreme thinking when I say that I 'always' get side effects."
"I will become dependent on the antidepressant."	"I have learned that people can have withdrawal symptoms if they try to come off antidepressants too quickly. However, these drugs do not cause dependency like narcotics or street drugs."
"I will lose control to the drug. I won't be myself."	"I am the one who decides to take the medication—to give it a try. If it does not agree with me or if I feel that it is changing me too much, I can stop it and discuss options with my doctor."
"They are trying to give me an experimental drug."	"This drug was experimental at one time, but it is now an approved drug. I think I understand the real risks and how the drug could help me."

lin was completely safe offered an opportunity for checking out his assumptions. A behavioral experiment to attend an aftercare group for patients who were taking clozapine was perhaps the most helpful part of the CBT intervention. Glenn was able to learn firsthand from other patients that clozapine has side effects and risks but that the overall results for many people are highly favorable. Glenn has been taking clozapine now for over 4 years and has not been rehospitalized. He lives in a halfway house and continues to see Dr. Wright for brief sessions about once monthly. His adherence to medication has appeared to be excellent.

Automatic thought:

"You are trying to give me an experimental drug. What I really need is penicillin."

Evidence for	Evidence against
Doctors only tell part of the story. I don't trust them.	*I trust my new doctor more than the old ones.*
They are recruiting for a research study at this hospital.	*The research study is for another drug, not clozapine.*
Penicillin is safe. It has been used for over 50 years.	*I have learned that penicillin also has side effects and allergies.*
Clozapine is a dangerous drug.	*Clozapine has been approved by the FDA. I met five people who are taking clozapine and say it is OK. The nurses here believe that clozapine helps more than any of the other medications. My doctor has explained the risks, the need for blood tests, and how clozapine might help me.*

Figure 5–1. Examining the evidence: Glenn's example.

FDA=U.S. Food and Drug Administration.

11. **Use motivational interviewing techniques.** Motivational interviewing has been shown to be a highly useful method of helping patients engage in effective treatment for addictions (see Chapter 13, "CBT for Substance Misuse and Abuse") and may have many other applications in psychiatric treatment, including the promotion of adherence to treatment recommendations (Barrowclough et al. 2001; Drymalski and Campbell 2009; Julius et al. 2009). To use this method for encouraging adherence, clinicians can ask questions such as these to stimulate the patient to think of positive reasons to take medication: What benefits might the medication provide? What risks or downsides might it prevent? How might the medication improve functioning at work, in relationships, or in other pursuits? The clinician can also help the patient identify and develop coping strategies for possible demotivators such as side effects or negative reactions of others.

12. **Develop a written adherence plan or coping card.** After discussing compliance behaviors and developing strategies based on the previous items

in this list of a dozen CBT methods, it can help to collate all of the recommendations in a written adherence plan or coping card. We especially recommend written adherence plans for patients who have had previous track records of noncompliance, who have severe symptoms that may interfere with following an adherence plan (e.g., psychosis, rapid-cycling or severe bipolar disorder, marked depression with psychomotor retardation), or who have problems with concentration or memory. Another strategy that we sometimes use is to ask patients to write and sign their own "prescription" for adherence on a prescription pad. This motivating technique can help certain patients make and keep a commitment to follow through with a rational plan for medication taking.

Examples of Using CBT Methods to Promote Adherence

In this section, we provide two detailed illustrations of how to implement CBT adherence-promoting strategies in brief sessions. The first case shows typical compliance problems in a woman who is starting treatment for bipolar disorder. The second case demonstrates CBT methods for improving adherence in a woman with active hallucinations and delusions.

Barbara, a Woman With Bipolar Disorder

Barbara's history of bipolar disorder was described in Chapter 2, "Indications and Formats for Brief CBT Sessions." She had been hospitalized for a manic episode and then started brief outpatient visits with Dr. Wright. In the second of these outpatient sessions, she listed two agenda items for discussion: 1) "Help me to stop 'losing it' when I get into arguments with my son" and 2) "Doing something about the tremor." Work on the first agenda item was detailed in Chapter 2.

When Dr. Wright began to ask Barbara questions about the second agenda item, he quickly found out that she had been "skipping and forgetting" some doses. Barbara estimated that she had missed about 50% of doses. Part of the difficulty was a tremor that was likely due to lithium. The tremor was a particular concern to Barbara because it was interfering with one of her favorite activities—quilting. As shown in Video Illustration 3, there were other reasons for her nonadherence. Uncovering some of Barbara's attitudes about having a diagnosis of bipolar disorder and having to take medication set the stage for a comprehensive CBT intervention to enhance compliance. This video demonstrates some of the CBT methods for adherence that were outlined earlier in the chapter.

> ◗ **Video Illustration 3.** CBT for Adherence I: Dr. Wright and Barbara

After Barbara says that she "just doesn't want to have the problem of bipolar disorder," Dr. Wright uses normalizing methods to help her understand that she is not alone in struggling to accept an illness and the need for treatment. Then he asks if there are any other reasons why she may be hesitant to take medication regularly. Her report that "sometimes I think it is just stress, and I don't need the medicine" leads to an exercise in examining the evidence. Dr. Wright and Barbara review her symptom summary worksheet (see Chapter 2, Figure 2–1), which lists many of the symptoms that occur when she has manic or depressive episodes, and Barbara concludes that there is much evidence that she actually does have bipolar disorder.

The vignette also demonstrates the use of motivational interviewing techniques. Dr. Wright suggests that they develop a coping card that builds up the case for taking medication by listing key motivators for adherence. Barbara becomes fully engaged in this process and is able to identify four strong motivators: staying out of the hospital, improving her relationship with her son, keeping straighter on finances, and helping avoid problems at work.

The next part of the intervention is directed at dealing with tremor, a side effect of lithium. Dr. Wright empathizes with her problem with tremor and the fact that the tremor makes quilting difficult, educates Barbara on the relationship between lithium levels and side effects, and is able to reach an agreement that Barbara will take medication fully for 1 week to help determine an accurate lithium level. If the level is still in the upper part of the therapeutic range, they will try to lower the level to see if this reduces the tremor. If dose adjustments do not work, an alternate plan for pharmacotherapy will be developed. One of the most important components of this section of the interview is their agreement to communicate openly about medication concerns and to work together as a team to find solutions.

As the session moves to its conclusion, some of the 12 CBT methods listed earlier in this chapter are employed to fill out and strengthen the adherence plan. When Dr. Wright asks Barbara about how well she is following a routine for taking medication, she notes that she has not been keeping her medication in a consistent place. In fact, she sometimes keeps the medication in her purse and leaves the purse at work. At these times, she has no access to medication when she needs to take it before bedtime. After exploring opportunities for pairing, they settle on a plan that Barbara will place the medication next to her toothpaste and toothbrush and will take the medication every evening immediately after she

> *Remind myself of motivators for taking medication regularly:*
>   *Stay out of the hospital.*
>   *Improve relationship with my son.*
>   *Keep straighter on finances.*
>   *Help avoid problems at work.*
> *Work with Dr. Wright on managing the tremor—communicate openly.*
> *Keep medication in consistent place—beside toothbrush and toothpaste.*
> *Take medication once a day, right after I remove makeup and brush teeth.*
> *Log medication taking, at least until my next treatment session.*

Figure 5–2.   Coping card: Barbara's example.

removes her makeup and brushes her teeth. The final part of the session is used to put the pieces of the plan together in written form on a coping card (Figure 5–2) and to arrange a homework assignment. Dr. Wright suggests that Barbara log her efforts to take medication reliably by making a check mark on a calendar. He also sets up possible future work on compliance by explaining that if they find barriers to taking medication routinely that they can work collaboratively to overcome these obstacles.

Helen, a Woman With Schizophrenia

Helen's treatment was first discussed in Chapter 4 ("Case Formulation and Treatment Planning"). She is a young woman with schizophrenia who was treated by Dr. Turkington for delusions and hallucinations (see Chapter 11, "Modifying Delusions," and Chapter 12, "Coping With Hallucinations"). In Video Illustration 4, Helen reports that she has not taken any medication in the past week and has missed many doses before then. Some of the reasons that she gives for nonadherence are difficulty remembering, weight gain, a sense that the medication is not helping, and a feeling that she is "dead in the head."

▶ **Video Illustration 4.** CBT for Adherence II: Dr. Turkington and Helen

The main strategy used by Dr. Turkington in this brief session is to build the therapeutic relationship by encouraging open communication and trust. When Helen asks how the medication could help, Dr. Turkington starts to explain that it will relax her. This seemingly gentle introduction to the possible benefits of taking medication backfires a bit. Helen's guard goes up, and she notes that she does not want to relax too much because she will not be able to keep track of what the "shadows" (part of her psychotic thinking) are doing. However, Dr. Turkington quickly regroups and gives a more detailed and acceptable explanation. A highly collaborative tone seems to put Helen at ease and helps her understand how medication could help her manage stress and cope with delusions and hallucinations.

A turning point in the session occurs shortly after Dr. Turkington emphasizes the importance of having an "honest dialogue." Soon Helen asks him what he would do about taking medication. Because they had already established an excellent working relationship, she is able to accept his recommendation to give the medication he had just prescribed a good try. Behavioral methods such as pill boxes and pairing are suggested as possible aids to remembering the medication. Although adherence could very well remain a major problem in the treatment of this woman with psychosis, efforts to promote communication and collaboration in this brief session could provide important building blocks for more consistent medication-taking behavior.

Practice Case: Using CBT to Promote Adherence

Learning Exercise 5–1   Using CBT to Promote Adherence

1. Imagine that you are treating Alonzo, a 27-year-old single man with bipolar disorder, who has had several relapses after stopping medications or taking them irregularly. You have started treatment with Alonzo recently, after he moved to your city to take a job as a computer programmer. Alonzo has had at least five manic or hypomanic episodes and has been depressed off and on since about age 18. Although he accepts the diagnosis of bipolar disorder and has taken the initiative to request a referral from his previous psychiatrist, you wonder if he might have some automatic thoughts that could interfere with routine medication taking. Therefore, early in treatment, you ask him some questions to try to identify automatic thoughts about taking medication. Write down some possible automatic thoughts and/or core beliefs that might lead to adherence problems for this young man who is trying to build his professional career and to find a life partner.

2. Next, list some CBT strategies that you could use to modify cognitions that you think could be involved in his adherence

problems. What is your plan for helping Alonzo develop adherence-promoting cognitions?

3. You find out that Alonzo has very irregular daily habits. His sleep and wake times can vary 4–5 hours from night to night. Although he has been getting up reliably at 6:30 A.M. on weekdays to get to work on time, he may go to bed anytime between 10:30 P.M. and 2 A.M., and on weekends he may stay up as late as 3–4 A.M. and sleep in until noon. His medication is prescribed for once-daily dosing at bedtime, but sometimes he gets "on a roll" with playing computer games or social activities and then "forgets" to take the medication before falling asleep. He stores his medication in his medicine cabinet in his apartment. However, he can get so worked up with his computer games and other evening activities that he eventually falls asleep with his clothes on and does not go into the bathroom where the medication is stored.

Although it seems obvious that a more regular routine could help with medication taking, you need to decide on a strategy for working on this problem with a 27-year-old man who wants to have an active social life, stay out late on weekends, and have the freedom to make his own choices of what to do with his time. What realistic goals would you have for using behavioral methods to enhance his compliance? Write down at least two barriers that you anticipate in implementing behavioral strategies. Then write out possible ways to overcome these obstacles to adherence.

Summary

Key Points for Clinicians

- The collaborative-empirical therapeutic relationship is the bedrock of the CBT approach to enhancing adherence.
- Even if there appears to be an excellent therapeutic relationship, it is important to routinely inquire about treatment compliance.
- Whenever possible, clinicians should try to simplify dosing schedules, minimize or effectively manage side effects, and help patients deal with practical concerns such as cost and availability of medication.
- Normalizing and educating methods are important components of CBT for adherence.
- Behavioral strategies include improving the consistency of the patient's daily schedule, storing medication in a memorable and routine

place, pairing medication taking with another activity, and reminder systems such as pill boxes or logs.

- Another highly useful behavioral method is to identify and then work out a plan to surmount barriers to full adherence to the medication regimen.
- Cognitive interventions for compliance problems use standard CBT methods such as assessing the meaning of events (in this case, a diagnosis of a mental illness and/or the taking of medication for psychiatric symptoms), eliciting automatic thoughts and core beliefs pertaining to the illness and medication, and examining the evidence and other thought modification techniques.
- Motivational interviewing can be used to help patients recognize positive features of taking medication and to identify possible issues or concerns that might interfere with taking medication regularly.
- A coping card or written adherence plan can be a good way to help patients remember and follow through with the CBT strategies for adherence developed in brief sessions.

Concepts and Skills for Patients to Learn

- Problems with taking medication commonly occur in the treatment of a wide variety of illnesses.
- Because difficulties in medication taking are a normal part of medical treatment, doctors expect that these problems will occur. They will not look down on you if you forget to take pills or have other problems with following the prescription. They just want to help you better understand your symptoms and develop a treatment plan that will work for you.
- If you have concerns about being diagnosed with an illness, are troubled with side effects, or have questions about medication, it is best to discuss these directly with your doctor.
- Working out a clear routine for medication taking and placing the medication in a spot where you will find it reliably can make it easier to remember to take doses as scheduled.
- Sometimes people can have negative thoughts about taking medication. For example, they might think that "taking an antidepressant means I'm weak…I should be able to handle this problem on my own." If you are having thoughts such as these, it can help to check them for accuracy.
- There can be many positive reasons to take medication for psychiatric illnesses. Listing some of these reasons could make it easier for you to

follow the plan that you and your doctor develop to overcome your symptoms.

References

Akincigil A, Bowblis JR, Levin C, et al: Adherence to antidepressant treatment among privately insured patients diagnosed with depression. Med Care 45:363–369, 2007

Barrowclough C, Haddock G, Tarrier N, et al: Randomized controlled trial of motivational interviewing, cognitive behavior therapy, and family intervention for patients with comorbid schizophrenia and substance use disorders. Am J Psychiatry 158:1706–1713, 2001

Drymalski WM, Campbell TC: A review of motivational interviewing to enhance adherence to antipsychotic medication in patients with schizophrenia: evidence and recommendations. J Ment Health 18:6–15, 2009

Fincham JE: Patient Compliance With Medications: Issues and Opportunities. New York, Haworth Press, 2007

Julius RJ, Novitsky AM, Dubin WR: Medication adherence: a review of the literature and implications for clinical practice. J Psychiatr Pract 15:34–44, 2009

Keck PE, McElroy SL, Strakowski SM, et al: Compliance with maintenance treatment in bipolar disorder. Psychopharmacol Bull 33:87–91, 1997

Kikkert MJ, Schene AH, Koeter MWJ, et al: Medication adherence in schizophrenia: exploring patients,' carers,' and professionals' views. Schizophr Bull 32:786–794, 2006

Rosa MA, Marcolin MA, Elkis H: Evaluation of the factors interfering with drug compliance among Brazilian patients with schizophrenia. Rev Bras Psiquiatr 27:178–184, 2005

Sajatovic M, Davies M, Bauer MS, et al: Attitudes regarding the collaborative practice model and treatment adherence among individuals with bipolar disorder. Compr Psychiatry 46:272–277, 2005

van Geffen EC, van Hulten R, Bouvy ML, et al: Characteristics and reasons associated with nonacceptance of selective serotonin-reuptake inhibitor treatment. Ann Pharmacother 42:218–225, 2008

Wright JH, Basco MR, Thase ME: Learning Cognitive-Behavior Therapy: An Illustrated Guide. Washington, DC, American Psychiatric Publishing, 2006

Zeber JE, Copeland LA, Good CB, et al: Therapeutic alliance perceptions and medication adherence in patients with bipolar disorder. J Affect Disord 107(1–3):53–62, 2008

CHAPTER 6

Behavioral Methods for Depression

LEARNING MAP

Behavioral model for depression

⇩

Monitoring of mood and activities

⇩

Behavioral activation

⇩

Graded task assignments

⇩

Behavioral rehearsal

⇩

Practice case: planning a behavioral intervention for depression

---

Behavioral procedures used to treat depression are an important component of cognitive-behavior therapy (CBT) and are prime methods for use in brief sessions. The behavioral techniques reviewed in this chapter can typically be taught in 10–15 minutes, or even less time in some circumstances. It is intended that patients practice these interventions as homework assignments and measure their impact on mood and targeted behaviors. After a brief overview of the behavioral model of depression, we detail four of the most commonly used behavioral methods: mood and activity monitoring, behavioral activation, graded task assignments, and behavioral rehearsal. Other behavioral strategies that are sometimes used to address associated symptoms of depression, such as anxiety and insomnia, are reviewed elsewhere in this volume (see Chapter 9, "Behavioral Methods for Anxiety," and Chapter 10, "CBT Methods for Insomnia").

Although for some patients behavioral interventions alone are sufficient, for most patients the behavioral strategies serve as but one component of a more comprehensive therapy plan that also includes cognitive restructuring (see Chapter 7, "Targeting Maladaptive Thinking"). When behavioral interventions are used within a more comprehensive therapy plan, they provide an important opportunity to elicit automatic negative thoughts and dysfunctional attitudes that typically emerge during homework assignments or within-session rehearsals.

Behavioral Model for Depression

Some theorists have likened the behavioral state of depression to an extinction paradigm, with the emotional disturbance resulting from the withdrawal of positive reinforcement. One reason for such "extinction" is a low rate of goal-directed behaviors: people who are depressed feel tired, have diminished appetitive drives, and do not respond with the same enjoyment from activities that used to give them pleasure. The last problem, which is often termed *anhedonia*, can also be viewed as a state of reduced reinforcer salience. In such cases, the person with depression usually has already noted that things just do not seem that much fun or that he merely seems to be "going through the motions."

Another problem for people with depression is their anticipation that such activities will not be worth their effort ("What's the use? Why bother?"). The problems are not simply perceptual, however, and at home and in the workplace, most people who are depressed have trouble completing effortful tasks, work at a slower pace, and tend to postpone or avoid more demanding tasks.

In addition to these examples of behavioral deficits, people with depression often show an excess of emotional behaviors that their friends, loved ones, and coworkers can find to be aversive, such as complaining or dominating the conversation with their own concerns (i.e., not showing a normal level of reciprocity). Over time, the likely consequences—declining invitations, avoiding interpersonal contacts, or behaving in a nonreciprocal way in interpersonal interactions—result in a reduction in the amount of companionship and support from others. Thus, people who are depressed do fewer of the things that make life worthwhile, get less pleasure and satisfaction from the activities that they do, evaluate these activities more negatively, and behave in a way that reduces the potential for reinforcement from their interpersonal milieu.

The behavioral goals for interventions in depression can be summarized as follows:

1. Increase level of pleasurable activities.
2. Decrease time spent alone.
3. Increase reciprocal behavior in interpersonal activities.
4. Increase ability to complete effortful or challenging tasks (e.g., problem solving at work and in more demanding activities of daily living).

The early sessions of conventional CBT for depression typically emphasize behavioral strategies to begin to address these problems, with a shift of therapeutic focus toward cognitive strategies after the patient begins to have some symptom relief. The orchestration of this approach, as well as the broader interrelationships between the behavioral, cognitive, and emotional symptoms of depression, has not changed dramatically since publication of Beck et al.'s (1979) treatment manual. Nevertheless, behavioral models of treatment for depression that do not directly address automatic negative thoughts or dysfunctional attitudes also have established efficacy (e.g., see the controlled study of Dimidjian et al. [2006] or the meta-analysis of Ekers et al. [2008]). For a fuller description of an expanded behavioral intervention, the interested reader is referred to the book by Addis and Martell (2004).

Figure 6–1 shows a mini-formulation for behavioral interventions with Darrell, a 33-year-old man who has sought treatment for a major depressive episode. We introduce Darrell in this chapter to illustrate behavioral methods for depression. Video illustrations in Chapter 8, "Treating Hopelessness and Suicidality," and Chapter 13, "CBT for Substance Misuse and Abuse," demonstrate CBT interventions that helped Darrell with hopelessness and a drinking problem. At this point in the therapy, Dr. Thase has just started to work with Darrell. Although Darrell initially reports drinking "one to two beers a couple times a week," Dr. Thase discovers later that alcohol abuse is a significant part of the problem.

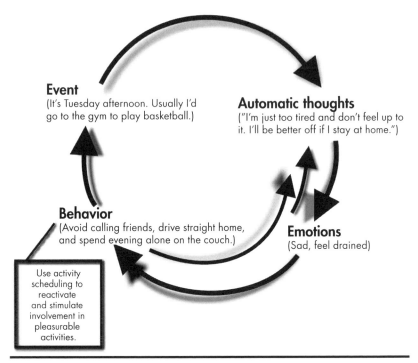

Event
(It's Tuesday afternoon. Usually I'd go to the gym to play basketball.)

Automatic thoughts
("I'm just too tired and don't feel up to it. I'll be better off if I stay at home.")

Behavior
(Avoid calling friends, drive straight home, and spend evening alone on the couch.)

Emotions
(Sad, feel drained)

Use activity scheduling to reactivate and stimulate involvement in pleasurable activities.

Figure 6–1.   A mini-formulation for behavioral interventions: Darrell's example.

Darrell is an African American man who has never married and has never had children. He has a history of one prior episode of major depression. The current episode of depression has been present at least 3 months and has appeared to have been triggered by the diagnosis of metastatic cancer in his mother. Her prognosis is grim, and Darrell knows that her condition is likely to be terminal. In addition to the current episode of depression, Darrell also reports chronic low self-esteem, a sense of stagnation in his job as a computer programmer, and disappointments in his relationships with women.

Darrell has a number of friends and interests, and normally he loves to play basketball and spend time with his friends watching and talking about sports. However, over the last few months, Darrell has been going out less, and he often feels too tired when he gets home from work to go back out to play basketball or spend time with his friends. Instead, most evenings he briefly visits with his mother and then stays home alone.

As diagrammed in Figure 6–1, there are several feedback loops between the negative cognitions, emotional responses, and behavior in depression that tend to worsen Darrell's illness state. Darrell feels down in the dumps and tired after work and, as a result, avoids engaging in one of the most reliably enjoyable activities in his adult life. Instead of getting exercise and interacting with friends, he ends up home alone and, more often than not, does little that gives him pleasure or satisfaction. It is little wonder that he feels even lonelier and more isolated by the end of the evening or that his mood the following day is even lower than before.

Monitoring of Mood and Activities

For most people with depression, behavioral strategies can be introduced in the first session. In fact, in the classic self-help pamphlet "Coping with Depression," Beck et al. (1995) suggest a behavioral exercise as the first step. This assignment is to complete a self-monitoring exercise using a weekly activity schedule, which is included in the pamphlet (see Appendix 1, "Worksheets and Checklists," for a weekly activity schedule). The most condensed version of this simple form is only one page long, displaying the hours of the day vertically and the days of the week horizontally. This form is too cramped for some patients, who prefer to use a loose-leaf or spiral-bound notebook, in which each page can be used to summarize a day's activities. Other patients may find it too taxing to log an entire week's activities. For such persons, an assignment to record activities for a single day or part of a day may be enough.

We recommend that clinicians illustrate how to fill out the form in the first session, drawing on the activities of the hours of the day of the current session. In each time block, the patient is asked to write down what she was doing, to rate her mood, and to describe the activities. Each activity in turn can be rated on two dimensions: mastery and pleasure. Most clinicians use a 0 (*none*) to 10 (*maximum possible*) scale to rate mastery and pleasure during activities, although other methods for scaling (e.g., 0–100) are sometimes preferred. It usually takes less than 10 minutes to introduce the rationale for monitoring mood and activities and to describe how to do the charting.

Self-monitoring has four very specific goals:

1. **To help improve mood and morale.** Although this improvement is perhaps part of a broader spectrum of so-called nonspecific therapeutic effects, people generally begin to feel better when they begin to take some action. As a first homework assignment, self-monitoring also explicitly begins the collaborative-empirical process of CBT.
2. **To help patients visualize the "cause-effect" relationships between what they are doing and how they are feeling.** Although it may seem

obvious that periods of solitary, sedentary activity are associated with low mood and that people generally feel better when they are engaged in interesting or stimulating activities, seeing the regularity of this association mapped out can help the person who is depressed decide to take action.

3. **To help patients make more finely tuned assessments of the activities that are associated with better moods and higher ratings of pleasure and mastery.** The cognitive biases of depression tend to cause people to think in a globally negative fashion and to overlook the fact that even when at their worst, they can exert some degree of influence over their conditions. Identifying these relationships helps to underscore this healthy, coping-oriented thought: "There are things that I can do that can improve my moods."

4. **To identify times of habitually low activity and mood that can be targeted for behavioral assignments.** Although Darrell does not feel particularly great most of the day, his mood and energy level are typically lower in the evening, after work, when he is home alone. Also, although a persuasive clinician might get Darrell to agree to target the early evening hours as a "high-yield" time for behavioral interventions without collecting these data, the process of doing the activity monitoring exercise can foster a sense of collaboration and help to illustrate the "personal scientist" aspect of CBT, particularly if Darrell is able to see the potential merits of this approach by collecting the evidence himself. This process is likely to increase the chances that he will collaborate more actively in devising subsequent homework assignments and may increase his ability to follow through with these exercises.

Usually, a self-monitoring homework assignment is necessary for only one or two visits. However, we have found that for some patients who are seen in brief sessions, activity scheduling, particularly pleasant events scheduling, is quite useful over the longer term.

Behavioral Activation

The term *behavioral activation* describes a series of strategies that employ planned activities to increase the amount of time that the person with depression spends doing things that are likely to increase feelings of pleasure and, to a lesser extent, mastery. Normally, the planned activities are things that the person has enjoyed doing in the past and were part of what helped to define a healthy, normal life.

We often implement a simple behavioral activation assignment in the first or second session, even before an activity schedule is completed. For example, the clinician might ask a patient this question: "Can you think of one thing that you could do in the next week that would make you feel better if you could get involved in this activity?" The clinician tries to help the patient choose an activity that is 1) specific, 2) likely to be achieved, and 3) likely to lift mood or bring at least a small modicum of pleasure. After an activity is chosen, some brief troubleshooting is done to help the patient identify potential barriers that may interfere with completing the planned activity and make plans to overcome such roadblocks. For example, a patient who says, "It would help to start cooking again—I've just been grabbing some fast food whenever I eat," might select a task that is not clearly defined or may be too challenging to complete at this point in the treatment. The clinician might say, "Could we come up with a realistic goal for cooking this week—something you are fairly sure that you can do? Then we can work out a specific plan for getting started." This line of questioning might lead to a plan to try to 1) go food shopping once to buy ingredients for two meals; 2) prepare one meal each on both Saturday and Sunday (or days when the person does not have to go to work); and 3) select meals that are relatively simple (i.e., something that is easy to prepare and does not take a whole lot of work but still tastes good).

In later sessions, after an activity schedule has been completed, clinicians can help their patients organize more comprehensive behavioral activation plans. Activities are usually planned to fill "holes" in the daily activity schedule—that is, those time slots that were previously associated with solitary or unstimulating activities. An especially important target for activity scheduling is to counter anhedonia with pleasant events scheduling. Many people who are depressed can readily identify a number of leisure-time activities or hobbies that they have stopped doing or spend much less time doing during the illness episode. For others, collaborative brainstorming may be needed to come up with activities that are feasible and will readily fit into their current lifestyle. On occasion, when brainstorming has not been successful, the clinician may ask the person with depression to complete a pleasant events schedule (e.g., see http://anxietydisorderscentrecom.nationprotect.net/Pleasant%20Events.doc, which contains a more comprehensive survey of the wide range of activities that at least some people find to be reinforcing).

One almost universal activity that can help with fighting depression is aerobic exercise. Epidemiological data suggest that people who exercise regularly have fewer depressive symptoms than people who do not (Daley 2008), and most people seeking treatment for depression have had some firsthand experience to suggest that they feel better when they exercise. Nevertheless, relatively few people with depression are doing exercise with any regularity. Results of several controlled studies of mild depression further indicate that approximately 30–60 minutes of light aerobic exercise can have an effect on depressive symptoms that is comparable to standard antidepressant medications (Blumenthal et al. 1999, 2007; Brenes et al. 2007).

When fatigue is particularly problematic or the person with depression is overweight or extremely out of shape, starting with 5 minutes a day of walking is an appropriate way to begin. Some clinicians suggest exercising outdoors in the morning hours after sunrise to also draw on the potential therapeutic effects of sunlight and stabilizing circadian rhythms. When the individual anticipates difficulty initiating an exercise program, the same type of analysis of barriers and solutions described above for simple behavioral activation may be helpful. Also, the clinician can use motivational interviewing methods that are described elsewhere in this book (see Chapter 5, "Promoting Adherence"; Chapter 13, "CBT for Substance Misuse and Abuse"; and Chapter 14, "Lifestyle Change: Building Healthy Habits").

More important than the particular tasks selected is the process used to choose the activities and to monitor the outcomes. Task selection should be collaborative, there should be strong agreement that the person will be able to complete the tasks during the allotted time, and it should be clear that the impact of the activity on mood and on mastery and pleasure ratings will be monitored and that the behavioral activation assignments will be revised accordingly on the basis of these data. In the event that the behavioral activation tasks are not completed or appear to make moods worse rather than better, the clinician may be able to elicit negative cognitions about what happened and address these within the session, prior to crafting the next assignment.

Setting initial expectations relatively low is important; these activities are intended as small steps toward recovery and are unlikely to fully ameliorate depression. Nevertheless, as suggested by the Zen aphorism about the longest journey beginning with a single step, small increases in activity and involvement in rewarding activities can have a reliable and meaningful impact that can set in motion the process of planned behavior change.

Video Illustration 5 shows Dr. Thase using activity scheduling and behavioral activation to help with Darrell's symptoms of low energy, anhedonia, and social isolation. The solid work that was done with these behavioral methods early in treatment was successful in reducing symptoms, gave Darrell firsthand evidence that therapy could help, strengthened the therapeutic relationship, and paved the way for later work on more difficult, emotionally charged issues.

▶ **Video Illustration 5.** Behavioral Methods for Depression:
Dr. Thase and Darrell

The vignette begins with Dr. Thase reviewing an activity schedule from the previous session. After Darrell reports that his energy has been low and says, "It is all I can do to get through the workday," Dr. Thase normalizes energy problems in depression and educates Darrell about the behavioral model. He then suggests that they try to find pleasurable activities for 2 days of the week that they can add to Darrell's schedule.

Darrell's first idea is to meet with his friends to watch a basketball game and get something to eat on a Sunday afternoon. Dr. Thase asks a number of questions to help Darrell increase the chances that this homework assignment will be a success. He asks Darrell, "What can you do to make sure that this happens and that you get there?" They also discuss when he will make a call to his friend to arrange the get-together and consider details on when he will wake in the morning, get a shower, and prepare for the social event. Further questioning centers on developing solutions to potential barriers that could interfere with following the plan.

Dr. Thase: Now can you think of anything that would, barring a setback with your mom, get in the way?

Darrell: I'm too tired…I just don't feel like doing it…It would be too much trouble.

Dr. Thase: Can you think of anything that you and I can work on right now that can minimize the chances that that would happen?

Darrell: Maybe I need to get up earlier…That might help. Instead of getting up right at the last minute, and then really feeling that it is too much trouble…I could get up earlier.

Dr. Thase: Can you think of anything else?

Darrell: Yeah, maybe I need a reminder like a note on the fridge or the calendar…or maybe something on my desk at work—something that is going to remind me to do it.

Dr. Thase: Can you think of any motivational message to yourself that would have an impact?

Darrell: One of the big things that is missing is fun…Maybe I could say something like…it would be fun…it would be good for you—something like that.

The extra effort that Dr. Thase made to troubleshoot possible difficulties in increasing activity levels only took a few extra minutes. However, this type of preparation can pay dividends in helping reactivate people who are stuck in behavioral ruts.

Graded Task Assignments

When depressive symptoms are severe, it is common for the individual to procrastinate or avoid attempting to perform more difficult or demanding activities. Both at work and at home, effortful chores and tasks go undone in part because the person who is depressed is aware that her functional capabilities are significantly decreased and that as a result, she may fail. Also, the patient may have a wistful hope that she may feel better in a day or two (or a week or two) and will be better able to draw on her usual faculties. As is obvious to even the person who is doing the procrastination, this self-deceptive strategy is rarely effective (i.e., beyond the brief sense of relief that one gets from postponing a difficult chore), and when the person is in the midst of a more long-standing bout of depression, the burden of work and the difficulty of actually catching up only increase over time.

The method used to make a graded task assignment basically follows the aphorism about how one person can move a 2,000-pound boulder that is blocking the road—namely, by breaking it down into fifty 40-pound rocks. This commonsense approach is applicable to almost all tasks or chores. Although the great majority of people already know this principle and in fact have used it in the past to solve problems, depression interferes with a person's ability to map out and implement a solution. Following the example of the boulder, the person who is depressed may feel as if she will not be able to find a sledgehammer, will feel too tired to move all those rocks, and—even if she could—will not have the time to do so. In such cases, the clinician helps coach people on how to put the graded task method to work in their lives.

The process of identifying the task, breaking it down into manageable chunks, and scheduling the time slots to work on the problem is a collaborative one. From start to finish, a graded task assignment can often be designed in 10 minutes or less in brief sessions. Often, this brief time is sufficient to get patients started with identifying some steps. They can then fill out a written plan for a graded approach as a homework assignment and can choose a few of the early steps to work on between sessions. Results are then logged (including effects on pleasure and mastery ratings) and reviewed at the next session.

During either the development or the implementation of a graded task assignment, the person with depression may encounter automatic negative thoughts about his predicament, most typically thoughts about the overwhelming magnitude of the problem (e.g., "I'll never get this done") or personal attributes that may have caused the problem (e.g., "I'm so lazy" or "I'm such a loser for getting this far behind"). This situation creates the opportunity to address these automatic negative thoughts with cognitive restructuring strategies (see Chapter 7, "Targeting Maladaptive Thinking").

Behavioral Rehearsal

Behavioral rehearsal strategies are an important way of helping patients with depression to prepare for and practice interactions in demanding or challenging situations that they have either avoided or have felt they have managed poorly in the past. Because these situations are typically interpersonal in nature, the clinician-patient dyad affords an excellent "studio" to rehearse new skills under less threatening circumstances. A particular event that did not go well in the past week or one that is looming on the horizon usually can be identified to provide the opportunity for rehearsal.

Drawing from the work of McCullough (2000), the clinician can pose these questions: "What do you want to get from this interaction?" and "What is likely to get in the way of achieving this goal?" Writing out a script for the planned interchange may also be worthwhile to guide the initiation of the behavior and provide a summary of key points and goals. Sometimes it is helpful for the clinician and patient to reverse roles for the first round of rehearsal to give the patient a chance to learn from observation. If role reversal is used, the patient can be encouraged to "turn up the heat" by behaving in a way that conforms to her fears about what might go wrong in the interaction.

Another useful application of behavioral rehearsal is to have the patient work on being a good listener in conversations with friends or loved ones. As noted earlier, a person who is depressed often gets caught up in his negative mood and cognitions and dominates a conversation with complaints and gloomy self-statements, without allowing time for the other person to talk about her concerns. In a behavioral rehearsal focused on this situation, the clinician coaches the patient to practice making specific statements of interest in the other person's life and to make reflective and nonjudgmental comments that encourage continued disclosure. It may be easiest to begin this type of behavioral exercise with telephone conversations with the other person so that possible incongruencies between affect and verbal behavior or occasional reliance on notes do not interfere with the success of the task. By explicitly demonstrating that one is again able to be a reciprocal member of a healthy relationship, the chances for further companionship and social support are enhanced.

Practice Case: Planning a Behavioral Intervention for Depression

The following learning exercise is provided to help clinicians build skills in using behavioral strategies. The practice case involves planning treatment interventions for Susan, a 37-year-old woman with a history of recurrent depression.

Learning Exercise 6–1   Planning a Behavioral Intervention for Depression

1. During the first session, you ask Susan how she is spending her time at home, and she sheepishly replies that most nights she goes to bed shortly after dinner and remains there until it is time to get ready for work in the morning. Write out some ideas for what you might do next.

2. Assume that the two of you agreed at the first session to do a self-monitoring exercise as a homework assignment and, at the next visit, the data essentially confirm her description, with clear deficits in both mastery and pleasure. While she is in bed, her mood is consistently low, with pleasure ratings ranging between 1 and 4 (a few favorite television shows lift her spirits), but with mastery ratings of 0–1. Although the deficits are clear, what else do you need to know about Susan's life?

3. You ask Susan how she spent her evenings when she was feeling less depressed, and she tells you that in addition to watching television, she enjoyed reading and "talking" (both by phone and instant messaging) with several friends who live in distant cities. At least once a week, Susan used to visit with her sister and on occasion would babysit her sister's three small children. At her best, Susan also would work out four or five times a week at the exercise room of her condominium complex, although she states that she cannot remember the last time that she exercised. Think about how you would approach a behavioral activation homework assignment, and write out some suggested activities that might increase Susan's pleasure ratings.

4. Over the next few weeks, Susan makes some headway with the behavioral activation assignments and is able to do more things that give her pleasure, is spending less time in bed, and is generally feeling better, with pleasure ratings now typically in the 4–6 range during the evening hours. Although her mastery ratings also have tended to increase during the day (while at work), these ratings remain low during the evenings. Susan confides that she would be embarrassed to have any company because she has not opened her mail for days and has not dusted or run the vacuum for "weeks." She also reports that her clothes hamper and laundry baskets are overflowing. Think about some appropriate exercises that may help Susan increase her mastery ratings, and write down your plan to introduce these assignments.

5. The graded task assignments that you and Susan developed were so effective that within 2 weeks, she had been able to open all of her mail, clean her condo, and catch up on her laundry. Susan's score on the Patient Health Questionnaire–9 (Kroenke et al. 2001; see Chapter 3, "Enhancing the Impact of Brief Sessions," for information on rating scales) is now only 9, which is 50% lower than before treatment. Susan has not yet resumed working out, however, and confides that after such a long layoff, she is likely to be embarrassed by what the regular attendees in the exercise room will think about her if she tries to go back. In particular, she is dreading running into one man she dated briefly several years earlier, who had once made a hurtful comment in the exercise room about how Susan could benefit from additional exercises aimed at improving the tone of her muscles. What plans do you have for the next homework assignment?

Summary

Key Points for Clinicians

- Depression is a state characterized by a low rate of activities that generate pleasure and self-appraisals of mastery and an increased likelihood of spending time in solitary, unstimulating activities.
- Strategies that specifically address these behavioral changes are an important component of CBT and are often emphasized early in the course of a comprehensive approach to therapy.
- Four behavioral strategies—self-monitoring, behavioral activation, graded task assignments, and behavioral rehearsal—can often be used effectively in brief sessions.
- Beyond the utility of these strategies for targeting key depressive symptoms and promoting healthier lifestyles, the process of introducing and implementing behavioral interventions can enhance the therapeutic alliance and create the opportunity for identifying negative automatic thoughts and testing out cognitive interventions.

Concepts and Skills for Patients to Learn

- Depression usually lowers energy levels and interferes with people's ability to experience pleasure. A natural reaction to these problems is to pull back from normal activities and to spend more time alone. Unfortunately, reducing your activity level often makes things worse.
- One of the most helpful strategies to fight depression and to restore your energy and interest is to log your daily activities on a chart. Then

you can see in "black and white" the effects of different activities on your sense of pleasure and your mastery of the things you do every day.

• Your doctor or therapist can coach you on ways of gradually resuming pleasurable, interesting, and meaningful activities. Taking action to build activity levels can be a very important part of an effective plan for recovery from depression.

• If you are facing a challenging task, it can help to break the task down into manageable pieces. A step-by-step approach can build your confidence and increase the chances of success.

References

Addis ME, Martell CR: Overcoming Depression One Step at a Time. Oakland, CA, New Harbinger, 2004

Beck AT, Rush AJ, Shaw BF, et al: Cognitive Therapy of Depression. New York, Guilford, 1979

Beck AT, Greenberg RL, Beck J: Coping With Depression (pamphlet). Bala Cynwyd, PA, Beck Institute, 1995

Blumenthal JA, Babyak MA, Moore KA, et al: Effects of exercise training on older patients with major depression. Arch Intern Med 159:2349–2356, 1999

Blumenthal JA, Babyak MA, Doraiswamy PM, et al: Exercise and pharmacotherapy in the treatment of major depressive disorder. Psychosom Med 69:587–596, 2007

Brenes GA, Williamson JD, Messier SP, et al: Treatment of minor depression in older adults: a pilot study comparing sertraline and exercise. Aging Ment Health 11:61–68, 2007

Daley A: Exercise and depression: a review of reviews. J Clin Psychol Med Settings 15:140–147, 2008

Dimidjian S, Hollon SD, Dobson KS, et al: Randomized trial of behavioral activation, cognitive therapy, and antidepressant medication in the acute treatment of adults with major depression. J Consult Clin Psychol 74:658–670, 2006

Ekers D, Richards D, Gilbody S: A meta-analysis of randomized trials of behavioural treatment of depression. Psychol Med 38:611–623, 2008

Kroenke K, Spitzer RL, Williams JB: The PHQ-9: validity of a brief depression severity measure. J Gen Intern Med 16:606–613, 2001

McCullough JP Jr: Treatment for Chronic Depression: Cognitive Behavioral Analysis System of Psychotherapy. New York, Guilford, 2000

CHAPTER 7

Targeting Maladaptive Thinking

LEARNING MAP

Cognitive targets for brief sessions

⇩

Cognitive pathology in depression and anxiety disorders

⇩

Efficient methods for identifying automatic thoughts

⇩

Problems with identifying automatic thoughts

⇩

Modifying automatic thoughts in brief sessions

⇩

Working with accurate thoughts

⇩

Promoting adaptive core beliefs

⇩

Developing a library of handouts

Changing maladaptive thinking is a hallmark of the cognitive-behavior therapy (CBT) approach. A rich and extensive research effort has characterized cognitive pathology in mood disorders, anxiety disorders, psychoses, eating disorders, substance abuse, and other psychiatric illnesses and has demonstrated that CBT methods are effective in reversing dysfunctional thinking in these conditions (Clark et al. 1999; Wright et al. 2008). In this chapter, we explain how to adapt CBT methods that modify pathological thinking for sessions that are briefer than the standard 50-minute hour.

Cognitive Targets for Brief Sessions

The primary cognitive targets for brief sessions—that is, automatic thoughts, cognitive errors, misattributions (i.e., assigning maladaptive meanings to events), and core beliefs—are the same as in standard sessions of CBT. However, the emphasis is typically on the more readily accessible automatic thoughts, cognitive errors, and misattributions than on deeply embedded core beliefs or schemas. Because this book is not an introductory text, we do not explain the different levels of cognitive processes in psychiatric disorders in detail. Readers who are not fully versed in this concept are referred to basic texts by Beck (1995), Sudak (2006), or Wright et al. (2006). Short definitions are supplied in Table 7–1.

Although work on identifying and revising core beliefs can be a very productive part of standard CBT, intensive efforts to modify schemas may be beyond the scope of most applications that use brief sessions. As noted in Chapter 2, "Indications and Formats for Brief CBT Sessions," persons with chronic low self-esteem, extensive histories of psychological trauma, significant Axis II pathology, or other evidence of long-standing, deeply entrenched pathology may not be the best candidates for CBT in brief sessions. Efforts to identify and change core beliefs and associated behavioral patterns are often a central part of longer-term and more extensive CBT for such persons. Nevertheless, we do think that efforts to recognize schematic patterns and to educate patients about cognitive methods to make these beliefs more adaptive may be worthwhile for some patients who are treated in brief sessions. Behavioral changes that occur as a result of briefer sessions can also provide new information that challenges long-held rules and assumptions for some patients.

Research on computer-assisted CBT, a method that uses brief sessions of about 25 minutes in combination with a computer program that teaches basic CBT principles, has found that core beliefs can change with relatively short contacts with a therapist (Wright et al. 2005). In a study

---

Table 7–1. Primary cognitive targets for brief sessions

Automatic thoughts: The stream of cognitive processing stimulated by events or memories of events that lie just below the surface of the fully conscious mind. Persons with psychiatric disorders often have large numbers of these types of thoughts that they do not subject to rational analyses. Negatively distorted or maladaptive automatic thoughts (e.g., "There's no use trying…I can't handle it…It will be a disaster") can often be modified with cognitive-behavior therapy techniques.

Cognitive errors: Logical errors that occur in automatic thoughts and schemas. Cognitive errors such as all-or-nothing thinking, personalization, magnifying and minimizing, and overgeneralization are very common in depression, anxiety disorders, and other psychiatric illnesses.

Misattributions: Attributions are the meanings that people attach to events. Misattributions occur when people assign maladaptive meanings to events. Depression is associated with a tendency for misattributions. For example, a depressed person may take excessive blame for a negative event, give the event global significance in her life, and view the event as having a fixed and unyielding impact on his entire future. Conversely, a person without depression who experiences the same event may take a balanced view of responsibility, make a circumscribed attribution about the significance of the event, and think "this too will pass." Cognitive-behavior therapy methods are used to help people move toward a rational attributional style.

Core beliefs (schemas): The basic rules for information processing that lie under the surface of more superficial and situation-specific automatic thoughts. Schemas can be adaptive (e.g., "Others can trust me"; "There's not much that can scare me"; "If I work at something, I can usually master it") or maladaptive (e.g., "I'm stupid"; "I'm unlovable"; "I must be perfect to be accepted").

---

of drug-free patients with major depression, persons treated with computer-assisted CBT had significantly greater reduction in dysfunctional core beliefs than those in a wait-listed control group, whereas those treated with standard CBT (50-minute sessions) did not show this benefit (Wright et al. 2005). The total amount of therapist time in computer-assisted CBT in this study was about 4 hours or less. Results of this study suggest that efforts to enhance brief sessions with computer-assisted therapy, or perhaps with other adjuncts that could stimulate learning and self-help, may be a useful approach for modifying core beliefs.

Cognitive Pathology in Depression and Anxiety Disorders

In planning cognitive interventions for brief sessions, clinicians can benefit from understanding the typical characteristics of maladaptive information processing in the various types of mental disorders. This knowledge can help clinicians gear their interventions toward the most important cognitive targets for each disorder. Table 7–2 lists some of the predominant features of cognitive pathology in depression and anxiety disorders.

Table 7–2.   Cognitive pathology in depression and anxiety disorders

Predominant in depression	Predominant in anxiety disorders	Common to both depression and anxiety disorders
Hopelessness	Excessive fears of harm or danger	Demoralization
Low self-esteem		Self-absorption
Negative view of environment	High sensitivity to information about potential threat	Heightened automatic information processing
Automatic thoughts with negative themes	Automatic thoughts associated with danger, risk, uncontrollability, incapacity	Cognitive errors in information processing
Misattributions		Maladaptive schemas
Enhanced recall of negative memories	Overestimates of risk in situations	
	Decreased estimate of ability to cope with the feared object or situation	
	Enhanced recall of memories for threatening situations	

Source.   Adapted from Wright JH, Beck AT, Thase ME: "Cognitive Therapy," in *The American Psychiatric Publishing Textbook of Psychiatry*, 5th Edition. Edited by Hales RE, Yudofsky SC, Gabbard GO. Washington, DC, American Psychiatric Publishing, 2008, p. 1217. Used with permission. Copyright © 2008 American Psychiatric Publishing.

As Aaron Beck noted, depression is characterized by negatively distorted thinking in three principal domains: the future (hopelessness), the self (low self-esteem, guilt, self-condemning cognitions), and the world around the individual (negative view of the environment) (Beck 1963, 1964, 1967; Clark et al. 1999). In addition to this "negative cognitive triad," persons with depression frequently have misattributions and often have a heightened recall of negative memories (Wright et al. 2008). In contrast, people with anxiety disorders usually have excessive fears of harm or danger from objects or situations (e.g., social encounters, triggers or reminders of previous traumatic events, crowds, driving, not completing a ritual), an increased estimate of the risk in these situations, and a decreased estimate of their ability to cope with or manage the situation (Mathews and MacLeod 1987; Wright et al. 2008). These patients also have heightened attention and vigilance about potential threats. Maladaptive automatic thoughts, cognitive errors, and problematic schemas are common in both depression and anxiety disorders.

Although this book focuses primarily on mood and anxiety disorders, we include chapters on working with psychotic symptoms, substance abuse, insomnia, and medical disorders. The typical forms of cognitive pathology for these conditions or applications are discussed in the respective chapters. Methods for identifying and modifying automatic thoughts are a central component of brief CBT sessions for all of these clinical problems.

Efficient Methods for Identifying Automatic Thoughts

The first steps in working with automatic thoughts are to help patients recognize that they are having these maladaptive cognitions and to identify specific automatic thoughts that are causing distress. However, before launching efforts to recognize automatic thoughts, the clinician should consider the timing and staging of interventions. For some patients who are severely depressed and who have considerable inertia, the best approach might be to begin with behavioral interventions to increase activity levels and counter low energy and anhedonia (see Chapter 6, "Behavioral Methods for Depression"). Also, patients with marked sleep and concentration problems may need assistance with improving sleep patterns to improve their capacity to monitor and change automatic thoughts. It is common to notice patients' maladaptive thoughts before they are ready to focus attention on thinking in a session. This is a good time to form hypotheses about the patient's cognitive style that will guide later interventions. Table 7–3 lists efficient methods for identifying automatic thoughts, each described in further detail in the following sections.

Table 7–3. Efficient methods for identifying automatic thoughts

Guided discovery

Identification of automatic thoughts that occur in a session

Brief explanations/mini-lessons

Readings and other educational resources

Thought records

Automatic thoughts checklists

Computer-assisted cognitive-behavior therapy

Guided Discovery

The most commonly used method for uncovering automatic thoughts in all formats of CBT is guided discovery, which involves asking good questions that help patients understand how their thinking patterns are part of their problem. Clinicians who are skilled in doing CBT in brief sessions can use guided discovery in a highly efficient and emotionally resonant manner to elicit and then modify automatic thoughts. Video illustrations throughout this book demonstrate how questions are asked in brief CBT to identify automatic thoughts and other cognitions. Characteristics of effective use of guided discovery in brief sessions are detailed in Table 7–4.

Identification of Automatic Thoughts That Occur in a Session

One of the most powerful ways of helping patients to quickly understand and identify automatic thoughts is to spotlight cognitions that have just occurred in a session. Therefore, clinicians should watch carefully for those moments when the patient experiences a "mood shift," marked by a sudden appearance of emotions such as anxiety, sadness, or anger. These mood shifts almost always are a sign that significant automatic thoughts have just occurred. The question "What thought just went through your mind?" will often help the patient access thoughts related to the distressing emotion.

In briefer sessions, the timing of these interventions is very important. Patients need to have adequate grounding in the principles of CBT to appreciate the need to uncover and evaluate automatic thoughts, and the therapeutic relationship must be strong enough for patients to trust the therapist to guide them safely through the process of exploring painful

---

Table 7–4. High-impact guided discovery methods for brief sessions

---

Focus on recent events of high significance. Generally, patients find it easier to recognize and accurately remember automatic thoughts that have occurred very recently and are highly significant to them. A less efficient approach is to have discourses about events or circumstances from long ago.

Be specific. Try to avoid discussions that are diffuse or poorly focused. Instead, find a specific situation or trigger and then ask targeted questions to identify automatic thoughts.

Stick with one line of questioning and one topic. It is especially important in brief sessions to stay focused on an area of questioning that has high potential for positive results. Remember that doing one thing well in cognitive-behavior therapy may be a better approach than attempting to cover a large number of topics and issues. If a patient learns cognitive-behavior therapy skills for one problem area or concern, these skills can then be used in many other situations.

Ask questions that stimulate emotion. Automatic thoughts of high relevance usually stimulate significant emotion. Thus, questions that draw out significant emotions will often lead to important automatic thoughts.

Use a mini-formulation to guide the questioning. The most effective questions are often ones that directly flow from a mini-formulation. Instead of a scattershot approach, use a mini-formulation to zero in on the most salient automatic thoughts.

Source. Adapted from Wright JH, Basco MR, Thase ME: *Learning Cognitive-Behavior Therapy: An Illustrated Guide.* Washington, DC, American Psychiatric Publishing, 2006, pp. 92–94. Used with permission. Copyright © 2006 American Psychiatric Publishing.

---

thoughts and emotions. Patients also need sufficient time to debrief and understand the reason for the interventions made by the therapist before the session is completed. Clinicians must be careful to explain that automatic thoughts are not always an accurate reflection of facts, but if the automatic thoughts are determined to be true, the therapist will help the patient to solve whatever problem exists.

Brief Explanations/Mini-Lessons

A good way to help patients learn to identify automatic thoughts is to give a brief explanation or mini-lesson on the cognitive-behavioral

---

Table 7–5.   Characteristics of automatic thoughts

Automatic thoughts usually are out of the person's awareness unless he focuses attention on them.

Automatic thoughts can come in several forms: verbal, visual (images), and "shorthand" (brief comments that indicate that a more expanded automatic thought is present).

When automatic thoughts come in the form of "shorthand" (e.g., "That figures," "Whatever," "Stuff happens") or rhetorical questions (e.g., "Why doesn't she like me?" "Can't he ever understand my feelings?" "What could I ever do to be accepted?"), clinicians need to help the patient expand the thought or answer the question to make it amenable to logical analysis.

The degree of distress caused by an automatic thought can be inversely proportional to how much it is evaluated.

Automatic thoughts are more likely to "feel" like facts when they are neither articulated nor written.

Automatic thoughts frequently recur and coalesce around central themes.

---

model. The clinician might follow the previous step of identifying some of the patient's cognitions that occur in a session with a short discussion that normalizes the occurrence of automatic thoughts, or the clinician could explain how automatic thoughts influence emotions and behavior. We often diagram the CBT model as a mini-formulation in a session and ask the patient to review the diagram for homework. Table 7–5 lists characteristics of automatic thoughts that can be helpful to teach to patients over time.

Another method of teaching patients about automatic thoughts is to give examples of how others might develop varied types of cognitions in response to a triggering event. One of the examples that we often use is to ask patients to try to identify automatic thoughts that might be common in a person with "road rage" compared with someone who calmly copes with a difficult driving situation.

Readings and Other Educational Resources

Readings and other psychoeducational materials that patients can use outside of sessions are particularly important when brief sessions are being used. For patients who want to learn about automatic thoughts and are willing to do some reading for homework, clinicians can suggest use-

---

Table 7–6. Readings and other educational resources for learning about automatic thoughts

---

Self-help books

Burns DD: Feeling Good. New York, Morrow, 1999

Greenberger D, Padesky CA: Mind Over Mood. New York, Guilford, 1995

Wright JH, Basco MR: Getting Your Life Back: The Complete Guide to Recovery From Depression. New York, Touchstone, 2002

Computer programs

Beating the Blues
www.beatingtheblues.co.uk

Good Days Ahead: The Multimedia Program for Cognitive Therapy
www.mindstreet.com

Internet resources

MoodGYM Training Program
www.moodgym.anu.edu.au

Note. These and additional recommendations are listed in Appendix 2, "CBT Resources for Patients and Families."

---

ful self-help books or other resources (Table 7–6). However, clinicians need to avoid overloading patients with readings or other learning tasks. For patients who are severely depressed or anxious, the best practice might be to recommend only a single book chapter, a portion of a chapter, or a pamphlet instead of an entire book or a list of books.

Thought Records

Methods of using thought records to identify and then change automatic thoughts are described in all basic texts (e.g., Beck 1995; Sudak 2006; Wright et al. 2006) and are not explained at length here. However, we want to emphasize that thought records are a fundamental element of CBT techniques for uncovering automatic thoughts and are well suited for use in brief sessions. The treatment of Grace, a woman with depression and anxiety, demonstrates how a thought record assigned for homework can very quickly lead to productive work in a brief session. We discuss a video illustration of Grace's use of a thought record later in this chapter. In this session, Dr. Sudak asked Grace to use a three-column thought record to identify automatic thoughts stimulated by a stressful work situation. Grace noted highly salient automatic thoughts on the

Event	Automatic thoughts	Emotions
	(Rate degree of belief 0%–100%)	(Rate intensity 0%–100%)
Preparing for new job	*I might get fired again. (95%)*	*Anxiety (90%)*
		Tension (75%)
	My boss might not like me. (85%)	
	I'll make a mistake and get fired. (90%)	

Figure 7–1. A three-column thought record: Grace's example.

record (Figure 7–1), and Dr. Sudak was able to jump-start the session by rapidly tuning in to these cognitions and getting to work on helping Grace cope better with her concerns about a new job.

> **Learning Exercise 7–1** Identifying Automatic Thoughts in a Brief Session
>
> 1. Use guided discovery and/or a mood shift to identify automatic thoughts with a patient you are seeing in a brief session.
>
> 2. Give a brief explanation/mini-lesson about automatic thoughts.
>
> 3. Suggest a thought record for a homework assignment.

Automatic Thoughts Checklists

Another method that may be useful in brief sessions is to ask the patient to complete an automatic thoughts checklist. This technique can help patients spot significant automatic thoughts that otherwise might go unrecognized. The most extensively researched inventory is the Automatic Thoughts Questionnaire (Hollon and Kendall 1980), which has 30 items rated on a 5-point scale from 0 (not at all) to 4 (all the time). A briefer 15-item checklist is used in the computer program *Good Days Ahead*, a form of computer-assisted therapy that has been shown to be effective in clinical practice (Wright et al. 2005). This checklist is shown in Table 7–7.

Table 7–7. Automatic thoughts checklist

Instructions: Place a check mark beside each negative automatic thought that you have had in the past 2 weeks.

_____I should be doing better in life.

_____He/she doesn't understand me.

_____I've let him/her down.

_____I just can't enjoy things anymore.

_____Why am I so weak?

_____I always keep messing things up.

_____My life's going nowhere.

_____I can't handle it.

_____I'm failing.

_____It's too much for me.

_____I don't have much of a future.

_____Things are out of control.

_____I feel like giving up.

_____Something bad is sure to happen.

_____There must be something wrong with me.

Note. This checklist is available in Appendix 1, "Worksheets and Checklists."
Source. Adapted from Wright JH, Wright AS, Beck AT: *Good Days Ahead: The Multimedia Program for Cognitive Therapy,* Professional Edition, Version 3.0. Louisville, KY, Mindstreet, 2010. Used with permission. Copyright © 2010 Mindstreet.

Computer-Assisted CBT

Computer programs and Internet-delivered psychoeducation can also help patients learn to identify automatic thoughts and may be especially useful for patients who are being seen in brief sessions and wish to use learning materials at home. Computer resources for CBT are listed in Appendix 2, "CBT Resources for Patients and Families."

Problems With Identifying Automatic Thoughts

When difficulties are encountered in accessing automatic thoughts (Table 7–8), several techniques, including imagery or role-play, can be help-

---

Table 7–8. Problems with identifying automatic thoughts

Patient has had insufficient time to learn the skill.

Patient has trouble identifying emotion or avoids emotion.

Patient has thoughts in the form of images.

Patient is frightened by the content of the thought.

Patient has difficulty relating the emotional experience to an external event.

---

ful tools in achieving good results (Wright et al. 2006). Clinicians who are accustomed to the use of imagery and role-play in traditional 45- to 50-minute sessions will need to modify these interventions to transfer them smoothly to a briefer format. After a short introduction or explanation, the clinician can ask the patient to imagine being back in a situation or to simulate the situation in a discussion with the clinician. Patients will need sufficient time to identify their thinking and to debrief with the therapist after the imagery experience or role-play. Clinicians must be sure that they have a sound therapeutic relationship and that the patient can reality-test prior to the use of role-play.

Patients may have trouble identifying automatic thoughts because they do not notice or identify emotions, or because they engage in emotional avoidance. In such a situation, discussing a mini-formulation with the patient can help. Also, the clinician can teach the patient skills to increase tolerance for experiencing emotion. Some patients will report the thoughts they have as emotional states—for example, "I feel worthless"—and need to be instructed as to what emotions are.

Patients may also have thoughts in the form of images and report "not having thoughts" at the time of distressing emotions. Educational efforts can assist these patients in reporting these images as the mental response they have to an event. Another problem can occur when patients are frightened by thoughts that seem objectionable or irrational. A good alliance and normalization statements about the ubiquitous nature of such thoughts can help ease barriers to expressing them. Sometimes patients do not identify a particular external event that causes dysphoria. Instead they "just begin to feel badly." One explanation for this type of experience is that the patient is having automatic thoughts about internal, privately held thoughts, emotions, or physiological sensations. Clinicians can sensitively help such patients identify these internal states as the precipitants of the automatic thoughts leading to dysphoric mood.

Table 7–9.	Methods for modifying automatic thoughts in brief sessions

Socratic questioning

Thought change records

Examining the evidence

Generating rational alternatives

Coping cards

Identifying cognitive errors

Reattribution

Cognitive rehearsal

Learning Exercise 7–2 Responding to Challenges in Identifying Automatic Thoughts

1. Ask a colleague to portray a patient who is having difficulty accessing automatic thoughts in a brief session.

2. Troubleshoot some potential reasons for the difficulty, and identify at least two ideas for helping the patient uncover automatic thoughts.

3. Practice at least one method for overcoming the difficulty in identifying automatic thoughts.

Modifying Automatic Thoughts in Brief Sessions

Most or all of the methods for modifying automatic thoughts that are used in longer 45- to 50-minute sessions can be adapted for briefer sessions (see Table 7–9). We describe adaptations for brief sessions in the following subsections. First, we discuss a case with video illustrations that demonstrates some key methods for modifying automatic thoughts.

Case Example: Grace

Grace's history and case conceptualization were presented in Chapter 3, "Enhancing the Impact of Brief Sessions," and Chapter 4, "Case Formulation and Treatment Planning." Video Illustration 2 was shown in Chapter 3 to provide a general sense of how to adapt CBT for brief sessions.

Here we use Video Illustration 2 to demonstrate methods for modifying automatic thoughts.

▶ **Video Illustration 2.** Modifying Automatic Thoughts I: Dr. Sudak and Grace

In this video, Dr. Sudak helps Grace identify and change her automatic thoughts related to the anxiety she has about her new job. Dr. Sudak obtains specific thoughts by using effective questions, asks Grace to write down the thoughts, and chooses the most troublesome thought as the target for the most attention. The primary methods for working with automatic thoughts that are demonstrated in this video illustration are Socratic questioning, thought change records (TCRs), examining the evidence, generating rational alternatives, and developing a written coping strategy. An interesting observation is how all of these procedures are used to good effect in a segment of the session that lasted only about 10½ minutes.

Socratic Questioning

Socratic questioning is an excellent way to teach patients to evaluate and restructure their thinking (Wright et al. 2006). Socratic questions encourage patients to subject their thoughts to logical analysis and often increase curiosity and therapeutic engagement. Ideally they stimulate patients to want to discover more about their own thinking. The clinician frequently has an endpoint in mind during this process of discovery but remains objective and attuned to patient leads.

In Video Illustration 2, Dr. Sudak demonstrates several productive strings of Socratic questions. In one of these, she helps Grace begin to modify an automatic thought that she is going to make a mistake and get fired.

Grace: I know I'm going to make mistakes.
Dr. Sudak: Would that [making mistakes] be something special about you?
Grace: No…no…A lot of people make mistakes when they're new on the job.
Dr. Sudak: What percentage of people who are new on the job make mistakes?
Grace: A lot of people—90%…Maybe 95%.
Dr. Sudak: How many of those people get fired?
Grace: Hardly any…People make mistakes when they're learning a new job.

Table 7–10. Tips for using Socratic questions in brief sessions

---

Ask high-yield Socratic questions.   Clinicians should target main points in asking Socratic questions. A cognitive-behavior therapy miniformulation can be used to identify key problems and opportunities that may respond to Socratic questions.

Ask questions that get patients involved in the learning process.   All forms of cognitive-behavior therapy are intended to help patients learn to become their own therapists. In brief sessions, it is especially important for the clinician to model a questioning style that will encourage patients to ask themselves questions to break through rigid and maladaptive thinking patterns.

Ask questions that provide openings for change.   Good Socratic questions often reveal opportunities for change in thinking and/or behavior. In brief formats for cognitive-behavior therapy, it may be best to select only one or two targets for change in a single session.

Choose questions that are matched to the patient's level of symptoms and cognitive capacities and are suitable for brief sessions.   Socratic questions should be pitched at a level that stimulates more adaptive thinking but does not confuse or overwhelm the patient. Preliminary goals in brief sessions may be to begin the Socratic questioning process and to succinctly demonstrate its value instead of engaging in extensive or taxing lines of questions.

Asking effective Socratic questions is one of the most useful CBT methods in sessions of all lengths. Tips for using Socratic questions in brief sessions are listed in Table 7–10.

Thought Change Records

In brief sessions, TCRs are often used to leverage the time available for working with automatic thoughts. If patients can record their thoughts for homework and then bring these logs to sessions, they may be able to proceed efficiently in generating a more adaptive thinking style. Writing thoughts down on paper (or on a computer) can serve a powerful function. Perceptions that seem quite "real" and accurate when they first pop into a person's mind may become much less believable when subjected to the objectivity of a written exercise.

Sometimes patients who are highly depressed can become more dysphoric when they begin to write down thoughts in the absence of objective evaluation. Such patients can believe strongly in the content of their highly negative thoughts and have difficulty revising them quickly. Clinicians must let patients know that if they feel worse after writing down negative thoughts, they should stop and wait. Later therapy sessions will teach them tools to evaluate the thought or to solve the problem to which the thought refers.

In using TCRs, the clinician may find it helpful to ask patients to rate the percentage of belief (0%–100%) they have in their automatic thoughts and the intensity of emotions (1%–100%) that are associated with the cognitions. Automatic thoughts may then become more accessible to objective evaluation and modification. A quantitative estimate of belief in the thought and degree of emotion experienced can help the therapist and patient identify which thoughts are more central and important. Dysfunctional thoughts that are strongly held and associated with a high degree of negative emotion are likely to be related to a substantial amount of symptom relief when examined and restructured. When patients experience this relief, they may function better and have increased motivation for treatment.

Video Illustration 2 shows a brief but effective use of the TCR technique. Because she had already taught Grace the basics of thought recording at a previous session, Dr. Sudak could rapidly introduce the TCR as a method of eliciting and changing automatic thoughts. Within the first 2 minutes of the vignette, Dr. Sudak and Grace worked with a TCR to identify three important automatic thoughts (i.e., "I might get fired again," "My boss might not like me," I'll make a mistake and get fired") related to her starting a new job (see Figure 7–1). These automatic thoughts provided important targets for the other interventions used in this session (Socratic questioning, examining the evidence, generating rational alternatives, and developing a written coping plan). By the end of the brief session, Grace is prepared for a homework assignment to use TCRs to record additional automatic thoughts and to use this method to reduce anxiety and depression associated with her life stresses.

A detailed explanation of the TCR method is available in Wright et al. (2006), and a blank five-column TCR is provided in Appendix 1, "Worksheets and Checklists," and can be downloaded in larger format from the American Psychiatric Publishing Web site (www.appi.org/pdf/62362). Some tips for using TCRs in shorter sessions are shown in Table 7–11.

Examining the Evidence

The therapy session shown in Video Illustration 2 also demonstrates an informal but useful approach to examining the evidence. Dr. Sudak does not set up a fully developed examining-the-evidence exercise in which the patient is asked to identify and write out lists of "evidence for" and "evidence

---

Table 7–11. Tips for using thought change records in brief sessions

---

Explain the method of using thought change records in a session, and record at least one sequence of "event → automatic thoughts → emotions" to demonstrate the technique.

Suggest reading materials to help patient learn the method of using thought change records.

Assign thought change records for homework. Always check the homework.

Adjust level of assignment to phase of therapy and patient capacity. Do not expect too much too soon.

Keep initial assignments fairly simple and easy to achieve.

Try to have most work with thought change records performed as self-help exercises between brief sessions.

Troubleshoot difficulties in using thought change records and give patient practical help in resolving these difficulties.

Ask patient to keep thought change records in a therapy notebook and to review them to reinforce learning.

Use thought change records to bridge between sessions, stick with important topics or problems, and stay focused on important goals for therapy.

---

against" an automatic thought (see Wright et al. 2006 for a description and video illustration of this technique). However, she does ask very effective questions that help Grace recognize that her fears about making a mistake and getting fired from a new job are largely unfounded. They also explore evidence about needing to be perfect to succeed in the new job.

Written, two-column, examining-the-evidence exercises also can be effective tools for brief sessions. For example, Luke, a 45-year-old man who was being treated with an antidepressant and brief CBT sessions for obsessive-compulsive disorder, was struggling with an obsessive automatic thought: "If I don't complete my rituals, something terrible will happen." Luke was beginning to make progress with the exposure and response prevention methods that are so important in treatment of obsessive-compulsive disorder (see Chapter 9, "Behavioral Methods for Anxiety"), but the obsessive thought was interfering to some extent with his progress. Over the course of two brief sessions, Luke and his psychiatrist developed the examining-the-evidence worksheet shown in Figure 7–2. Notably the worksheet includes identification of cognitive errors and generation of a rational alternative, two related methods for modifying automatic thoughts that are described later in this chapter.

Automatic thought:

"If I don't complete my rituals, something terrible will happen."

Evidence for:

My father is elderly and very frail, something could happen to him at any time.

When I try to stop counting, I get really nervous and bad things could happen.

I've done well at my job—the rituals seem to help me avoid trouble.

Evidence against:

Because my father is getting very old, it's likely that he will get sick or even die.

This will happen whether I do the rituals or not.

I've been reducing my counting, and nothing bad has happened.

There is no scientific evidence that doing rituals can protect me or my loved ones from harm.

Cognitive errors in evidence for:

Magnifying the risk and magnifying my control over bad things that could occur.

Ignoring the evidence—there is loads of evidence that counting has no ability to prevent trouble.

Jumping to conclusions—thinking the worst thing will happen just because I don't do my counting.

All or nothing thinking—If I don't do the entire ritual, something terrible is sure to happen.

Alternative thoughts:

I have OCD, which makes me think I have to do the rituals.

The counting is just a habit that is related to the way my brain functions.

I need to train my brain to stop the counting—CBT and medication will help me do this.

Figure 7–2. Examining the evidence in brief sessions: Luke's example.

CBT=cognitive-behavior therapy; OCD=obsessive-compulsive disorder.

Generating Rational Alternatives

As illustrated in the interventions with Grace and Luke, the development of rational alternatives to a maladaptive automatic thought is a projected outcome of the examining-the-evidence method. If the patient cannot generate alternatives, it may be because the thought is linked to closely held belief systems that will require a different means of change, such as a behavioral experiment. When patients have difficulties generating alternative thoughts, therapists should normalize these difficulties by noting that effort and practice are necessary for most people to learn how to evaluate and restructure their thinking.

Examining the evidence is only one of a variety of CBT methods that can be used in brief sessions to help patients generate rational alternatives. All of the other techniques listed in Table 7–9 (e.g., Socratic questioning, TCRs, coping cards, identifying cognitive errors, reattribution) can be used effectively. Also, when automatic thoughts appear to be firmly held rules that patients have for themselves, it can be useful to explore whether the patient would hold others to the same rule or standard of behavior. Recognizing the existence of a "double standard" can often help patients to generate a new response to the situation.

Another good method to generate rational alternatives is to ask the patient to put himself or herself in the place of another person. The clinician can ask questions such as these: "If your friend were thinking this way, what would you tell her?" "If you had an effective and supportive coach, what would this person say about your thinking?" Other techniques include decatastrophizing a situation by asking the patient to predict the best, worst, and most likely outcomes, and by generating coping strategies for "worst-case scenarios." The goals of all of these interventions are to improve the patient's cognitive flexibility and increase the likelihood that the patient will consider other possible meanings to ascribe to the situation.

> **Learning Exercise 7–3** Modifying Automatic Thoughts in a Brief Session
>
> 1. Use Socratic questioning to work on automatic thoughts with a patient you are seeing in a brief session.
>
> 2. Introduce a TCR as a method of changing automatic thoughts.
>
> 3. Examine the evidence for automatic thoughts in a brief session.
>
> 4. Generate at least one rational alternative to an automatic thought in a brief session.

> - *People don't get fired for making a single mistake.*
>
> - *I don't have to be perfect to keep the job.*
>
> - *I don't expect others to be perfect.*
>
> - *I can do it!*

Figure 7–3.   A coping strategy: thoughts Grace posted on her bathroom mirror.

Developing Coping Cards and Other Coping Strategies

Therapy sessions, particularly briefer sessions, often involve rapid exchanges of information in an emotionally charged setting. Patients may have difficulty remembering rational alternatives or other positive changes in their cognitions unless they are reinforced in sessions and/or in homework assignments. At the end of Video Illustration 2, Dr. Sudak works with Grace to solidify a coping strategy of posting a series of revised thoughts on her mirror to remind her to use these healthy modifications to cope with her fears about a new job. These thoughts are listed in Figure 7–3.

Index or business-sized cards can also be used to write down a coping strategy. The therapist and/or patient can write these coping cards during a session, or the patient can be assigned the task for homework. We recommend that clinicians keep a supply of blank cards in their offices to use to provide patients with bullet points of the essential elements learned in therapy. Therapists can enhance the effectiveness of the coping card strategy by making sure that the cards are brief, practical, and viewed frequently. Even the best coping card will not be very useful if it is kept buried at the bottom of a patient's purse. One of the productive strategies that we have used is to make a series of coping cards that are placed on a key ring that is readily accessible.

In a session not shown in the video illustrations, Dr. Sudak worked with Grace to produce the coping card shown in Figure 7–4. Grace agreed to keep the card in her daily appointment book.

> **Learning Exercise 7–4**   Developing Coping Cards
>
> 1. Generate a coping card for one of your current patients.
>
> 2. In creating this card, focus primarily on reinforcing the patient's use of rational alternatives to automatic thoughts.

> **Situation: In the kitchen at night, thinking about making mistakes at work and the possibility of losing the job.**
>
> 1. *Take out a piece of paper and write down the evidence for and against poor work performance.*
>
> 2. *Watch for unrealistic standards. Remind myself it is normal to leave some things undone at the end of the day.*
>
> 3. *Don't sit there! Review the list of rational alternatives, do a thought record, or plan for tomorrow.*
>
> 4. *Then turn off the worries, do something effective to relax (tea, book).*

Figure 7–4. A coping card developed in a brief session: Grace's example.

Identifying Cognitive Errors

Although Dr. Sudak does not demonstrate the method of identifying cognitive errors in the video illustrations with Grace, this technique can be a very efficient way of helping patients change automatic thoughts in brief sessions. This process has three stages. First, the clinician uses the mini-lesson technique to instruct the patient on the nature of cognitive errors. It can be helpful to provide the patient with a list of common cognitive errors, similar to that shown in Table 7–12. During this educational phase of the intervention, it is also useful to normalize the occurrence of cognitive errors. Patients who see thinking errors as universal can begin to view their own thoughts as less abnormal and unusual.

After the clinician educates the patient about cognitive errors, the second step is to spot cognitive errors in at least one of the patient's own automatic thoughts, preferably one that has recently been identified in the current session. The third step is to ask the patient to complete a homework assignment to identify cognitive errors in automatic thoughts. A good way to do this is to have the patient write down these cognitive errors in the fourth column of a five-column TCR (the column labeled "Rational response"). As patients identify which error is being made, automatic thoughts typically become more amenable to rational analysis.

Reattribution

Another valuable technique not shown in the video illustrations is reattribution. Because mood disorders and other psychiatric illnesses are

Table 7–12. Definitions of cognitive errors

Ignoring the evidence: When you ignore the evidence, you make a judgment (usually about your shortcomings or about something you think you cannot do) without looking at all the information. This cognitive error has also been called the *mental filter* because you filter, or screen out, valuable information about topics such as 1) positive experiences from the past, 2) your strengths, and 3) support that others can give.

Jumping to conclusions: If you are depressed or anxious, you might jump to conclusions. You might immediately think of the worst possible interpretations of situations. Once these negative images come into your mind, you might become certain that bad things will happen.

Overgeneralizing: Sometimes you might let a single problem mean so much to you that it colors your view of everything in your life. You can give a small difficulty or flaw so much significance that it seems to define the entire picture. This type of cognitive error is called overgeneralizing.

Magnifying or minimizing: One of the most common cognitive errors is magnifying or minimizing the significance of things in your life. When you are depressed or anxious, you might magnify your faults and minimize your strengths. You also might magnify the risks of difficulties in situations and minimize the options or resources that you have to manage the problem.

An extreme form of magnifying is sometimes called *catastrophizing*. When you catastrophize, you automatically think that the worst possible thing will happen. If you are having a panic attack, your mind races with thoughts such as these: "I'm going to have a heart attack or stroke" or "I'm going to totally lose control." Depressed persons may think they are bound to fail or that they are about to lose everything.

Personalizing: Personalizing is a classic feature of anxiety and depression in which you get caught up in taking personal blame for everything that seems to go wrong. When you personalize, you accept full responsibility for a troubling situation or problem even when there is no good evidence to back your conclusion. This type of cognitive error undermines your self-esteem and makes you more depressed.

Of course, you need to accept responsibility when you have made mistakes. Owning up to problems can help you start to turn things around. However, if you can recognize the times that you are personalizing, you can avoid putting yourself down unnecessarily, and you can start to develop a healthier style of thinking.

Table 7–12. Definitions of cognitive errors *(continued)*

All-or-nothing thinking: One of the most damaging of the cognitive errors—all-or-nothing thinking—is demonstrated by the following types of thoughts: "Nothing ever goes my way." "There's no way I could handle it." "I always mess up." "She's got it all." "Everything is going wrong." When you let all-or-nothing thinking go unchecked, you see the world in absolute terms. Everything is all good or all bad. You believe that others are doing great and you are doing just the opposite.

All-or-nothing thinking also can interfere with your working on tasks. Imagine what would happen if you thought that you had to achieve 100% success or you should not even try at all. It is usually better to set reasonable goals and to realize that people are rarely complete successes or total failures. Most things in life fall somewhere in between.

Note. These definitions are available in Appendix 1, "Worksheets and Check-lists."

Source. Adapted from Wright JH, Wright AS, Beck AT: *Good Days Ahead: The Multimedia Program for Cognitive Therapy,* Professional Edition, Version 3.0. Louisville, KY, Mindstreet, 2010. Used with permission. Copyright © 2010 Mindstreet.

associated with misattributions, a reasonable target for some brief sessions is to help patients recognize and correct these damaging cognitions. We often use the pie-chart method to rapidly assist patients who are blaming themselves excessively for negative events (an internally skewed attribution). When a depressed person is first asked to divide a pie chart into sectors to assign blame for a negative event (e.g., divorce, job loss, financial reversal, difficulty with a child), he often can identify only two or three contributors and places an irrational amount of blame on himself. However, after Socratic questioning, a number of other possible influences can usually be identified, and the degree of blame or responsibility can be shifted to a more balanced perspective. This method can also be used with patients who make attributions in a maladaptive, external direction (i.e., placing too much blame on others and not accepting enough personal responsibility for actions). Patients with hypomania or substance abuse are prone to make these types of attributions.

The ruler technique can also be used to speed the reattribution process. For example, when attributions are distorted in an overgeneralized direction (giving negative events general or global significance instead of seeing them as localized or compartmentalized experiences), the clinician might draw a ruler with markings from 0 to 100 on a sheet of paper.

Then the patient can be asked to place marks on the ruler to indicate answers to questions such as these:

1. At this moment, how much does it seem that this event damages your life (defines who you are, affects how others view you, and so forth)?
2. What do you think is a healthy view of how much this event damages your life (defines who you are, affects how others view you, and so forth)? How would a person who isn't depressed view the event?
3. What is your goal for the meaning you want to give this event?

Cognitive Rehearsal—Sealing the Deal

Patients can learn new skills, such as reattribution and examining the evidence, in brief sessions with the coaching of the clinician. However, a necessary additional step is to help them use these skills in real-world situations. Patients must be able to apply what they learn in therapy outside of sessions and in the presence of strong emotion. Without this transfer of skills, the work of modifying automatic thoughts is unfinished.

Implementing new learning can be quite difficult when emotions are highly active. Clinicians must help patients understand the challenge of implementing skills in highly charged situations. Other adult learning situations, such as learning a new sport, can be helpful examples of the time required to modify old behaviors or learn new skills. We have already discussed several core CBT methods, such as homework assignments and coping cards, that can help patients transfer lessons from therapy to their daily lives. Cognitive rehearsal is another method that can be especially effective in solidifying the gains from brief sessions.

Many clinicians are familiar with how useful it is to imagine an important or difficult situation and to rehearse methods of improving their efforts or of preparing for adverse circumstances. This same process can be extremely helpful in preparing patients to use techniques to contend with negative automatic thoughts outside of therapy. Patients can be asked to imagine situations that will evoke automatic thoughts and negative emotions. They can then be instructed to imagine using the techniques they have learned in therapy to deal with these thoughts, and ultimately to change their behavior. This is a good exercise to give patients for homework between sessions.

An example not shown in the video illustrations comes from a brief session that Dr. Sudak had later with Grace. They recognized that a situation that could cause Grace considerable difficulty was when her boss would comment about a task that was left undone or perhaps was not performed to his expectations. They rehearsed 1) identifying the automatic thoughts that Grace might have in such a situation (e.g., "I really messed up"; "I'm not good enough for this job"; "I will lose the job and end up on the street"); 2) countering the automatic thoughts with a more rational perspective (e.g., "Don't overreact—he is just bringing a problem to my attention"; "My overall work performance has been fine"; "He has been supportive and has thanked me for doing a good job"; "Stay focused on listening to the problem and working on a solution"); and 3) using the rational alternatives to cope effectively with the situation.

Working With Accurate Thoughts

Obviously, not every automatic thought that a patient has will be maladaptive. Patients may face situations that present real dilemmas and generate strong emotions. Unsolved problems may exist because of depression or anxiety. Losses are endemic to life experience. Frequently, however, patients have belief systems that make them uniquely vulnerable to loss and disappointment. Significant events that occur in the lives of many people may have idiosyncratic meanings that can increase their predisposition to affective or anxious complaints. For example, patients who believe that true happiness is only possible in the context of a committed relationship will be uniquely vulnerable to interpersonal rejection. Therefore, when a thought is true or partly true, clinicians need to evaluate if the patient needs help to solve problems or if the situation has a particular meaning to the patient that leads to symptoms.

Patients may also have thoughts that are accurate but not useful and that increase their dysphoria under adverse circumstances. A resident who is on call and required to stay up all night, for example, may feel angry about the situation and consider it unfair to be kept awake (despite all educational rationales presented). If this thought recurs during the 2 hours when the resident can rest, and the subsequent emotion keeps the individual awake, the thought is not useful. Often, armed with the knowledge that thoughts can be true and not useful, patients can more easily defuse and put aside accurate thoughts that work to produce more symptoms and dysfunction.

Promoting Adaptive Core Beliefs

As noted earlier in this chapter and in Chapter 2, "Indications and Formats for Brief CBT Sessions," patients who require intensive efforts to identify and modify schemas may be best treated with standard CBT in 45- to 50-

---

Table 7–13. Tips for promoting adaptive core beliefs in brief sessions

---

Pick up on spontaneously verbalized core beliefs.

Look for schemas in themes or patterns of automatic thoughts.

Question the validity of beliefs with obvious damaging effects (e.g., "I'm a failure"; "I'm unlovable"; "I'm stupid").

Identify and reinforce positive schemas (e.g., "I'm a good friend"; "If I try hard, I can usually figure out a solution"; "I'm a survivor") that may help patients cope with their problems.

Use treatment adjuncts (e.g., readings, computer-assisted therapy) to supplement in-session efforts.

Suggest practical tools for putting adaptive core beliefs to work (e.g., coping cards).

Emphasize the positive effects of adaptive core beliefs on behavior (e.g., building and maintaining relationships, problem solving, sticking with tasks).

---

minute sessions, or at least in several longer meetings mixed with brief sessions. However, clinicians who are seeing patients for brief sessions do not need to ignore the importance of schemas or pass up opportunities to encourage patients to use and more fully develop adaptive core beliefs. In many respects, the CBT methods for working with core beliefs parallel those already described for modifying automatic thoughts (e.g., Socratic questioning, examining the evidence, generating rational alternatives). Readers who are unfamiliar with CBT methods for schemas or who wish to brush up on their knowledge and skills can consult Wright et al. (2006) or other texts noted in the Recommended Reading List (see Appendix 3, "CBT Educational Resources for Clinicians"). In this section, we provide a few suggestions on adapting CBT methods for working with core beliefs in brief sessions and discuss a video illustration of this type of work. Some ideas for using CBT methods for core beliefs are given in Table 7–13.

In standard CBT, longer sessions can be used to systematically identify a series of maladaptive and adaptive schemas. In brief sessions, however, schema-level interventions may be most useful if they are focused on working with the most potent core beliefs that are revealed during the course of Socratic questioning or are observed in patterns of automatic thoughts. For example, if a patient reports, "No matter what I do, I'm bound to fail," the clinician might pause to note that holding this type of belief can deal a serious blow to self-confidence and also interfere with expending productive effort on tasks. The clinician and patient could then use CBT methods described in this chapter (e.g., identifying cognitive errors, examining the evidence, generating rational alternatives) to attack this negative core belief and could arrange a homework assignment to practice a revision in the schema.

We recommend that clinicians who are seeing patients in brief sessions be always on the lookout for adaptive schemas that can be used to fight symptoms and cope with problems. Clinicians have a natural tendency to place most weight on the negative or maladaptive features of patients' thinking, resulting in the risk that positive beliefs can be missed or be given insufficient attention. One strategy that might be used is to give patients a brief checklist of adaptive beliefs (Figure 7–5) to stimulate their thinking about this domain of cognitions.

Because time is limited in brief sessions, treatment adjuncts (e.g., readings about core beliefs, computer-assisted therapy) can be considered when work on schemas seems important. Also, use of practical tools such as coping cards and written homework assignments can be especially important to reinforce concepts and help patients put needed changes into effect. We also recommend that clinicians make a special effort to underscore the positive effects of adaptive schemas on behavior. When patients realize that they have failed to appreciate adaptive beliefs that help them behave in a more productive or effective manner, they can have significant breakthroughs in accepting and utilizing their strengths.

Video Illustration 6 shows a follow-up to the work done by Dr. Sudak and Grace on automatic thoughts in Video Illustration 2. Even though the segment of the session in Video Illustration 6 is quite brief (about 7½ minutes), it demonstrates a highly collaborative effort to help Grace cope with the death of her husband; reduce self-condemning automatic thoughts; and pay adequate attention to a core belief that she is a strong person who was able to keep working, care for a husband with terminal cancer, take care of household chores and family finances, and keep her family intact in the face of a massive stress. Although Dr. Sudak did not undertake a formal and detailed effort to uncover and test schemas, the video demonstrates how she blended an empathic approach to Grace's emotional pain with effective CBT methods for identifying, shoring up, and utilizing an adaptive core belief. We think that this type of therapeutic intervention can be helpful in CBT sessions of any length.

▶ **Video Illustration 6.** Modifying Automatic Thoughts II: Dr. Sudak and Grace

Developing a Library of Handouts

In this chapter, we have discussed a large array of methods that can be used in brief sessions to target maladaptive thinking. To enhance the un-

____ I'm a solid person.

____ If I work hard at something, I can master it.

____ I'm a survivor.

____ Others trust me.

____ I care about other people.

____ People respect me.

____ If I prepare in advance, I usually do better.

____ I deserve to be respected.

____ I like to be challenged.

____ I'm intelligent.

____ I can figure things out.

____ I'm friendly.

____ I can handle stress.

____ I can learn from my mistakes and be a better person.

____ I'm a good spouse (and/or parent, child, friend, lover).

Figure 7–5. Brief checklist of adaptive core beliefs.

Note. This checklist is also available in Appendix 1, "Worksheets and Checklists."
Source. Adapted from Wright JH, Wright AS, Beck AT: *Good Days Ahead: The Multimedia Program for Cognitive Therapy*, Professional Edition, Version 3.0. Louisville, KY, Mindstreet, 2010. Used with permission. Copyright © 2010 Mindstreet.

derstanding and effective use of these methods, it may be helpful to organize a series of handouts to give patients. We have found that patients benefit greatly by having written materials to take away from the sessions to reinforce what they have learned. Handouts may be particularly important when the patient is anxious or depressed, because these conditions frequently alter information processing and retention. Several potentially useful handouts have been included as tables and figures in this chapter and can also be downloaded in larger format at the American Psychiatric Publishing Web site (www.appi.org/pdf/62362).

> **Learning Exercise 7–5**   Developing a Library of Handout Materials
>
> 1. Review the tables and figures in this chapter. Make copies of these tables and figures for handouts or download these items from the American Psychiatric Publishing Web site (www.appi.org/pdf/62362).
>
> 2. Supplement these materials with any other handouts that you believe will be helpful for using CBT to target maladaptive thinking.
>
> 3. As you read other chapters in this book, add handouts for other CBT methods and applications.

Summary

Key Points for Clinicians

- Clinicians who wish to use CBT methods in brief sessions to modify cognitions need to have a good basic understanding of cognitive pathology in major mental disorders, efficient methods of identifying automatic thoughts, and CBT techniques for changing automatic thoughts and core beliefs.
- Adaptations of CBT methods for changing maladaptive thoughts in brief sessions emphasize succinct and clear psychoeducation, use of mini-formulations to direct interventions at the most important targets, selection and artful use of techniques that can be delivered in relatively short sequences, and use of homework to extend and reinforce learning.
- Some of the commonly used methods for changing automatic thoughts in brief sessions are Socratic questioning, thought change records, examining the evidence, generating rational alternatives, coping cards, identifying cognitive errors, reattribution, and cognitive rehearsal.
- Although extensive efforts to change schemas may be beyond the scope of most formats for brief sessions, productive work can be conducted on promoting use of adaptive core beliefs.
- It is advantageous to prepare a file of CBT readings and worksheets to use as handouts for targeting maladaptive cognitions in brief sessions.

Concepts and Skills for Patients to Learn

- The immediate thoughts (automatic thoughts) that people have in situations may be distorted or inaccurate and may lead to painful emotions.
- It is possible in relatively brief treatment sessions to learn CBT methods for identifying these dysfunctional automatic thoughts, changing them, and thus relieving symptoms.
- Writing automatic thoughts on paper or on a computer and then checking them for accuracy can be a very useful way of fighting depression and anxiety.
- To get the most benefit from brief sessions on changing maladaptive thinking, it helps to do "homework" to identify and modify automatic thoughts between visits to your doctor or therapist.
- Everybody has positive core beliefs, but these beliefs can be forgotten when people become very depressed or anxious. It is often helpful to try to spot your positive core beliefs and to use them effectively to cope with problems.

References

Beck AT: Thinking and depression. Arch Gen Psychiatry 9:324–333, 1963

Beck AT: Thinking and depression, II: theory and therapy. Arch Gen Psychiatry 10:561–571, 1964

Beck AT: Depression: Clinical, Experimental, and Theoretical Aspects. New York, Harper & Row, 1967

Beck J: Cognitive Therapy: Basics and Beyond. New York, Guilford, 1995

Burns DD: Feeling Good. New York, Morrow, 1999

Clark DA, Beck AT, Alford BA: Scientific Foundations of Cognitive Theory and Therapy of Depression. New York, Wiley, 1999

Hollon SD, Kendall PC: Cognitive self-statements in depression: development of an automatic thoughts questionnaire. Cognit Ther Res 4:383–395, 1980

Mathews A, MacLeod C: An information-processing approach to anxiety. J Cogn Psychother 1:105–115, 1987

Sudak D: Cognitive Behavioral Therapy for Clinicians. Philadelphia, PA, Lippincott Williams & Wilkins, 2006

Wright JH, Basco MR: Getting Your Life Back: The Complete Guide to Recovery From Depression. New York, Touchstone, 2002

Wright JH, Wright AS, Albano AM, et al: Computer-assisted cognitive therapy for depression: maintaining efficacy while reducing therapist time. Am J Psychiatry 162:1158–1164, 2005

Wright JH, Basco MR, Thase ME: Learning Cognitive-Behavior Therapy: An Illustrated Guide. Washington, DC, American Psychiatric Publishing, 2006

Wright JH, Beck AT, Thase ME: Cognitive therapy, in The American Psychiatric Publishing Textbook of Psychiatry, 5th Edition. Edited by Hales RE, Yudofsky SC, Gabbard GO. Washington, DC, American Psychiatric Publishing, 2008, pp 1211–1256

Wright JH, Wright AS, Beck AT: Good Days Ahead: The Multimedia Program for Cognitive Therapy, Professional Edition, Version 3.0. Louisville, KY, Mindstreet, 2010

CHAPTER 8

Treating Hopelessness and Suicidality

LEARNING MAP

The damaging effects of hopelessness

⇩

Methods for building hope

⇩

Managing suicide risk in brief sessions

⇩

Developing antisuicide plans

Hopelessness, a core symptom of depression, as well as a frequent problem in many other psychiatric illnesses, can erode confidence and undermine patients' efforts to change. In its most malignant form, hopelessness can be a driving force behind suicide. Because psychiatrists and other prescribing clinicians often see patients who express hopeless and suicidal thoughts, effective tools are needed to address these problems. This chapter details cognitive-behavior therapy (CBT) methods that can be used to build hope and fight suicidal thinking in brief sessions.

The Damaging Effects of Hopelessness

From the time of some of the earliest writings on CBT, hopelessness has been considered a particularly destructive form of maladaptive thinking (Beck 1963; Beck et al. 1975). Persons who have low levels of hope may exert less effort in participating in activities of daily life and on solving tasks. They may withdraw socially and drop out of meaningful pursuits. They also may give up trying to use treatment options to fight depression or other psychiatric problems (Wright 2003). If persons act in helpless and defeated ways, their negative predictions (e.g., "My wife will leave me," "I will lose my job," "No one will want to spend any time with me") may be more likely to come true.

A large number of investigations have confirmed that hopelessness is a major predictor of suicide risk (Beck et al. 1975, 1985; Fawcett et al. 1987). In one study, Beck et al. (1975) found that scores on the Beck Hopelessness Scale were much more strongly associated with suicidal thinking than a rating of overall level of depressive symptoms. In a later investigation, Beck et al. (1985) observed that high Beck Hopelessness Scale scores by depressed patients at the time of discharge from the hospital were highly predictive of future risk for suicide.

Of the many risk factors for suicide, hopelessness presents an especially important target for CBT interventions. If a person has given up all hope, can see no reasons to live, and is suffering from deep despair, suicide may appear to be the best or only option. However, if the clinician can help the patient generate some genuine hope for the future and some positive reasons to keep going, the risk for suicide may be lessened. CBT has been shown to have a robust effect on building hope and in reducing suicidality (Brown et al. 2005; Rush et al. 1982). A highly influential study performed by Brown et al. (2005) found that patients who received a course of CBT after a suicide attempt had about 50% fewer subsequent suicide attempts than those who received standard treatment. Specific methods for coping with suicidality are detailed later in the chapter, but first we describe some general CBT strategies for treating hopelessness.

Methods for Building Hope

A number of CBT interventions can be used in brief sessions to help restore hope (see Table 8–1). The first item in the table, "use the thera-

---

Table 8–1. Cognitive-behavior therapy methods for building hope

---

Use the therapeutic relationship to instill hope.

Educate about reasons for an optimistic outcome.

Structure treatment.

Set realistic goals.

Suggest behavioral assignments that demonstrate ability to change.

Challenge hopeless cognitions.

Identify strengths and positive core beliefs.

Use cognitive methods to develop a more optimistic thinking style.

Use coping cards.

Source. Adapted from Wright JH, Turkington D, Kingdon DG, et al: *Cognitive-Behavior Therapy for Severe Mental Illness: An Illustrated Guide.* Washington, DC, American Psychiatric Publishing, 2009, p. 147. Used with permission. Copyright © 2009 American Psychiatric Publishing.

peutic relationship to instill hope," is a key element in all effective psychotherapies. Jerome Frank (1978) noted that "most persons who seek psychotherapy suffer from a single condition that assumes protean forms…demoralization, and the effectiveness of all forms of psychotherapy depends on ingredients that combat this state of mind" (p. 10). In CBT, the remoralization process begins with the therapeutic relationship. If patients have reached the point at which they cannot find solutions on their own, they need a lifeline from a clinician who is genuine and empathic, and who offers a sensible path toward recovery.

The collaborative-empirical relationship of CBT (described in Chapter 3, "Enhancing the Impact of Brief Sessions") can offer considerable hope to patients who are demoralized, discouraged, or beaten down. In Video Illustration 7, Dr. Thase demonstrates a sensitive and caring approach to a man who is facing the terminal illness of his mother. Darrell is a young man who has just heard that his mother has only 6–12 months to live. The clinician uses an empathic style, which resonates with Darrell's sadness and grief, but still adopts an empirical, problem-solving approach to help Darrell cope with the impending loss and the ramifications of this life-changing event. We think this video shows the special blend of well-dosed empathy and action-oriented interventions that are characteristic of the CBT approach. We recommend that while watching this video illustration, readers focus on the therapeutic relationship and try to spot specific CBT methods that are used to generate hope.

▶ **Video Illustration 7.** Generating Hope: Dr. Thase and Darrell

In the first part of the session (not shown in the video illustration), Dr. Thase collaborated with Darrell to set an agenda and perform a symptom check. Although Darrell noted that he had become more depressed since his last visit and wanted to work on how he was coping with some bad news about his mother, he did not have any significant suicidal ideation and made it clear that he had many reasons to keep living.

After they started to discuss Darrell's problems coping with his mother's illness, Dr. Thase noted that Darrell's "gloomy state of mind" might be causing him to look at other areas of his life more pessimistically.

> Darrell: It's all been a struggle, and it just seems that nothing is going to turn out at this point…It seems like my life is going to amount to nothing (pause). What woman is going to want to date a guy who lives with his mom?…You end up being a momma's boy…and they think you are going to have to take care of her and there will be nothing left for me.

Darrell then goes on to talk about getting passed over for promotion in his job and concludes that nothing is going to work out for him. Dr. Thase is aware of Darrell's emotional pain but points out that the negative state he is in seems to be coloring his perception of just how pessimistic or hopeless these things might be. After he asks Darrell about the possibility that there could be other ways of looking at these circumstances, Darrell agrees to try. Some of the methods used include psychoeducation about the influences of negative thinking in depression, keeping a structure and focus for treatment, challenging hopeless cognitions, using cognitive methods to develop a more optimistic thinking style, identifying strengths, and using coping cards.

A frequently used, high-yield method for modifying hopeless cognitions is to engage patients in a very direct attempt to generate reasons to have hope. As we explain later, a parallel technique of asking for reasons to live is one of the most powerful CBT interventions that can be used to counter suicidal thinking. In Video Illustration 7, Dr. Thase gets right to the point with the next question.

> Dr. Thase: What about reasons to hope?
> Darrell: That's hard to come by, Dr. Thase. It really is…It's going to be terrible when her end comes. I'll really have to struggle with it. It will be terrible for everybody…But it can't last forever. That's kind of the other side of it…It can't last forever.
> Dr. Thase: As bad as this could be, this will pass? This is limited to this time in your life right now?
> Darrell: Yeah…Yeah.

Darrell was able to generate an alternative way of seeing things that gave him somewhat more hope that his life would not always be burdened with so much sorrow and pain. Dr. Thase then built on this effort by asking some Socratic questions to uncover additional reasons to have a better outlook for the future.

> Dr. Thase: You mentioned that some women might think of you as a momma's boy for doing this. I'm wondering if you could also see a different description of a man who would move in to care for his dying mother.
> Darrell: You know, I think this is what you've got to do…when you've got a mom that's sick. Maybe some women would think,…"This is a good guy, and maybe this is a guy who would treat me as good as he treats his mom."
> Dr. Thase: This would be an incentive…A good thing?
> Darrell: Yeah…Yeah.
> Dr. Thase: Along the way, it sounded like you thought you might have to put your personal life completely on hold during the next 6–12 months. Was that your sense—that things you were looking forward to trying to do, you just couldn't do at all?
> Darrell: How does it look when your mom is sick and you are going out dating people and having fun…It's just terrible.
> Dr. Thase: There is this tendency for people who are depressed to see things in—like all or none…And I wonder if what you are feeling now might be pulling you into that trap…Either you would have no dating life whatsoever, or if you did you might be irresponsible and cavalier, and running around carefree when your terminally ill mother is at home. I think there is quite a bit of room between those two. Do you see any?
> Darrell: It's hard to see…but I guess some people could do both.

Dr. Thase then explains that Darrell's mother probably will have better days and worse days and that on some better days she may need less of him.

> Dr. Thase: And I'll ask you this: What would your mom want of you?
> Darrell: She wouldn't want me to just sit around and be unhappy.

Darrell then agrees that it is reasonable to strike a balance between his caring for his mother and still having a life outside this situation. He and Dr. Thase explore other positive aspects or "silver linings" of the situation and discover that Darrell can use this opportunity to reduce expenses and straighten out his finances. As a capstone to this intervention, Dr. Thase introduces a coping card directed at building hope.

> Dr. Thase: While you were talking, I began to construct a way of coping with pessimism…It's called a coping card. And I wrote down the four reasons for hope that you just came up with [see Figure 8–1].

Reasons to Have Hope for the Future

- *No matter how bad it is, this circumstance is time limited, and it will pass.*
- *I won't be seen by others as a "Momma's boy." I'm being a conscientious man...some women would find this attractive.*
- *I can still date...this problem doesn't have to completely close down that portion of my life.*
- *Giving up my apartment will allow me to straighten up my financial situation and get out of debt.*

Figure 8–1.   A coping card to build hope: Darrell's example.

The final portion of this video illustration shows Dr. Thase 1) explaining that the coping card will work best if it is kept handy so that it can be used to interrupt negative monologues and 2) noting that Darrell's mood seems improved since they have worked on identifying reasons for hope. The entire video illustration takes about 10 minutes—an amount of time that seems reasonable to expend to build hope in a brief session.

The video does not directly illustrate goal setting or using behavioral assignments to demonstrate ability to change (items listed in Table 8–1). However, Dr. Thase and Darrell did have clear overall goals for their work together, and behavioral methods were used consistently throughout the treatment (as shown in Video Illustration 5, which was discussed in Chapter 6, "Behavioral Methods for Depression"). Keeping reachable and specific goals in mind (and making progress toward these goals) can be an effective antidote to hopelessness. Also, if behavioral methods start to yield gains (e.g., activity scheduling to enhance interest and energy, graded assignments to help accomplish tasks, hierarchical exposure to reduce anxiety and avoidance), the patient's confidence in the positive benefits of therapy and hope for recovery are likely to improve.

We think that all of the methods listed in Table 8–1 can be appropriately implemented in brief sessions to build hope. Clinicians can work to develop highly attentive and collaborative relationships that can have a positive impact on patients in a limited amount of time. Mini-lessons or other succinct educational techniques can help patients see that change is possible. A structured approach can be used to set goals and agendas that get results and that reduce the sense of being overwhelmed or unable to cope. Targeted and well-focused CBT methods—such as Socratic questions, thought change records, and examining the evidence—can be employed in brief visits to modify hopeless cognitions. Behavioral assignments and coping cards can assist patients with making changes that defuse hopelessness.

We have found that these methods often work well in brief sessions. However, if the patient remains hopeless and appears to need a more intensive approach, longer or more frequent sessions can be scheduled, or the dual-therapist format can be used to bring more resources into play. Also, changes in the pharmacotherapy regimen can be considered. Readers who want to learn more about CBT methods for hopelessness and to view additional video illustrations on this topic are referred to Chapter 7, "Depression," in *Cognitive-Behavior Therapy for Severe Mental Illness: An Illustrated Guide* (Wright et al. 2009).

> **Learning Exercise 8–1**   Building Hope
>
> 1. Identify at least one patient you are seeing in brief sessions who could potentially benefit from CBT methods to build hope.
>
> 2. Review the therapeutic relationship. Is there anything you can do to enhance the hope-stimulating aspects of the relationship? Are you being appropriately hopeful? Are you getting discouraged about the treatment, and is this possibly affecting the patient's attitude?
>
> 3. Review the goals and structure of the treatment. Is there an opportunity to give the sessions more focus and structure? Could these efforts have a positive effect on the patient's hopefulness?
>
> 4. Try to identify at least one cognition and one behavior that are contributing to hopelessness. Use CBT methods in an attempt to reverse these problems.
>
> 5. Reinforce several of the patient's strengths and core beliefs.
>
> 6. Write out a coping card that is designed to stimulate hope.

Managing Suicide Risk in Brief Sessions

The 2002 National Survey of Psychiatric Practice found that the average time psychiatrists spent with patients dropped to 34 minutes in 2002, compared with 55 minutes in 1988–1989 (Scully and Wilk 2003). Although more recent data were not available at the time this book was

---

Table 8–2.   Questions to ask when suicidal thoughts are expressed in brief sessions

---

What kinds of suicidal thoughts does the patient have?

What are the patient's risk factors for suicide?

What positive reasons does the patient have to keep living?

What personal strengths does the patient have to fight suicidal thoughts?

What supports does the patient have?

What are the patient's capacities to modify hopeless and self-destructive cognitions?

What are the patient's capacities to engage in positive behaviors that can counter suicidal thoughts?

How solidly can the patient commit to and adhere to an antisuicide plan?

---

written, we expect that the trend for reduced time in sessions has continued. Thus, psychiatrists and other prescribing professionals are likely to see in brief sessions many patients who have been suicidal, are currently having suicidal thoughts, or will have such thoughts in the future.

General methods for assessing and managing suicide risk have been detailed in a number of excellent publications (see, e.g., Jacobs and Brewer 2004; Simon 2004; Simon and Hales 2006) and are not repeated here. A full evaluation of suicide risk and implementation of reasonable precautions and interventions are expected for responsible clinical management. We think that when evaluating suicidality and applying CBT methods in brief sessions, clinicians need to ask several key questions, which are discussed in the following subsections and listed in Table 8–2.

What Kinds of Suicidal Thoughts Does the Patient Have? What Are the Patient's Risk Factors for Suicide?

The first two questions in Table 8–2 are standard parts of the assessment of suicide risk. Clinicians need to determine the intensity, frequency, and mutability of suicidal thoughts and plans. Also, clinicians must consider risk factors for suicide (e.g., hopelessness, age, gender, ethnicity, history of previous attempts, lethality of suicidal plans if present, substance abuse, psychosis, family history of suicide).

What Positive Reasons Does the Patient Have to Keep Living?

Asking a patient, "What positive reasons do you have to keep living?" is pivotal for both the assessment and cognitive-behavioral treatment of suicidality (Ellis and Newman 1996; Linehan et al. 1983; Malone et al. 2000). If the patient reports several highly meaningful reasons to live, and in doing so has a lift in mood and a decline in the intensity of suicidal thoughts, the clinician can usually rest easier that actions can be taken to build an effective antisuicide plan. On the other hand, if the patient can identify no reasons or very weak reasons to live, much greater concern is warranted. The most ominous response to this type of question occurs when the patient not only reports no reasons to live but also seems convinced that others would be better off if she were dead.

Questions about reasons to live can help clinicians evaluate suicide risk, as well as provide an opportunity to break through intense hopelessness and begin to turn the patient's thinking in a more positive direction. Sometimes patients will easily verbalize solid reasons to live with little prompting. Other times they may need assistance from the clinician to uncover and detail reasons to live. We give two examples here.

> Dan was a 54-year-old man with a history of bipolar disorder who was currently depressed. Dan had recently had some problems at his work as a trucking supervisor. His boss had criticized his handling of a personnel matter and had asked if Dan needed any help in handling a recent promotion to be the chief supervisor of all the drivers in their fleet.

In a session with Dr. Sudak, Dan reported that he was very fearful that he might lose his job, and he wasn't sure he could live with the humiliation of being fired. After asking about standard elements of suicide risk, Dr. Sudak engaged Dan in a series of questions.

> Dr. Sudak: Dan, you've been telling me about your reasons for being fearful and discouraged, but what if we looked at a more positive side of your thinking? What reasons do you have for surviving a job loss if it were actually to happen? What reasons would you have to keep living no matter what happened to you?
>
> Dan: My family—my wife and my kids, and my mother. I could never do anything to hurt them. I would have to suck it up somehow and keep going.
>
> Dr. Sudak: What is it about your family that would make you want to fight off any thoughts of suicide?
>
> Dan: I love them, and they love me. They are the most important thing in my life. And I want to have grandchildren someday.
>
> Dr. Sudak: I can see that your family really means a lot to you. How about any other positive reasons to keep living?
>
> Dan: (pause) My brothers—we're close buddies. We get a big kick out of spending time together at our cabin.
>
> Dr. Sudak: I'm making a list of some of these positive reasons to live. (She writes out list.) Anything else to add to the list?

- *My family—I don't want to hurt them.*

- *Hopes of having grandchildren someday.*

- *My brothers—all the good times we have together.*

- *My volunteer work with "Habitat for Humanity."*

Figure 8–2.   Dan's list of positive reasons to live.

Dan: Yes, the work I do with Habitat for Humanity means a lot to me. This is something I could do for a long time, even after I retire. (Dan volunteers in this effort to build housing for those who can't afford it.)

Dr. Sudak: You are thinking of lots of strong reasons to keep living. If I gave you this list, do you think you could add some more things later?

Dan: I probably could do that.

Dr. Sudak: When you balance all these reasons to live with your negative thoughts about work and the ideas about suicide that came into your mind, what happens?

Dan: I could never harm myself. There is too much to lose…too much hurt to cause others.

Because Dan did not have a deep and fixed sense of hopelessness, had no history of previous suicide attempts, did not have any suicidal plans, and had many reasons to live, Dr. Sudak was reasonably confident that she could help him develop an effective antisuicide plan as noted later in this chapter. Figure 8–2 displays Dan's list of reasons to live.

Another case presented somewhat more difficult terrain for the therapist.

Allie was a 38-year-old woman with schizophrenia who reported hearing voices telling her to swallow poison. Allie had once had a very promising future. She had been doing well as a sophomore at a college where she had received a full scholarship to study music. However, a psychotic episode at the end of that school year had initiated a downward slide. Now she was unemployed, living on disability, and staying with her parents and a brother who has a developmental, neurological disorder. Despite aggressive treatment with antipsychotic medications, Allie continued to have auditory hallucinations. There was a history of two previous suicide attempts by overdose and a total of five psychiatric admissions.

As part of the assessment and management of suicide risk, Dr. Wright asked Allie two important questions.

Dr. Wright: Allie, you have been telling me that the voices have gotten stronger and they are telling you to hurt yourself. What has kept you from doing anything to harm yourself? Are there some reasons that you want to keep living and fight off the message from the voices?

Allie: I don't know…My whole life has been going downhill…I can't even work at fast food places anymore…and I don't see any of my old friends. I can't face seeing any of those people…They all have husbands and kids…I don't have anything.

Because Allie still appeared hopeless and had not responded with any positive reasons to live, Dr. Wright tried again to draw out a more hopeful set of cognitions.

Dr. Wright: (in an empathic tone) I know it has been very hard for you. This illness has taken its toll. But you have still kept going…You came to the appointment today. So, I suspect there is something about your life—something positive—that makes you want to live and to not give in to the voices. Just take your time and think about that question. Let's try to start a list of your reasons to live.

Allie: (pause) I guess my brother needs me. I take him to his doctor appointments and help him get around…He doesn't have any real friends except me.

Dr. Wright: That's a good point…I know that you are very close with your brother and that you help him a lot. Can you think of any other positive reasons to keep living?

Allie: Just that I have been struggling for so long and haven't given up yet. I really don't want to kill myself. I just get overwhelmed sometimes, and it's hard to keep going.

Dr. Wright: You have been trying very hard, and I think you have been making real progress. I was thinking of a recent example of a positive move that you've made. Didn't you say something about getting involved with a benefit art show that the mental health association is having?

Allie: Yeah. I'm playing guitar in the little band that is giving a concert at the show…It's sort of neat to play the guitar again. (Her mood begins to lift somewhat, and she smiles.)

Dr. Wright: I can tell that playing the guitar and helping out at the show means a lot to you.

Allie: Yes, it feels good to actually do something constructive.

Even though Allie identified some reasons to live with Dr. Wright's assistance, she still did not appear to have identified a strong counterbalancing argument to the message of the voices. Therefore, Dr. Wright asked more questions to help build the case for living.

Dr. Wright: OK, I have written these things down on the list of reasons to keep living. Now that we have gotten started, can you think of some other reasons?

Allie: (pause) Maybe I could have a relationship someday. I've just dated a couple of guys, and nothing ever went anywhere. But I've seen other people with my kind of problems find someone…And I would like to do more with my music.

Dr. Wright: I'm really glad to hear you talking about hopes for the future. We can put them on the list and also spend time working on your plans in our sessions…Before we finish working on the list for now, I wonder if there are any relationships of any sort in your life right now that give you some reason for wanting to keep living.

Allie: I don't do much with Mom and Dad anymore. But they are still important to me. I know that if I died, they would take it real hard. They already feel guilty because I have this illness.

Deciding what to do about Allie's suicide risk was more of a challenge than developing a plan to manage Dan's lower-grade suicidal thoughts. Although she denied having a suicidal plan, Allie had overdosed twice before. Also, she was hearing voices telling her to poison herself and had encountered many disappointments that could be fuel for despair. Additionally, she needed a fair amount of assistance in generating a list of reasons to live (see Figure 8–3). On the positive side, she had developed a meaningful list, had a good therapeutic relationship with Dr. Wright, and appeared willing to continue to work on developing ways of coping with suicidal thoughts. Could she be managed as an outpatient with brief sessions, or was a more intensive treatment plan required? Answers to some of the additional questions in Table 8–2 helped to solve this dilemma.

What Personal Strengths Does the Patient Have to Fight Suicidal Thoughts? What Supports Does the Patient Have?

In Chapter 4, "Case Formulation and Treatment Planning," we discussed the importance of identifying and capitalizing on a patient's positive assets. When suicidal thoughts are present, clinicians can try to help patients penetrate through the dark veil of hopelessness to recognize and tap their personal strengths and supports. Some examples might include religious or other spiritual beliefs, activities or interests that are highly meaningful, supportive relationships with family or friends, habits of participating in physical exercise and/or sport, commitments to people or causes, and a sense of humor. If patients have such strengths and can mobilize plans to use them to manage suicidal thoughts and counter despair, the likelihood of a good outcome may be increased.

Dan had a very good basic track record at work, and it appeared that his chance of being fired was actually quite low. He also was a deeply spiritual man who reported that committing suicide would be "against my religion." He had already noted that volunteer work in the community was very im-

- *My brother—he needs me, and I am his only friend.*

- *I have been trying hard to fight my problems—I really don't want to die.*

- *I enjoy music and getting back into playing the guitar.*

- *I have hope that I could have a relationship some day.*

- *It would hurt my parents if I died.*

Figure 8–3. Allie's list of positive reasons to live.

portant to him. He also told Dr. Sudak that he could commit to calling his wife or one of his brothers if suicidal thoughts ever intensified to the point where he gave them any serious consideration. If such resources and supports could not have been identified, Dr. Sudak would have needed to exert a greater degree of vigilance for possible suicidal behavior.

Allie did not have as much family support. Her father was ill with advanced cardiac disease, and both parents were often stressed, irritable, and depressed themselves. Also, she had a more difficult time recognizing her strengths. Nevertheless, there were significant assets that could be used to combat suicidality. Although her parents had disengaged somewhat from Allie over the years and were often preoccupied with their own problems, Dr. Wright had learned from a family session held several months earlier that they remained interested in helping Allie whenever possible and still cared deeply about her. Also, Allie identified concern for her parents as one reason to keep living.

Dr. Wright had a longer-range goal of trying to help Allie improve her communication with her parents. At this point, however, the more accessible social supports that could be used to build an immediate safety plan appeared to be at Bridgespring, a day program that Allie typically attended three times a week. Bridgespring had a full-time social worker who was quite concerned about Allie and could serve as an on-site resource for helping her cope with suicidal thoughts and to carry out other elements of an antisuicide plan. Also, Allie had friends at Bridgespring whom she could ask for support.

In the search for other strengths that could be used to manage suicidality, Allie's musical interests stood out as a definite asset. She had some talent in this area, clearly enjoyed participating in these activities, and was getting positive feedback for getting involved in a benefit concert. She also enjoyed working in a garden at her parents' home and reading magazines and novels. Dr. Wright was able to draw on these strengths as he helped Allie build an antisuicide plan (see Figure 8–5, later in this chapter).

What Are the Patient's Capacities to Modify Hopeless and Self-Destructive Cognitions?

The malleability of negative cognitions is an important factor in gauging the effectiveness of CBT interventions to reduce the risk of suicide. Do Socratic questions help the patient see healthier perspectives? Do the interventions described earlier in this chapter (see Table 8–1) help reduce the level of hopelessness? If psychotic features are present, as in Allie's case, is the patient able to develop an understanding of the symptoms that allows for effective reality testing? Is the patient able to use CBT methods to develop coping strategies for delusions or hallucinations (see Chapter 11, "Modifying Delusions," and Chapter 12, "Coping With Hallucinations")?

Fortunately, both Dan and Allie were able to use CBT methods in the brief session format to moderate cognitions that could be associated with self-destructive behaviors. Dan readily generated a list of reasons to live and was able to recognize that he was probably magnifying the risk of getting fired. He also was able to collaborate with Dr. Sudak on developing a coping strategy for the "worst-case scenario" if he actually did lose his job. Allie was able to recognize and give more value to some of the assets of her current life (e.g., activities and supports at Bridgespring, potential to improve communication with parents, relationships with friends) instead of continuing to dwell heavily on the losses that were associated with her illness. Also, she was able to work with Dr. Wright to reinforce a healthy explanation for her command hallucinations (i.e., "I have a chemical imbalance that isn't my fault…Stress can make the voices worse…I can learn to cope with the voices and not allow them to have power over me").

Another case from Dr. Wright's practice showed much less of a shift in potentially dangerous cognitions. Carl was being seen for his second visit in the brief session format. He was a 67-year-old man with a history of recurrent depression who had just retired and moved with his wife to a new town to be closer to his only child and three grandchildren. Carl had requested to see Dr. Wright for long-term medication management because he had needed to transfer care from his previous psychiatrist after the move. Dr. Wright had seen Carl for an initial evaluation about 4 weeks previously. At the time of the initial evaluation, Carl had reported a history of at least five previous episodes of major depression, one hospitalization after a suicide attempt at about age 45, and over 30 years of treatment with antidepressant medication.

Carl had appeared to be in remission at the time of the initial evaluation and denied any suicidal ideation, so Dr. Wright decided to continue the previous pharmacotherapy regimen and to schedule brief visits for pharmacotherapy and CBT. The initial goals of the CBT were to help Carl adjust to his move and to work on relapse prevention. However, by the time of the first follow-up session 4 weeks later, the situation had clearly deteriorated. Carl appeared severely depressed and noted that suicidal thoughts had returned after having been absent for many years.

A relapse of depression with a rapid surge in hopelessness appeared to have been triggered by his retirement and move to a new city. The following are examples of some of Carl's extremely negative cognitions: "This was the biggest mistake of my life…I should have never moved… I don't have anything to do here…All I can see is boredom and grinding out my days until there's nothing left…I just want to end it now and not prolong the agony." Carl was having rather intense suicidal thoughts and had a plan to shoot himself.

Dr. Wright attempted to help Carl modify these cognitions in the brief visit and prolonged the session as much as possible to try to reduce Carl's despair. However, only modest gains were possible. Even though Carl apparently had strong support from his wife, son, and son's family, he continued to think that he was a "waste and that they would be better off if I exited the stage now and saved them all the trouble." Also, attempts to have him look at possibilities of adapting to life in the new environment were not very successful (e.g., "I suppose I could start going to some classes or try to meet some people, but I really don't think anything like that will work"). Because the suicide risk was quite high and efforts to change his hopeless cognitions were not having much impact, a decision was made to hospitalize Carl. After a productive hospital stay, a detailed antisuicide plan was developed, and an outpatient plan was implemented for a more intensive dual-therapist program with Dr. Wright and a nonmedical cognitive-behavior therapist.

What Are the Patient's Capacities to Engage in Positive Behaviors That Can Counter Suicidal Thoughts?

If patients can take actions that show them that positive changes are possible, they may become more optimistic about their future. The behavioral changes do not have to be earthshaking or profound to make a difference. For example, Allie agreed to spend more time with two of her friends playing music in a small group at Bridgespring and to participate more heavily in several other activities at this facility. Although this was a simple behavioral change, it did reduce her preoccupation with the command hallucinations (see Chapter 12, "Coping With Hallucinations," for more details on behavioral methods for hallucinations) and relieved some of her distress. Dan reported that spending more time exercising would probably help him feel more hopeful. He also noted that no Habitat for Humanity projects were on the near horizon, but there were several opportunities for volunteer work through his church.

Other examples of simple behavioral plans that could play a role in an overall strategy for reducing suicidality include devoting a specified amount of time to pleasurable activities (e.g., cooking a new recipe, getting a therapeutic massage, scheduling time for talking on the phone with an old friend); listening to a relaxation tape; using behavioral methods for insomnia; and asking a sibling to visit. Although these efforts are unlikely to be full antidotes for hopelessness and suicidality, they can add to other initiatives in building a comprehensive strategy for reducing suicide risk.

How Solidly Can the Patient Commit to and Adhere to an Antisuicide Plan?

If the clinician and patient have a strong, highly collaborative relationship, and if the patient can make a firm commitment to carrying out a CBT-generated antisuicide plan, there can be a reasonable expectation that the plan will be helpful. However, these measures only have the potential to reduce risk, not to eliminate it. Clinicians need to be wary of being overly secure about the patient's safety simply because CBT methods have been used to stimulate hope and to cope with suicidal thoughts. In a study of the effectiveness of CBT in preventing repeat suicide attempts, Brown et al. (2005) reported that the subsequent rate of suicide attempts over an 18-month period was reduced to 24% in the CBT group, compared with 43% in patients who received treatment as usual. In situations where patients appear unable to carry out an effective antisuicide plan or express significant ambivalence about the plan, an even greater level of concern is warranted. In the next section of the chapter, we outline common ingredients of antisuicide plans and give examples of how they are used in clinical practice.

Developing Antisuicide Plans

Some of the basic elements of effective antisuicide plans are listed in Table 8–3. The importance of identifying reasons to live and finding adaptive cognitions and behaviors to combat despair have been detailed previously. Specific safety precautions are also important components of many antisuicide plans. Although Dan appeared not to have a high risk of suicide, he was a hunter and had guns in the house. As part of his antisuicide plan, he

Table 8–3. Key features of effective antisuicide plans

Identify specific reasons to live.

Collaboratively agree to safety precautions.

  Commit to contact/call a specific person(s) (list contact information).

  Commit to contact therapist or get other help (list contact information).

  Block or reduce access to guns or other dangers (e.g., have a family member lock up all medications and supply only one day's dose at a time).

Identify adaptive cognitions and behaviors that may help patient fight despair, anxiety, or other symptoms.

Develop coping strategies for possible triggers for increased suicidal thinking.

Write out plan and review it frequently.

Source.   Reprinted from Wright JH, Turkington D, Kingdon DG, et al: *Cognitive-Behavior Therapy for Severe Mental Illness: An Illustrated Guide.* Washington, DC, American Psychiatric Publishing, 2009, p. 150. Used with permission. Copyright © 2009 American Psychiatric Publishing.

agreed to ask one of his brothers to take all of his guns and lock them in a gun cabinet that Dan could not access. He also agreed to contact Dr. Sudak (or the doctor on call for her office) and to phone his brother if suicidal thoughts ever intensified to the point that he was seriously considering self-harm. Allie decided that she would call the social worker at Bridgespring if her suicidal thoughts got worse. As a backup, she listed phone numbers for Dr. Wright and two of her friends from the day program. Another item in her safety plan was to take all of the rodent poison and garden insecticides that were kept at her house to an aunt's house for storage.

    The adage, "Even the best laid plans can go astray," has a precautionary message that clinicians need to heed. Even if an antisuicide plan seems to be well thought out, practical, and full of good strategies, patients can have difficulties following through with some of the elements. New stresses or triggers can also derail patients and send them spiraling back toward suicide. Thus, it can often be useful to spend some time preparing patients for possible future obstacles.

    Cognitive-behavioral rehearsal can be a useful method for helping patients develop coping strategies for worst-case scenarios or other potential problems. For example, Dr. Sudak worked with Dan to prepare him for the possibility that his fears about being fired could come true.

    Dr. Sudak: Before we end the session today, I want to go back to some of the statements you made earlier. Do I recall that you said, "I don't think I could live with the humiliation of getting fired?"

Dan: Yeah, I said something like that. But I still don't think I would do anything to hurt myself.

Dr. Sudak: Just in case your worst fears came true and you lost your job, I think it might help to think through in advance how you could cope. Could we try to do this?

Dan: OK.

Dr. Sudak: I'm sure it would be a real blow and would hurt a lot. Even if this bad thing happened, I wonder what you could say to yourself to hold onto your self-esteem and not see this as an intolerable humiliation.

Dan: I'd be thinking about how ashamed I'd be to tell my wife and my family…But I guess I could try to remember the successes I had at work—at this job and some others. I did get the promotion, so they must have thought I have what it takes to handle the job. And I could probably get another job fairly soon. Even with a bad economy, someone with experience in trucking usually can find work. I could even go back to driving a truck if it came to that.

Dr. Sudak: You're coming up with some great ideas. The key thing in situations like these is to take a problem-solving attitude. You would feel the pain of losing the job, but your next task would be to build up your self-esteem and to start working on solutions. Any other positive thoughts that could help shore you up through this rough time? Could you think about some of the things you still have, instead of concentrating only on the loss?

Dan: Nobody could take away my faith, and I would still have my family …and my health.

Dr. Sudak: For homework, could you write down some of the negative automatic thoughts that might pop into your mind if you did get fired? And then write out a coping card with some of the ideas we just discussed?

Dan: Sure.

We have asked the types of questions listed in Table 8–2 and have developed written antisuicide plans in many brief sessions (see examples in Figures 8–4 and 8–5). However, we want to underscore the importance of doing a thorough evaluation of suicidality and devoting sufficient time to developing antisuicide plans. If the brief session does not provide enough time, or if the risk of suicide appears to be too high to deal with in the limited time available, several options can be considered: 1) extend the session; 2) ask an associate (e.g., a nurse or social worker) in your practice who has more time available to see the patient immediately; or 3) arrange for hospitalization.

Another point that we want to emphasize is the value of reviewing antisuicide plans regularly. At the next session, the clinician can ask the patient how the plan worked. What suicidal thoughts, if any, occurred since the last session? How were the thoughts handled? What parts of the plan

- *Remind myself of my many reasons to live:*
  - *My family—I don't want to hurt them.*
  - *Hopes of having grandchildren someday.*
  - *My brothers—all the good times we have together.*
  - *My volunteer work with "Habitat for Humanity."*

- *Self-harm is against my religion.*

- *If I ever have any significant thoughts of suicide, tell my wife and/or my brother and ask them to help me.*

- *Have my brother store my guns in his locked cabinet.*

- *Realize that I am probably magnifying the risk of getting fired.*

- *Do some positive things to make myself feel better:*
  - *Exercise*
  - *Volunteer work at church*

Figure 8–4.   Dan's antisuicide plan.

- *Think of reasons I want to live and not to do what the voices say:*
  - *My brother—he needs me, and I am his only friend.*
  - *I have been trying hard to fight my problems—I really don't want to die.*
  - *I enjoy playing the guitar.*
  - *I have hope that I could have a relationship some day.*
  - *It would hurt my parents if I died.*

- *If I am thinking of actually hurting myself, I will call Linda—the social worker at Bridgespring—or Dr. Wright. I can also tell my two best friends, Miranda and Letitia.*

- *Play my guitar in the group at Bridgespring.*

- *Remind myself that the voices are from a chemical imbalance in my brain. I don't need to pay attention to them or to let them have power over me.*

- *Stay involved in activities that calm the voices:*
  - *Work in the garden*
  - *Read a magazine*
  - *Listen to some soft music*

Figure 8–5.   Allie's antisuicide plan.

were used? What seemed to be helpful? Were there problems in carrying out any parts of the plan? Are any changes needed to make the plan more useful? Answers to these questions will help the clinician reevaluate suicide risk and troubleshoot any difficulties in using the plan.

> **Learning Exercise 8–2**   Developing an Antisuicide Plan
>
> 1. The next time you have a brief session with a patient who reports suicidal thoughts, ask the patient for her reasons for living.
>
> 2. If the suicide risk assessment indicates that the patient can still be managed with outpatient treatment (i.e., does not require hospitalization), develop an antisuicide plan with these elements:
>
>   • Reasons to live
>
>   • Specific safety precautions
>
>   • Adaptive cognitions and behaviors
>
> 3. Use cognitive-behavioral rehearsal to prepare the patient for future triggers for increased hopelessness or suicidal thoughts.

Summary

Key Points for Clinicians

- Hopelessness is an especially damaging cognition. It is associated with helplessness, defeated behavior, and suicidality. When hopelessness is present, it becomes a primary target for CBT interventions.
- A variety of general and specific CBT methods can instill hope. These methods include 1) drawing strength from the therapeutic relationship; 2) providing psychoeducation about reasons for hope; 3) keeping sessions focused on achievable goals and agendas; 4) involving patients in behavioral exercises that demonstrate an ability to change; 5) modifying hopeless cognitions; 6) identifying strengths and positive core beliefs; and 6) developing coping cards that build hope.
- Clinicians can use CBT methods to treat suicidality in brief sessions of combined CBT and pharmacotherapy. However, if suicide risk cannot be effectively managed in the available time, the clinician should extend sessions or refer the patient for more intensive treatment.

- Asking for positive reasons for living often provides an effective method of both assessing and treating suicide risk.
- In developing antisuicide plans, clinicians need to identify patient strengths and supports that can become components of the plan. They also need to consider the patient's capacities to modify hopeless and self-destructive cognitions and to engage in healthy behaviors that can help counter suicidal thoughts.
- Cognitive-behavioral rehearsal can assist patients in coping with possible stressful events in the future that could heighten suicidal thinking.

Concepts and Skills for Patients to Learn

- Depression and other psychiatric illness can breed a sense of hopelessness. Try not to give in to the hopelessness—it is a symptom of the disease. Work with your clinician to see beyond current negative thinking and find reasons for hope.
- Depression and other psychiatric illnesses are treatable. As symptoms improve, people usually become more hopeful about the future.
- One way to build hope is to identify and pay attention to your positives. List some of your strengths and healthy core beliefs. Review this list frequently.
- Cognitive-behavior therapy teaches people how to spot and reverse negative thinking. Learning these methods can help people to become more optimistic and to look forward to life.
- If you are having any suicidal thoughts, make sure to tell your clinician. Also, ask for help from your family, friends, or anyone else who could give you support.
- Suicidal thinking is temporary. Treatment works to reduce emotional pain and help people overcome suicidal thoughts.
- One of the most important questions you can ask yourself is, "What are my positive reasons for living?" When people get deeply depressed and think of suicide, they often lose track of their reasons for living. Getting back in touch with this positive side of your life can lift your mood and give you more hope for the future.
- Your clinician can work with you to develop an antisuicide plan. These plans usually work best if you collaborate with the clinician and give lots of input. If you develop an antisuicide plan, be sure to review it regularly and tell your doctor or therapist about your successes and problems, if any, in using the plan.

References

Beck AT: Thinking and depression. Arch Gen Psychiatry 9:324–333, 1963

Beck AT, Kovacs M, Weissman A: Hopelessness and suicidal behavior—an overview. JAMA 234:1146–1149, 1975

Beck AT, Steer RA, Kovacs M, et al: Hopelessness and eventual suicide: a 10-year prospective study of patients hospitalized with suicidal ideation. Am J Psychiatry 142:559–562, 1985

Brown GK, Ten Have T, Henriques GR, et al: Cognitive therapy for the prevention of suicide attempts: a randomized controlled trial. JAMA 294:563–570, 2005

Ellis TE, Newman CF: Choosing to Live: How to Defeat Suicide Through Cognitive Therapy. Oakland, CA, New Harbinger, 1996

Fawcett J, Scheftner W, Clark D, et al: Clinical predictors of suicide in patients with major affective disorders: a controlled prospective study. Am J Psychiatry 144:35–40, 1987

Frank JD: Psychotherapy and the Human Predicament: A Psychosocial Approach. Edited by Dietz PE. New York, Shocken Books, 1978

Jacobs D, Brewer M: APA practice guideline provides recommendations for assessing and treating patients with suicidal behaviors. Psychiatr Ann 34:373–380, 2004

Linehan MM, Goodstein JL, Nielson SL, et al: Reasons for staying alive when you are thinking of killing yourself: the Reasons for Living Inventory. J Consult Clin Psychol 51:276–286, 1983

Malone KM, Oquendo MA, Hass GL, et al: Protective factors against suicidal acts in major depression: reasons for living. Am J Psychiatry 157:1084–1088, 2000

Rush AJ, Beck AT, Kovacs M, et al. Comparison of the effects of cognitive therapy and imipramine on hopelessness and self-concept. Am J Psychiatry 139:862–866, 1982

Scully JH, Wilk JE: Selected characteristics and data of psychiatrists in the United States, 2001–2002. Acad Psychiatry 27:247–251, 2003

Simon RI: Assessing and Managing Suicide Risk: Guidelines for Clinically Based Risk Management. Washington, DC, American Psychiatric Publishing, 2004

Simon RI, Hales RE (eds.): The American Psychiatric Publishing Textbook of Suicide Assessment and Management. Washington, DC, American Psychiatric Publishing, 2006

Wright JH: Cognitive-behavior therapy for chronic depression. Psychiatr Ann 33:777–784, 2003

Wright JH, Turkington D, Kingdon D, et al: Cognitive-Behavior Therapy for Severe Mental Illness: An Illustrated Guide. Washington, DC, American Psychiatric Publishing, 2009

CHAPTER 9

Behavioral Methods
for Anxiety

LEARNING MAP

CBT model for anxiety disorders

⇩

Relaxation training

⇩

Positive imagery

⇩

Breathing retraining

⇩

Exposure therapy

Behavioral methods for anxiety disorders offer an especially appealing opportunity for using cognitive-behavior therapy (CBT) in brief sessions.

The techniques described in this chapter can often be taught to patients in short periods of time and can be practiced and implemented in homework assignments. Patients who are willing to take responsibility for building anxiety management skills and following exposure and response prevention protocols can perform a good deal of the work outside therapy sessions.

We begin the chapter with a brief overview of the basic CBT model for anxiety disorders. Then we outline three behavioral methods—relaxation training, positive imagery, and breathing retraining—that are commonly used for reducing anxiety and physical tension. Although these coping strategies can be used alone to treat anxiety symptoms, they are most often used as components of a comprehensive package that also includes exposure therapy and cognitive restructuring (see Chapter 7, "Targeting Maladaptive Thinking"). In the final part of the chapter, we give a detailed accounting of methods for using exposure and response prevention techniques in brief sessions. Several examples of exposure-based approaches are given to illustrate ways to treat different forms of anxiety disorders.

CBT Model for Anxiety Disorders

The cognitive elements of anxiety disorders were outlined in Chapter 7, "Targeting Maladaptive Thinking." The following are the key features of cognitive pathology in these conditions:

1. Excessive fears of danger, harm, and/or vulnerability (e.g., in response to objects or situations such as elevators, driving, crowds, social encounters, triggers or reminders of previous traumatic events, not completing a ritual)
2. Increased estimate of risk in these situations
3. Decreased estimate of ability to manage these situations
4. Heightened attention and vigilance about potential threats

The interrelationships between these types of cognitions and the emotional responses and behavioral patterns in anxiety disorders can be understood by using the basic CBT model that was described in Chapter 4, "Case Formulation and Treatment Planning." Figure 9–1 shows an example of the CBT model in a mini-formulation format for Rick, the patient with social phobia who was introduced in Chapter 4. We recommend viewing the two video illustrations of Rick's treatment with CBT later in this chapter.

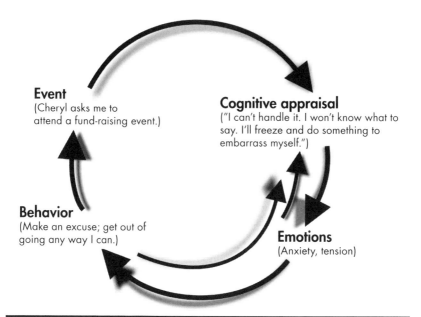

Figure 9–1. Cognitive-behavior therapy model for anxiety disorders: Rick's example.

Rick is a 37-year-old man who works as a supervisor in a construction company. He has never married but is now engaged to Cheryl, a socially outgoing woman who works as a fund-raiser for a local college. Cheryl, who has lots of friends and interests, has been pushing Rick to get more involved with social activities and to participate in her work-related social engagements (e.g., lunches with coworkers and friends, concerts and plays, fund-raising events). Rick has always been shy and socially avoidant, but has been able to largely hide this problem by working in a job that is task oriented and spending much of his leisure time in outdoor activities (e.g., fishing and hiking) with a few close buddies. His previous dating relationships had primarily been with women who were also socially retiring. However, now that he has fallen in love with Cheryl and wants to spend the rest of his life with her, his problem with social phobia has come to the forefront.

As diagrammed in Figure 9–1, multiple feedback loops exist between maladaptive cognitions, emotional responses, and the avoidance behaviors of anxiety disorders. When patients avoid feared situations, their maladaptive cognitions (e.g., "I can't handle it"; "I won't know what to say"; "I'll freeze and do something to embarrass myself") are reinforced, and a vicious cycle ensues in which the cognitive and behavioral components of the anxiety disorder feed on one another to perpetuate symptoms. CBT interventions for anxiety disorders can be directed at any of the four components of the basic model: 1) events (e.g., problem solving), 2) cognitive appraisal (e.g., modifying automatic thoughts and schemas), 3) emotions (e.g., relaxation training to reduce anxiety and physical tension), and 4) behavior (e.g., exposure therapy).

For most of the anxiety disorders (e.g., simple phobia, social phobia, panic disorder, posttraumatic stress disorder [PTSD], obsessive-compulsive disorder [OCD]), the crux of the behavioral component of CBT is engaging patients in one form or another of exposure therapy. These methods can help them break out of long-standing avoidance patterns and develop constructive coping skills (Klosko and Barlow 1996; Sanderson and Wetzler 1995).

Avoidance can be seen on at least three levels:

1. **The patient either completely or partially avoids a feared object or situation.** Examples include walking many flights of stairs to circumvent the need to take elevators; limiting driving to very short distances in a "safety zone"; not visiting shopping malls or other crowded areas; and following a compulsive ritual because of fear of what may happen if it is not completed.

2. **The patient utilizes "safety behaviors" to participate in a feared situation.** Although it may appear that the patient is confronting a feared situation or is taking steps to change avoidance behaviors, he is using safety maneuvers that may play a role in maintaining the anxiety disorder. Examples include getting drunk or taking tranquilizers to cope with taking an airplane flight; managing fear of driving by recruiting a friend or family member to serve as an assistant; and sticking close by a partner when in social situations, letting this person do the vast majority of the work in carrying on social discourse. Unless safety behaviors are identified and reduced, the patient will not gain full benefit of exposure-based therapies.

3. **The patient does not engage in activities that would help with learning ways to cope better with feared situations.** When Rick has automatic thoughts, such as "I won't have anything to say to them" or "I'm no good at going to parties," these cognitions could be partially true. He may have avoided social situations for so long that his skills in engaging others and carrying on conversations may not be well developed. Because he has concluded that he cannot do well in social situations, he also has avoided taking any positive steps to learn these types of skills. As we illustrate later in the chapter, CBT for anxiety disorders can be complemented by efforts to build the patient's capacity to effectively manage feared situations (e.g., coaching and/or readings on ways of making small talk; taking classes in effective pub-

lic speaking; practicing assertiveness, boundary setting, and rational safety precautions by persons who have been assaulted and suffer from PTSD). It is important to note that these types of skill-building exercises are designed to enhance effective coping, not to promote the kinds of safety behaviors that are associated with the patient's continued avoidance.

Exposure therapy can be rapid (as in flooding therapy for a simple phobia, in which a patient may be asked to confront a feared object or situation in a single session), but it is most commonly implemented in a gradual manner (Klosko and Barlow 1996; Sanderson and Wetzler 1995). In our brief sessions with persons who have anxiety disorders, we collaboratively design hierarchies in which we start with exposure activities that are rated fairly low in degree of difficulty and then progress upward through the list of activities as patients gain confidence and skills.

A variety of other behavioral techniques are available for reducing anxiety and tension levels and helping patients participate in exposure exercises. In the following sections, we detail three of the most useful and frequently applied methods: relaxation training, positive imagery, and breathing retraining. In addition to being helpful in promoting a tolerable and effective use of exposure therapy, these techniques can be quite beneficial in treating generalized anxiety disorder, damping physiological arousal in panic disorder and performance anxiety, correcting patterns of hyperventilation, relieving insomnia, and helping with a number of other anxiety-associated clinical problems.

Relaxation Training

The relaxation response has been part of the behavioral treatment of anxiety since the early history of this approach. In *The Practice of Behavior Therapy*, Wolpe (1969) argued that if patients could achieve a state of physical relaxation, psychic anxiety would be reduced because relaxation and anxiety are fundamentally incompatible. He recommended teaching patients progressive relaxation before engaging in hierarchical exposure so that they could have an effective tool for managing anxiety while gaining experience in facing feared objects or situations. Subsequently, relaxation training has been studied extensively in the treatment of anxiety disorders and in helping patients cope with stress-related physical illnesses such as migraine headaches, hypertension, and coronary artery disease.

A meta-analysis of 27 studies of relaxation training conducted between 1997 and 2007 found an overall moderate effect size for the benefits of this method in reducing anxiety (Manzoni et al. 2008). As expected, results were better for those who spent time practicing the technique at home. Two other studies (Arntz 2003; Ost and Breitholtz 2000) found that relaxation training alone was as effective as a full package of CBT for generalized anxiety disorder. Also of note, Clark et al. (2006) observed that relaxation training led to substantial improvement in social phobia. These findings suggest that efforts to adapt relaxation training methods for brief sessions could have a positive impact on clinicians' ability to help patients with anxiety disorders.

The classic form of relaxation training, described by Jacobsen (1938), is sometimes termed *Jacobsen's progressive relaxation*. In more recent years, some investigators and clinicians have used terms such as *applied relaxation* or *autogenic training*. However, the central element of this method—the practicing of sequential steps to relax voluntary muscles—is used in all such protocols. Readers who want to learn more about progressive relaxation may want to consult texts by Bernstein and Borkovec (1973), Jacobsen (1938), or Payne (2005). In Table 9–1, we provide a method from one of our earlier books that we think can be adapted nicely for use in brief sessions (Wright et al. 2006).

If not enough time is available in a brief session to thoroughly teach patients the principles of progressive relaxation, or if the clinician and therapist believe the session should focus on other topics, any or all of the instruction can be provided in alternative ways. Table 9–2 lists several resources (including audio guides) that provide a full grounding in this technique. Also, the clinician can suggest that patients see another therapist who has expertise in this approach. For example, we have worked on inpatient units where nurses or activity therapists provide excellent education in progressive relaxation. If the psychiatrist is working in the dual-therapist mode for combined CBT and pharmacotherapy, the non-medical therapist can offer relaxation training. A novel approach that may have considerable potential is using virtual reality to help patients achieve and utilize relaxation responses (for example, see relaxation programs offered by Virtually Better). Although this high-tech method is not yet available in many clinical settings, mental health offices of the future may be more likely to have computer tools such as virtual reality to assist clinicians and patients.

> **Learning Exercise 9–1**   Coaching Progressive Relaxation in Brief Sessions
>
> 1. Review the instructions in Table 9–1 and practice coaching one or more of your patients in relaxation techniques using 10 minutes or less of a brief session.

Table 9–1. Method for relaxation training in brief sessions

---

1. **Teach patients about the potential benefits of relaxation training.** Prepare the patient for the relaxation exercise by explaining how it can be used to reduce tension and help cope with anxiety or other symptoms. A short mini-lesson should suffice. Emphasize the self-help component of this technique. The clinician will get the process started in a session, but it will be up to the patient to practice the skills at home.

2. **Explain how to rate levels of muscle tension and anxiety.** Use a 0–100 scale, where a rating of 0 is equivalent to *no tension or anxiety* and 100 represents *maximum tension or anxiety*.

3. **Demonstrate voluntary control over muscle tension.** To show the patient that he has the capacity to reduce muscular tension, ask him to try to tighten one fist to the maximum level and then to let it completely relax to a rating of zero or to the lowest level of tension he can achieve. Then, ask him to perform the tightening and relaxing exercises with the opposite hand.

4. **Help the patient learn to reduce muscle tension.** Starting with the hands, help the patient relax muscles as much as possible (rated as a zero or close to zero). Methods to facilitate this process can include a) exerting conscious control over muscle groups by monitoring tension and telling oneself to relax the muscles; b) stretching the targeted muscle groups through their full range of motion; c) gentle self-massage to sooth and relax tight muscles; and d) use of calming mental images (the "Positive Imagery" section of this chapter provides more details on how to use this technique).

5. **Ask the patient to progressively relax each of the major muscle groups of the body.** After achieving a state of deep relaxation of the hands, ask the patient to allow the relaxation to spread through the entire body, one muscle group at a time. A commonly used sequence is hands, forearms, upper arms, shoulders, neck, head, eyes, face, chest, back, abdomen, hips, upper legs, lower legs, feet, and toes. However, any sequence can be chosen that you and the patient believe will work best for her. During this phase of the induction, all of the methods from step 4 that have proved helpful can be repeated. We often find that stretching allows the patient to find especially tense muscle groups that may require extra attention.

6. **Assign progressive relaxation for homework.** Reinforce the value of practicing relaxation between sessions. Also, consider using audio, video, or computer aids (Table 9–2) so that the patient does not have to rely completely on the clinician to learn and rehearse this skill.

Source. Adapted from Wright JH, Basco MR, Thase ME: *Learning Cognitive-Behavior Therapy: An Illustrated Guide.* Washington, DC, American Psychiatric Publishing, 2006. Used with permission. Copyright © 2006 American Psychiatric Publishing.

Table 9–2.   Resources for relaxation training and practice

Benson-Henry Institute for Mind Body Medicine (audio CD)
www.massgeneral.org/bhi

Letting Go of Stress: Four Effective Techniques for Relaxation and
Stress Reduction (audio CD by Emmett Miller and Steven Halpern)
Available from various music vendors

Progressive Muscle Relaxation (audio CD by Frank Dattilio, Ph.D.)
www.dattilio.com

Time for Healing: Relaxation for Mind and Body (audio set by
Catherine Regan, Ph.D.)
Bull Publishing Company
www.bullpub.com/healing.html

Virtual reality program for relaxation by Rothbaum and associates
http://virtuallybetter.com

Note.   These resources are also listed in Appendix 2, "CBT Resources for
Patients and Families."

2. Either use the resources listed in Table 9–2 for aids to
relaxation training or develop your own list. Make
suggestions to one or more patients for using one of these
aids as a self-help tool.

Positive Imagery

Imagery techniques are often used in combination with other CBT methods, such as progressive relaxation, breathing retraining, and exposure
therapy, as part of a comprehensive effort to treat anxiety disorders
(Simpson et al. 2008; Singer et al. 1999; Wolpe 1973; Wright et al.
2006). There are two principal ways to use imagery to facilitate behavioral methods for reducing anxiety and tension. The first, guided imagery, is a method in which a clinician works to induce a state of relaxation
by giving detailed and soothing instructions for the patient to imagine being in a calming environment. We do not typically use this type of guided
imagery in our CBT sessions because the clinician has to do most of the
work in creating the image, and thus patients are not encouraged to build
their own skills in using imagery. Also, fully developed guided imagery
exercises can be rather time consuming and may not offer enough yield
to justify their use in brief sessions. We think a good solution for use of
full protocols for guided imagery is to recommend that patients use one
of the resources listed in Table 9–2 to practice these sorts of exercises.

A more commonly used imagery technique is to simply ask the patient to imagine a calming scene to shift attention away from distressing cognitions or to reduce physiological arousal. For example, a patient with panic disorder might be taught to use positive imagery (e.g., imagining oneself walking along a beach or being in a favorite vacation spot) along with breathing retraining to interrupt the escalation of panic attacks. This application is illustrated in the next section of this chapter, "Breathing Retraining." Also, imagery could be used to augment progressive relaxation methods (e.g., imagining being "loose as a goose" or letting "your tensions melt away and drip off your fingertips and onto the floor like ice melting slowly" [Wright et al. 2006]).

Some patients take readily to the use of imagery, but others may have difficulty using this technique. As with many other CBT interventions, it can help to start with a mini-lesson to explain imagery and give an example or two. In Table 9–3, we give some suggestions for effective use of positive imagery techniques.

We use positive imagery techniques in our own lives for many purposes—to help get back to sleep after middle-of-the-night awakenings; to reduce muscle tension when stressed by work demands; or to take a "mini-break" from pressured days, health concerns, or worries about family or friends. We sometimes tell patients about our own use of imagery to normalize this technique and to let them know that it can be OK to take a few moments to evoke a pleasant and calming image—to have a short "daydream" that is a healthy coping mechanism.

Some examples of images that we or our patients have found useful are listed in Table 9–4. Scenes that may work best are those that are clearly relaxing, do not involve memories of troubled relationships or other disappointments, do not trigger elaborations of thought that will drive tension back up again, and can be entered and exited fairly quickly.

> **Learning Exercise 9–2** Using Positive Imagery
>
> 1. Identify at least two relaxing positive images that you can use to manage stress in your own life.
>
> 2. Practice using these images.
>
> 3. Ask at least one of your patients to work on identifying and using positive imagery as a coping mechanism for anxiety.

Breathing Retraining

Efforts to coach patients on breathing have been shown to be a valuable element of CBT for panic disorder (de Beurs et al. 1995; Taylor 2001)

Table 9–3.   Tips for using positive imagery methods for anxiety
disorders

---

1. **Begin with a brief explanation of how imagery can be helpful in
    combating anxiety.** Whenever possible, relate this explanation
    directly to a problem that the patient is currently facing and that is
    being targeted in this session (e.g., panic attack, insomnia aggravated
    by excessive worry, chronic tension and anxiety in generalized
    anxiety disorder).

2. **Ask the patient to describe his previous experience (or lack of
    experience) in using imagery.** If the patient already uses this
    method, support and reinforce its value. Offer to coach the patient
    on productive use of imagery. If the patient has little or no
    experience with imagery or reports being unable to evoke calming
    images, explain that this is a skill that can be developed.

3. **Elicit the patient's own images that can be used to reduce anxiety and
    tension.** The clinician may need to "prime the pump" by giving
    examples (see Table 9–4), but the emphasis should be primarily on
    uncovering and elaborating images from the patient's own experience.

4. **Model and/or try out the positive imagery method in a session.**
    Clinicians can show the patient how a positive image might be used
    in breaking a panic attack or in managing some other anxiety-related
    problem (see "Breathing Retraining" section and Video Illustration
    8) or get the patient directly involved in using imagery to reduce
    symptoms.

5. **Assign imagery practice for homework.** Repeated practice of this
    technique is likely to help patients solidify their ability to use
    imagery as an effective coping tool.

---

because this condition is frequently associated with hyperventilation. A
typical evolution of a panic attack might include 1) a surge in catastrophic cognitions (e.g., "I'm having a heart attack or a stroke…I'll
faint…I'm losing control") in response to a triggering situation; 2) intense
anxiety and physiological arousal, including fast, irregular, or excessively
deep or shallow breathing; 3) hyperventilation-induced numbness, tin-
gling, or other physiological changes, which lead to an increased sense of
being out of control; and 4) an escalation of catastrophic cognitions and
intensification of physiological arousal.

Breathing retraining can interrupt this cascade of maladaptive cognitions and behaviors by giving patients a positive focus that can distract
them from the disturbing cognitions, providing a method to gain control
of the situation, and stopping the physiological effects of hyperventila-

---

Table 9–4. Images used to cope with anxiety

Beach and ocean scenes (attending to the sounds of the waves, the feel
of the sand and water on one's feet, blue skies, comfortable
temperature of the air and water, etc.)

A favorite vacation spot (e.g., walking along a street at Disney World,
sitting on the front porch of a family cabin on a pleasant night when
the crickets are singing and the air is sweet with the smells of summer)

Hearing a song or other piece of music (listening to soothing music in
imagination)

Mountain scenes (e.g., strolling around a lake that is in the mountains
and is surrounded by majestic peaks)

A pleasant memory of a person or situation (reexperiencing in
imagination a comfortable, nonconflicted moment that evokes warm
feelings)

Casting a fly rod (with a rhythmic and graceful motion and a soft
delivery of the fly on a gentle stretch of water)

Replaying a relaxing image from a movie or book (with choice of an
image that is interesting but not overstimulating)

---

tion. Some authors have cautioned that breathing retraining could possibly detract from the cognitive restructuring elements of CBT for panic
disorder if it is misused as a method of avoiding feared situations
(Schmidt et al. 2000; Taylor 2001). However, when this technique is explained carefully and is integrated with other parts of a comprehensive
CBT approach, we have found that it is typically used as an adaptive behavior.

In our consultations with patients who have had previous treatment
but are still experiencing panic attacks, we typically inquire about the
coping methods they have tried (e.g., "What do you do when you have a
panic attack? How do you try to stop it?"). A surprisingly large number
of patients report, "I was told to start taking lots of deep breaths so that
I could catch my breath." Others describe being taught "diaphragmatic
breathing." This latter term has been somewhat mystifying to us as physicians because all breathing uses the diaphragm to some extent, unless
this muscle is paralyzed. Unfortunately, patients sometimes misunder-
stand the instructions of well-meaning therapists or information on Web
sites and conclude that the answer is to breathe very deeply in a rather
exaggerated and labored manner. In many cases, this strategy seems to
make things worse.

The breathing retraining method shown in Video Illustration 8 emphasizes normalizing the breathing pattern to help patients break out of states of hyperventilation. Although many different strategies of breathing retraining have been suggested for patients with panic disorder, we have found that the general methods used in the video illustration can rapidly teach patients a helpful technique to get panic attacks under control. Breathing retraining of this type is often one of the first initiatives that we choose when patients have panic disorder with hyperventilation because it can be taught in brief periods of time and can yield quick and impressive results.

▶ **Video Illustration 8.** Breathing Retraining: Dr. Wright and Gina[†]

In the video illustration, Dr. Wright is working with Gina, a woman with panic disorder. The treatment of Gina is a central feature of one of our earlier books (Wright et al. 2006). She has multiple fears, including creating a scene in public places such as a cafeteria, driving by herself, and riding in elevators. Several other videos on the DVD that accompanies our earlier text demonstrate cognitive restructuring, use of hierarchical exposure, and in vivo exposure therapy with Gina. The breathing retraining video illustrates a pragmatic and straightforward method to help her manage her panic attacks. The key steps in this approach are summarized in Table 9–5.

Exposure Therapy

In Vivo and Imaginal Exposure

The most commonly used method for exposure therapy is *systematic desensitization*—a stepwise progression through a hierarchy of feared encounters in a series of sessions. The exposure can be done *in vivo* (i.e., the patient uses either self-directed exposure or therapist-guided exposure to actually participate in a feared activity, such as driving, shopping in a crowded mall, or attending social events) or by *imaginal exposure* (i.e., the patient imagines being in the feared situation).

Because in vivo exposure involves full immersion in the experience, it

---

[†]Video Illustration 8 is used with permission from Wright JH, Basco MR, Thase ME: *Learning Cognitive-Behavior Therapy: An Illustrated Guide.* Washington, DC, American Psychiatric Publishing, 2006. Copyright © 2006 Jesse H. Wright, M.D., Ph.D.

Table 9–5. A method for breathing retraining

Teach the patient about overbreathing in panic attacks.

Model hyperventilation behavior in panic attacks.

Show the patient how to gain control of breathing when in a panic attack.
- Suggest taking a few deep breaths to start gaining control.
- Then slow breathing to a normal rate of about 15–16 breaths per minute (one cycle in and out about every 4 seconds).
- Recommend watching the second hand of a clock to help get back into a normal pattern and also to provide a brief distraction from catastrophic cognitions.

Implement positive imagery to further reduce anxiety and calm the breathing pattern.

Advise the following practice strategy to build mastery: 1) overbreathe to induce the beginning of a panic attack, 2) then implement the procedures above to stop the panic attack.

usually offers the best opportunity for therapeutic gain. Whenever possible, we try to help patients engage in real-life situations that are triggering anxiety and avoidance. However, in many clinical situations, imaginal exposure offers advantages. For example, a person who has a fear of flying may not be able to get on a plane or take a flight of any length until imaginal exposure is used to reduce anxiety levels and build a modicum of confidence in her ability to manage a plane trip. Similarly, a patient with PTSD who has total avoidance of the workplace after a work-related accident might benefit from some imaginal exposure exercises in advance of attempts to gradually reenter the job environment.

Using Hierarchies for Exposure Therapy

Whether exposure therapy is done in vivo or in imagination, a hierarchy is usually constructed to help the patient take gradual steps toward reaching ultimate goals of being able to participate comfortably in activities that have stimulated excessive anxiety. We offer some suggestions for developing effective hierarchies in Table 9–6.

Rick, the man with social phobia, was a good candidate for taking responsibility for doing exposure therapy assignments outside brief sessions. He was functioning well in his job as a construction supervisor, did not have any significant comorbid problems with Axis II disorders or substance abuse, was involved in a healthy relationship with his fiancée, and

Table 9–6.   Tips for developing graded exposure hierarchies

Be specific. Help the patient write out clear, definitive descriptions of the stimuli for each step in the hierarchy. Examples of overgeneralized or ill-defined steps are "learn to drive again," "stop being afraid of going to parties," and "feel comfortable in crowds." Examples of specific, well-delineated steps are "drive two blocks to the corner store at least three times a week," "spend 20 minutes at the neighborhood party before leaving," or "go to the mall for 10 minutes on a Sunday morning when very few people are there."

Rate the steps for degree of difficulty or amount of expected anxiety. Use a 0- to 100-point scale. These ratings will be used to select the steps for exposure and to measure progress. The usual effect of progressing through a hierarchy is to have significant reductions in the ratings for degree of difficulty or anxiety as each step is mastered.

Develop a hierarchy that has multiple steps of varied degree of difficulty. Coach the patient on listing a number of different steps (typically 8–12) that range in degree of difficulty from very low (ratings of 5–20) to very high (ratings of 80–100). Try to list steps throughout the entire range of difficulty. If the patient only lists steps with a high rating or can think of no mid-range steps, assist him in developing a more gradual and comprehensive list.

Choose steps collaboratively. As with any other cognitive-behavior therapy assignment, work with the patient as a team to select the order of steps for graded exposure therapy.

Design hierarchies that lend themselves to work outside sessions. To effectively leverage your time in brief sessions, try to develop hierarchies that provide reasonable steps that the patient can take between therapy sessions. Where possible, minimize exposure steps that require the clinician to do a good deal of work in engaging the patient in imaginal exposure.

Source.   Adapted from Wright JH, Basco MR, Thase ME: *Learning Cognitive-Behavior Therapy: An Illustrated Guide*. Washington, DC, American Psychiatric Publishing, 2006. Used with permission. Copyright © 2006 American Psychiatric Publishing.

was motivated by this relationship to change his behavior of social avoidance. In one of the early sessions with Dr. Wright, he sketched out several items for a hierarchy and then completed this exercise for homework. Figure 9–2 shows the hierarchy that Rick used to overcome his social phobia.

Rick was seen for a series of 10 brief sessions after an initial evaluation. He preferred the brief session format because he could arrange visits during his lunch hour and did not have to take off from work to participate in CBT. Although treatment with a selective serotonin reuptake inhibitor (SSRI) was considered, Rick preferred not to take any medications, at least in part because of fear of sexual side effects. Dr. Wright suggested that Rick keep open the possibility that medication might help and that side effects would not occur. However, Rick made good progress using CBT and successfully completed treatment without requiring pharmacotherapy. Video Illustration 9 shows an early session with Rick. He had already been instructed on how to develop a hierarchy and had written out the list of items in Figure 9–2 for a homework assignment. He had also agreed to start doing the first two items on the hierarchy.

▮ **Video Illustration 9.** Exposure Therapy I: Dr. Wright and Rick

In the beginning of the video illustration, Rick reports on his homework—he had been able to answer all phone calls with potential for socially oriented conversation. Previously, he had looked at caller ID and had not answered calls that were from people, other than close friends, who might challenge him to carry on discussions of any significant length. Because Rick seemed to be getting the idea behind graded exposure and was having some initial success, Dr. Wright decided to press forward with work on the hierarchy. They first discussed Rick's experiences with an item that was ranked fairly low on the hierarchy—having dinner with his fiancée's parents. Then they began to work on a more challenging task—attending a fund-raising event and carrying on conversations with people that he did not know well.

> Dr. Wright: What's [attending a fund-raising event] like for you?
> Rick: That's pretty hard. I don't do very well in that situation, I don't think.
> Dr. Wright: And I hear you've been pretty much avoiding all of that if you can.
> Rick: Whatever I can avoid, I try. It's not easy because Cheryl wants me to be there and to participate, but it's hard.
> Dr. Wright: What was the rating on going to one of the events with Cheryl and you have to stick it out and stay for a fair amount of time?

Situation	Rating
Accept phone calls from people I don't know very well (e.g., some of Cheryl's friends or people from church) that I think might want to carry on a conversation.	*10–15*
Go out after work with some of the other guys (not my closest buddies) who work with me.	*10–15*
Go to Cheryl's parents' for dinner and stay for at least an hour after dinner.	*20*
Have dinner in a restaurant with Cheryl and have a discussion with the waiter about how a dish is prepared, or complain if something isn't done well.	*25*
Go to a restaurant that doesn't take reservations—stand around and socialize with other people who are waiting for a table.	*30–35*
Meet Cheryl and a bunch of her coworkers for lunch—carry on conversations with these people.	*40*
Go early or stay late after church—carry on conversations with other members I am meeting for the first time.	*55*
See a movie with two or three other couples we don't know very well—stop for coffee or a beer after the movie.	*60*
Attend a concert or play—initiate conversations before the production or at intermission with people I hardly know.	*70*
Attend a fund-raising event with Cheryl—make a real effort to meet and talk with others. Stay for at least 2 hours.	*80–85*
Invite two or three couples we don't know very well to have dinner with us at Cheryl's house—be social and stick it out for about 3 hours.	*90*
Take the lead in hosting a party at my house for at least 20 people, including some I don't know too well. Be a good conversationalist and host.	*100+*

Figure 9–2.   Rick's hierarchy for social phobia.

Rick: That's 80, 85.

Dr. Wright: Pretty high.

Rick: Yeah. If I have to start a conversation with somebody, that's like really high…which is what I tend to have to do in that sort of situation.

After targeting this type of social event as an eventual goal for hierarchical exposure, Dr. Wright suggested that Rick might need to work on his ability to initiate and maintain social conversations. Because of his long-standing pattern of avoidance, he had underdeveloped skills in talking with people he did not know well or in building social relationships. Two methods for building these skills were suggested: 1) role-playing in sessions and 2) reading about how to make small talk. Rick agreed to acquire a book on this topic after checking available resources using an Internet search. Role-playing exercises were planned for future sessions.

The last part of the video illustration shows Rick and Dr. Wright deciding on exposure assignments to be conducted for homework before the next session. Rick was not yet ready to take on the task of attending the fund-raiser, but he was able to commit to three activities rated at 40 or lower (going to a restaurant that does not take reservations and conversing with others waiting in line, having a detailed discussion with a waiter, and having lunch with Cheryl and some of her coworkers whom he did not know well).

Later sessions with Rick were directed at moving upward through the hierarchy to participate in increasingly more demanding exposure activities. At each visit, Dr. Wright and Rick collaboratively selected targets for next steps, did troubleshooting if there were problems in carrying out any of the tasks, and practiced skills in managing social situations. As Rick made progress in taking on more challenging activities, items on the lower end of the hierarchy became much easier to accomplish. At about the midpoint of therapy, Rick reported that he was trying to participate in fund-raisers and other similar activities with his fiancée, but he was having difficulty. Dr. Wright turned this problem into an opportunity by helping Rick understand and manage the phenomenon of safety behaviors.

Working on Safety Behaviors

Safety behaviors can subtly undermine the attempts of clinicians and patients to overcome anxiety disorders. If patients use such behaviors, they can appear to be making strides in surmounting a problem but they are still avoiding a full experience of the feared situation. Thus, the anxiety symptoms may continue in one form or another. In Video Illustration 10, Dr. Wright asks questions that uncover several of Rick's safety behaviors.

After reporting that he would sometimes "freeze" in social situations, Rick tells Dr. Wright about some ways that he had found to manage the dilemma.

▶ **Video Illustration 10.** Exposure Therapy II: Dr. Wright and Rick

> Dr. Wright: Now this freeze thing. Are you actually freezing?...Like you can't say anything. Would people know this?
>
> Rick: People wouldn't always know that this is what is happening, but I kind of run out of stuff to say...It's kind of like my mind goes blank.
>
> Dr. Wright: You get that sense of real anxiety. And what do you do next?
>
> Rick: If it doesn't go away and I can't think of anything, then I usually say, "Hey, I need to go take a phone call," or I usually excuse myself.
>
> Dr. Wright: I see. So, you have some way of getting out of the situation... Any other things you do?
>
> Rick: Sometimes I say, "Hey, Cheryl needs me. I need to go check on her."
>
> Dr. Wright: And I'm wondering if sometimes it's a little easier to hang around Cheryl and let her do the talking.
>
> Rick: Oh yeah. She can always talk.
>
> Dr. Wright: OK. Now what I think we're identifying here are things that are called safety behaviors.

Dr. Wright then goes on to explain safety behaviors and their role in continuing a pattern of avoidance. Next he helps Rick set goals for maintaining conversations for longer periods of time. Video Illustration 10 ends with a brief discussion of another important topic—beginning to plan for activities that would expose Rick to the higher-ranked situations on the hierarchy. It appears to be a good sign that Rick is considering the idea of hosting a cookout or some other type of party.

Another example of work with safety behaviors is demonstrated in the treatment of Consuela, a woman with agoraphobia (especially fear of driving) and PTSD who was first described in Chapter 2, "Indications and Formats for Brief CBT Sessions." Consuela was treated in the dual-therapist format. Her other therapist was a pastoral counselor who was not trained in CBT and was helping Consuela with grief issues after the death of a close friend in a traffic accident. Consuela had agoraphobic symptoms before being in a car accident that resulted in her friend's death; however, the symptoms had escalated greatly after the traumatic incident. Although Consuela seemed to be making some progress in her treatment with Dr. Sudak, which included treatment with an SSRI, she typically performed about two-thirds of the exposure activities they agreed on at the previous session, and she continued to insist that one of her parents accompany her when she was driving. She was driving longer distances and was experiencing more congested highways, but it was almost always with the safety net of having a parent or friend with her.

To reduce these safety behaviors, Dr. Sudak worked with Consuela to develop exposure logs. Figure 9–3 shows an exposure log from later in therapy, after they had already achieved some success in decreasing Consuela's use of safety behaviors.

Exposure logs are valuable tools for helping patients set targets for working through hierarchies and for fine-tuning exposure protocols. In Consuela's case, Dr. Sudak suggested a particular focus on designing and monitoring attempts to have driving experiences without having a supportive person on board. In the beginning of this effort, they had to drop back to lower ends of the hierarchy to find driving activities that she could tolerate alone. Over the course of several sessions, however, Consuela was gradually able to increase her capacity to drive significant distances by herself.

Brief Exposure Therapy Sessions for PTSD

Consuela's treatment illustrates one possible use of brief sessions of combined CBT and pharmacotherapy for PTSD. However, many cases of PTSD may require longer sessions if severe traumas have been experienced and there is a need for extensive discussions to understand and circumvent avoidance of triggers or reminders of traumatic incidents. For example, JoAnne, a patient with PTSD, was seen by one of us for 50-minute CBT sessions plus treatment with an SSRI. Joanne was a 34-year-old woman who was sexually traumatized in her first year of college by "acquaintance rape." Since that time, she developed a complicated set of symptoms including avoidance of intimacy, depression, very low self-esteem, and severe obesity (which she openly admitted helped her avoid being an object of attraction from men).

Another patient seen in 50-minute sessions was Sergio, a 47-year-old telephone lineman who fell off a high utility pole when he was working at night during a power outage after a storm. Sergio injured his back severely, was hospitalized for over 2 weeks for the back injury, and had been unable to work for the subsequent 3 years. Part of his problem was PTSD. He became highly anxious whenever he thought of returning to his job and doing any climbing or even being raised above the ground with a hydraulic lift. Sergio also was depressed, had some element of chronic pain, and was experiencing a marked deterioration in his marriage since the accident. He was treated in the dual-therapist format by one of the authors (who saw Sergio for brief sessions to manage medications, support and facilitate the CBT, and provide overall direction for the treatment) and a nonphysician cognitive-behavior therapist who was part of the treatment team.

Exposure goals: *Drive alone at least five times a week.*
Drive alone in congested areas at least three times a week.

Day	Driving activity	Not alone	Alone	Comments
Sunday	To mall with friend Marcy	X		It's getting easier to drive to the mall.
	Drove about 8 blocks to take some books to a neighbor		X	It wasn't too hard to drive this short distance alone.
Monday	To grocery store with mother	X		I thought of going by myself, but mother wanted to go shopping with me.
	Took clothes to cleaners about ½ mile away after rush hour was over		X	This was more difficult—had to go on four-lane road, but it wasn't very congested at the time.
Tuesday	To bookstore with parents	X		It went OK. There was a fair amount of traffic in early evening.
Wednesday	To mall by myself		X	I was very nervous. Felt tense and sweaty but stuck with it. Drove on expressway to mall.
Thursday	To movie with friends	X		I picked them up and drove to movie at another mall about 4 miles away—was tense and very watchful of other drivers.
	Short trip to sandwich shop to pick up lunch		X	Did fine with this one—only about 10 blocks each way on neighborhood streets.
Friday	No driving this day, stayed home and worked in garden			
Saturday	Drove into city to shop		X	I went on expressway, even though I could have gone only on city streets. Not quite as tense. Went on Saturday so traffic wasn't as bad.
	Went out to dinner with friends	X		I am pushing myself to be the driver. I drove back and forth to the restaurant, which was about 3 miles away.

Figure 9–3.   An exposure log with attention to safety behaviors: Consuela's example.

Because CBT procedures for PTSD often require prolonged, intensive, and repeated efforts to have the patient reexperience traumatic events and to modify overt and subtle forms of avoidance (Ehlers et al. 2005), we rarely attempt to treat this condition with brief sessions alone. However, some patients with uncomplicated or relatively mild PTSD symptoms might be reasonable candidates for the brief session, sole-clinician format. An example from our practices is Terry, a 40-year-old man with a history of irritable bowel syndrome, who sought treatment after having an "accident" with his bowels while attending one of his son's soccer games. He had been far away from any bathroom facilities and had been "trying to hold it." The loss of bowel control had been terribly embarrassing for him, and now he had intrusive memories and images of this event and intense fears that it would happen again. As a result, he was avoiding any outdoor activities with his family, was trying to evacuate his bowels at least four times a day, and was spending up to an hour sitting on the toilet before going to work.

Dr. Thase, who was treating this patient, called Terry's gastroenterologist to coordinate their efforts and to better understand the effects of irritable bowel syndrome on Terry's behavior. The gastroenterologist noted that she was pleased that Terry had consulted Dr. Thase because she had recognized that Terry's anxiety was leading to massive overreactions. For example, the gastroenterologist believed that there was no physiological reason why Terry needed to spend more than a few minutes on the toilet in the morning or to schedule attempts to move his bowels at least four times a day. Fortunately, Terry did not appear to have other psychiatric or social problems. He had a successful career as an accountant and reported excellent family relationships. Although there was an obsessive character to some of his bowel-related behaviors, he had no other symptoms suggestive of OCD.

Terry was a very busy accountant who had a rather autonomous and self-controlling personality style. When Dr. Thase discussed several options for treatment, including referral for 50-minute sessions with a nonmedical therapist, Terry chose to start an SSRI and to do brief sessions with exposure therapy assignments for homework. Over the course of about 3 months, Dr. Thase and Terry worked together to implement a rational plan for being close enough to toilet facilities in case Terry had an actual need to evacuate his bowels quickly, but also began to use systematic desensitization to gradually resume outdoor activities with his family and to tolerate increasing distances from bathrooms. They used an exposure log, such as the ones detailed in the next section, to sequentially reduce the amount of time he spent on the toilet. By the end of treatment, Terry was able to regularly attend soccer games, take at least short hikes of an hour or less with his family, and participate in other outdoor activities. His intense fear about loss of bowel control abated considerably, and he accepted a normalizing explanation that a rare "bowel accident" occurs in many people and can be tolerated without undue shame. He was spending less than 5 minutes sitting on the toilet in the morning before work.

Exposure Therapy for Obsessive-Compulsive Disorder

In exposure therapy for OCD, the clinician typically involves the patient in a process of agreeing to stop specified obsessive behaviors while tolerating anxiety associated with not completing a ritual until the fear is significantly reduced or extinguished entirely (Foa et al. 2005). The term *response prevention* is often used to describe the stopping of compulsive behaviors. As in treatment of other anxiety disorders, a hierarchical approach is usually employed. We have found that brief sessions of combined CBT and pharmacotherapy can have a solid place in the treatment of patients with OCD. A frequently used method is for us to prescribe an SSRI, raise the dose to effective levels, monitor and manage possible side effects, and engage the patient in a straightforward exposure therapy protocol. This therapy is usually done in the sole-clinician mode, especially if the patient has circumscribed OCD without any other severe comorbidities and is motivated for use of CBT. Our sense of security in treating such patients in brief sessions is bolstered by studies that have shown good results for treatments that primarily utilize self-directed exposure for OCD and demand little therapist time (Marks et al. 1988; Mataix-Cols and Marks 2006).

The treatment of Prakash provides a good example of this type of work. Prakash consulted Dr. Turkington for treatment of long-standing obsessive-compulsive symptoms characterized by ritualistic counting. Prakash had worked in the United Kingdom for over 20 years as a paralegal assistant and reported good job satisfaction and a supportive family environment. However, his days were occupied by many rituals that consumed much time and effort. At the first visit, Prakash estimated that he spent about 30%–35% of his waking hours completing rituals such as counting windowpanes in his office, counting books on the shelves of offices that he entered, counting numbers that appeared on automobile license plates, and counting utility poles. His overall goal for treatment was to reduce the counting so that it took no more than 5% of his waking time.

Dr. Turkington's treatment plan included an exposure therapy protocol that engaged Prakash in a 6-month effort to gradually winnow down his counting behaviors. Brief sessions were scheduled initially at 2-week intervals but were extended to 4-week intervals in the last 2 months of the active CBT component of treatment. After 6 months of therapy, Prakash had reached his goal and declared that the counting was so minimal that it had an inconsequential effect on his life. He continued treatment with an SSRI and follow-up visits with Dr. Turkington every 3 months. Sample exposure logs from the second and fifth months of his treatment are shown in Figure 9–4 to illustrate the types of activities that were integral to the success of the behavioral component of treatment.

> **Learning Exercise 9–3**   Using Hierarchical Exposure Therapy
>
> 1. Try to identify a simple phobia or fear that you may have. Most people have a pattern of excessive fear and avoidance in response to at least one stimulus (e.g., stinging insects, heights, public speaking or other performance situations, social anxiety). Although this avoidance may not be causing any real distress, it still offers an opportunity to learn to apply exposure therapy principles.
>
> 2. Construct a hierarchy to increase your ability to face this anxiety-producing stimulus. Then put the hierarchy to work.
>
> 3. Select at least one patient from your practice who might benefit from exposure therapy in brief sessions. Develop a hierarchy and implement the exposure-based treatment approach.

Summary

Key Points for Clinicians

- Behavioral methods for anxiety disorders can be quite useful in brief sessions because they often can be taught in a succinct manner and can be carried out in homework assignments between visits to the clinician.
- Cognitive pathology in anxiety disorders (e.g., excessive fears, decreased estimate of ability to manage anxiety-provoking situations, heightened attention and vigilance about potential threats) stimulates patterns of avoidance, which in turn confirm and amplify maladaptive cognitions.
- Behavioral interventions in CBT can break the "vicious cycle" between fearful cognitions and avoidance.
- Avoidance can be manifested in several ways: 1) complete or partial

A log from month 2

Behavioral target	Goal	Results	Comment
Counting windowpanes	When entering a room, allow myself to count the panes in only one window and do this only once. Spend no more than 2 minutes doing this.	About 75% successful with this task. Sometimes found myself coming back to recount the panes in a window.	The counting is so automatic that it takes a real effort to resist it.
Counting numbers on license plates	Try not to do this at all.	Probably counted numbers on license plates about 15% of time.	I thought this would be easier to do, but I kept slipping back into the old routine.
Counting books in all the offices I visit	Count books in no more than three of the offices I enter each day. Count books only on the first shelf, then stop.	The first-shelf plan worked well—was able to stop there over 90% of time. But when I was in and out of many offices in a day, I usually counted books in more than three offices.	Just need to keep trying with this one.

Figure 9–4.   Exposure logs for treatment of obsessive-compulsive disorder: Prakash's example.

A log from month 5

Behavioral target	Goal	Results	Comment
Counting windowpanes	*Allow myself to look at windows with multiple panes, but do not do any counting of the panes. Only glance at the window for 10 seconds or less.*	*About 95% successful with this goal. Only very rarely do I start to count, and then I can usually stop it in a few seconds.*	*Much relief. I can give my full attention to work or other tasks.*
Counting utility poles and numbers on license plates	*No counting of utility poles. License plate number counting: less than 10% of plates.*	*Met all goals here. Very minimal license plate counting—I only glance at about 1 out of 100 plates.*	*This is no longer a problem.*
Counting books in all the offices I visit	*Look at bookshelf, appreciate the collection of books. Maybe glance at a few titles if close enough to read. Try to avoid all counting, but if counting starts, stop it within 15 seconds.*	*I am focusing more on the books that might be on the shelves instead of mindless counting. I am always able to stop within 15 seconds. Start counting only about 10% of time.*	*Getting close to getting this in really good control.*

Figure 9–4. Exposure logs for treatment of obsessive-compulsive disorder: Prakash's example (continued).

avoidance of a feared object or situation, 2) safety behaviors, and 3) lack of efforts to learn ways to cope better with feared situations.

- Relaxation training, positive imagery, and breathing retraining can be used alone in some applications (e.g., generalized anxiety disorder) but are most commonly delivered as parts of an overall CBT approach. These methods can facilitate participation in exposure therapy.

- Several useful aids (e.g., audio CDs, computer programs) are available for teaching and implementing progressive relaxation. These aids can conserve time in brief visits by helping patients develop relaxation skills on their own.

- Positive imagery can be a useful method for treating anxiety disorders in brief sessions. Patients can be instructed on use of relaxing mental images and encouraged to practice these methods between visits to the clinician.

- Breathing retraining is one of the core behavioral strategies for panic disorder. Implementing this method in brief sessions usually entails a mini-lesson, followed by modeling of a panicked breathing style and normal breathing. Patients are taught to slow breathing down to a normal rate and use adjunctive positive imagery to further calm anxious emotions and physical tension.

- Exposure therapy methods typically involve construction of a graded hierarchy that is used for systematic desensitization to triggers for anxiety. Effective hierarchical exposure can be promoted by selecting specific, measurable steps and designing a hierarchy with activities that have a wide range of difficulty levels (i.e., low, medium, and high degrees of difficulty).

- Therapeutic work with safety behaviors will usually provide additional benefit for patients who are following exposure therapy programs. When safety activities are identified, these behaviors can become targets for further exposure interventions.

- Exposure logs can be very useful ways of monitoring and supporting change. Assigning these logs for homework can help clinicians maximize the time available for brief sessions while increasing patient involvement in the self-help component of CBT.

Concepts and Skills for Patients to Learn

- People who have anxiety disorders often avoid feared objects or situations. Each time the situation is avoided, it just builds up the amount of fear and deepens a person's belief that she cannot cope with the situation.

- A key to overcoming anxiety disorders is developing a gradual plan to break patterns of avoidance.
- CBT for anxiety disorders usually involves developing a hierarchy—a stepwise list of ways to expose yourself to feared situations. By starting with activities that cause low levels of anxiety or distress, you can build your confidence and skills in managing the triggers for your fear.
- Clinicians coach and support you as you work through a hierarchy, but much of the work has to be done outside treatment sessions as you put lessons to work in everyday life.
- A number of behavioral methods can reduce anxiety and tension and help people overcome their fears. Some of the techniques that the clinician may teach you are relaxation exercises (ways of reducing muscle tension and stress), positive imagery (bringing calming images to mind), and breathing retraining (learning to focus on a relaxed style of breathing to stop panic attacks and other anxiety spells).
- Setting targets for change is a collaborative process in CBT. You and your clinician will use teamwork in designing hierarchies and planning the way to reach your goals.
- Logging your efforts to change is a very important part of CBT for anxiety. Try to monitor and write down your experiences as homework exercises, and bring these written accounts to your therapy sessions.

References

Arntz A: Cognitive therapy versus applied relaxation as a treatment of generalized anxiety disorder. Behav Res Ther 41:633–646, 2003

Bernstein DA, Borkovec TD: Progressive Relaxation Training: A Manual for the Helping Professions. Champaign, IL, Research Press, 1973

Clark DM, Ehlers A, Hackman A, et al: Cognitive therapy versus exposure and applied relaxation in social phobia: a randomized controlled trial. J Consult Clin Psychol 74:568–578, 2006

de Beurs E, Lange A, van Dyck R, et al: Respiratory training prior to exposure in vivo in the treatment of panic disorder with agoraphobia: efficacy and predictors of outcome. Aust N Z J Psychiatry 29:104–113, 1995

Ehlers A, Clark DM, Hackmann A, et al: Cognitive therapy for post-traumatic stress disorder: development and evaluation. Behav Res Ther 43:413–431, 2005

Foa EB, Liebowitz MR, Kozac MJ, et al: Randomized, placebo-controlled trial of exposure and ritual prevention, clomipramine, and their combination in the treatment of obsessive-compulsive disorder. Am J Psychiatry 162:151–161, 2005

Jacobsen E: Progressive Relaxation. Chicago, IL, University of Chicago Press, 1938

Klosko JS, Barlow DH: Cognitive-behavioral treatment of panic attacks, in Handbook of the Treatment of the Anxiety Disorders, 2nd Edition. Edited by Lindemann CG. Lanham, MD, Jason Aronson, 1996, pp 221–231

Manzoni GM, Pagnini F, Castelnuovo G, et al: Relaxation training for anxiety: a ten-years systematic review with meta-analysis. BMC Psychiatry 8:41, 2008 (online publication). Available at: http://www.biomedcentral.com/1471-244X/8/41. Accessed February 25, 2010.

Marks IM, Lelliott P, Basoglu M, et al: Clomipramine, self-exposure and therapist-aided exposure for obsessive-compulsive rituals. Br J Psychiatry 152:522–534, 1988

Mataix-Cols D, Marks IM: Self-help with minimal therapist contact for obsessive-compulsive disorder: a review. Eur Psychiatry 21:75–80, 2006

Ost LG, Breitholtz E: Applied relaxation vs. cognitive therapy in the treatment of generalized anxiety disorder. Behav Res Ther 38:777–790, 2000

Payne RA: Relaxation Techniques: A Practical Handbook for the Health Care Professional, 3rd Edition. London: Churchill Livingstone, 2005

Sanderson WC, Wetzler S: Cognitive behavioral treatment of panic disorder, in Panic Disorder: Clinical, Biological, and Treatment Aspects. Edited by Asnis GM, van Praag HM. Oxford, UK, Wiley, 1995, pp 314–335

Schmidt NB, Woolaway-Bickel K, Trakowski J, et al: Dismantling cognitive-behavioral treatment for panic disorder: questioning the utility of breathing retraining. J Consult Clin Psychol 68:417–424, 2000

Simpson, HB, Foa EB, Liebowitz MR, et al: A randomized, controlled trial of cognitive-behavioral therapy for augmenting pharmacotherapy in obsessive-compulsive disorder. Am J Psychiatry 165:621–630, 2008

Singer JL, DiFillippo JM, Overholser JC: Cognitive-behavioral treatment of panic disorder: confronting situational precipitants. Journal of Contemporary Psychotherapy 29:99–113, 1999

Taylor S: Breathing retraining in the treatment of panic disorder: efficacy, caveats and indications. Scandinavian Journal of Behaviour Therapy 30:49–56, 2001

Wolpe J: The Practice of Behavior Therapy. New York, Pergamon Press, 1969

Wolpe J: The current status of systematic desensitization. Am J Psychiatry 130:961–965, 1973

Wright JH, Basco MR, Thase ME: Learning Cognitive-Behavior Therapy: An Illustrated Guide. Washington, DC, American Psychiatric Publishing, 2006

CHAPTER 10

CBT Methods for Insomnia

```
┌─────────────────────────────────────────────┐
│                 LEARNING MAP                  │
│                                               │
│        CBT conceptualization of insomnia      │
│                      ⇩                        │
│     Evidence for efficacy of CBT for insomnia │
│                      ⇩                        │
│        Steps to manage insomnia with CBT      │
└─────────────────────────────────────────────┘
```

Insomnia is a costly and common condition, occurring as a chronic and persistent problem in 10%–15% of the population (Morin 2004). Forty-four percent of adults report a sleep problem every night or nearly every night (National Sleep Foundation 2008). In patients with medical and psychiatric illnesses, insomnia is more likely to be persistent and to have negative impacts on quality of life and work performance (Ford and Kamerow 1989; Simon and Von Korff 1997). Sleep disturbance is an independent risk factor for depression recurrence in older adults (Cho et al. 2008) and can predict relapse in alcoholics (Currie et al. 2004). In elderly persons, sleep problems can decrease health function and increase mortality (Newman et al. 1997; Pollak et al. 1990).

Studies of cognitive-behavior therapy (CBT) for insomnia have shown durable increases in sleep times and decreased sleep latency (Morin

2004), even in patients with medical or psychiatric comorbidity (Smith et al. 2005). In this chapter, we give an overview of the CBT conceptualization for insomnia, discuss some of the evidence for effectiveness of this approach, and then detail practical methods that are well suited for work in brief sessions.

CBT Conceptualization of Insomnia

Morin and Espie (2004) described a vicious cycle that occurs in insomnia and provided a conceptual framework for guiding cognitive-behavioral treatment (Figure 10–1). The essence of this view of insomnia is as follows:

1. Once insomnia is established, whatever the cause, cognitions about the sleep disturbance can play a role in worsening and/or perpetuating the problem. Examples of dysfunctional cognitions include worry about getting to sleep, hypervigilance about sleep, and inability to turn off worries from the day that intrude upon sleep.
2. Maladaptive cognitions about sleep may increase arousal and thus interfere with sleep patterns.
3. Behavioral sleep disturbances, such as poor sleep hygiene, irregular sleep and wake times, and daytime naps, often play a role in insomnia. These behavioral problems can be influenced by dysfunctional cognitions.
4. Insomnia is not only a problem at night. Patients with sleep disruption also have insomnia-related symptoms during the day. These include emotional symptoms (irritability, lability, anxiety), cognitive symptoms (memory and concentration difficulties, worry, and rumination), behavioral symptoms (naps, absenteeism), and interpersonal symptoms (withdrawal from relationships).

Evidence for Efficacy of CBT for Insomnia

In two meta-analyses, behavioral interventions for insomnia were shown to be durable and to produce significant change in 70%–80% of patients who used them (Morin et al. 1994; Murtagh and Greenwood 1995). The evidence base for CBT interventions clearly indicates that the components of CBT for insomnia, particularly stimulus control and sleep restriction, have a high degree of success in multiple populations with sleep disturbances (Edinger and Mears 2005). Also, studies have demonstrated that CBT interventions can be learned when taught in brief sessions by phone (Bastien et al. 2004) and in groups (Espie et al. 2001).

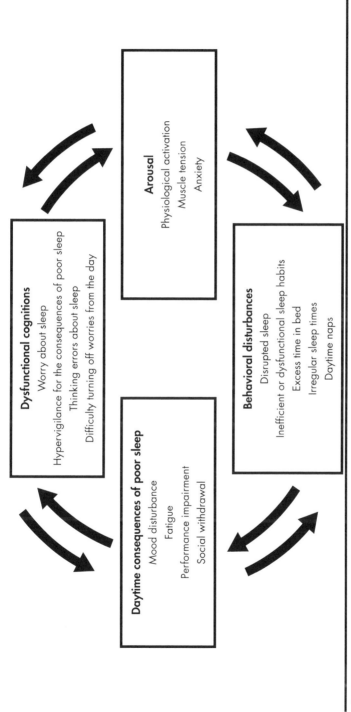

Figure 10–1. Cognitive-behavior therapy conceptualization of insomnia.

Source. Adapted with permission from Morin CM: *Insomnia: Psychological Assessment and Management.* New York, Guilford, 1993. Copyright © 1993 The Guilford Press. Used with permission of The Guilford Press.

Combining sleeping medications with CBT for insomnia is less clearly beneficial for patients. Only a few studies have evaluated combined treatment. In the short term, combined treatment has a slight advantage over either treatment alone, but in long-term follow-up, CBT alone is far more durable (Morin et al. 1999). Taking medication for sleep might produce dysfunctional thoughts about CBT interventions (e.g., "I can only do this because I am on medication") that make change less likely. Results of several studies (Morin et al. 2004; Zavesicka et al. 2008) point to the possibility that CBT may facilitate tapering and withdrawal from hypnotics and improve the sleep quality of patients taking benzodiazepines and similar drugs. We emphasize that we are referring here to patients whose primary condition is not likely to deteriorate with a brief period of significant lack of sleep. Patients who have bipolar disorder, for example, may require the use of sleeping medication in the short term to help reduce the chances for a worsening of their mood symptoms.

Steps to Manage Insomnia With CBT

The primary interventions used in CBT for insomnia are listed in Table 10–1. Each has been validated as a useful tool for sleep disturbance. Clinicians should determine the sequence and use of each intervention based on the case conceptualization. Many psychiatrists and other prescribing clinicians who use CBT in briefer sessions will be using these techniques with patients who do not have insomnia as the primary presenting complaint but who develop insomnia secondary to another psychiatric disorder. In these instances, sleep hygiene, lifestyle management, and relaxation training may be sufficient on their own to help patients sleep well. However, for patients with primary chronic insomnia, a more comprehensive approach may be needed.

Table 10–1. Steps to manage insomnia

Assess sleep habits

Psychoeducation

Sleep hygiene and lifestyle modification

Stimulus control

Sleep restriction

Relaxation training

Positive imagery

Cognitive restructuring

Assess Sleep Habits

A good first step to help patients sleep better is to have them keep a diary or log of their sleep habits. A typical example of a sleep diary is shown in Figure 10–2. This tool can help patients in a number of ways: it provides detailed data on sleep patterns for use in planning treatment; yields evidence about the effects of certain behaviors on sleep (e.g., going to the kitchen for a snack or going to another bedroom after awakening); helps with gauging the success of CBT interventions for sleep; helps patients be better detectives about factors that interfere with adequate rest; and helps in changing cognitions about sleep—patients frequently overestimate the time it takes to fall asleep, underestimate the time they spend asleep, and catastrophize about the results of poor sleep. Sleep logs can be excellent between-session homework assignments and are a prime example of efficient CBT methods that can enhance the quality of brief sessions.

Dr. Sudak asked Grace, who was introduced in Chapter 3, "Enhancing the Impact of Brief Sessions," to complete a sleep diary for one of her homework assignments. Grace completed the diary for 2 weeknights (Monday and Tuesday) and the weekend (Figure 10–3). This allowed them to review the typical sleep habits she had and modify those that interfered with good sleep. As you can see, Grace had the common pattern of altering her sleep on weekends, by getting up and going to bed later than usual and by napping during the day. This behavior, in addition to her anxiety about the start of the workweek, set the stage for sleep problems. After Grace kept this record and saw the evidence for herself, she made an effort to relinquish her naps and late bedtimes on weekends.

We recommend that you complete the next learning exercise to learn more about how sleep diaries can be helpful in managing insomnia. If you have sleep problems yourself, you can complete the log for 3 nights of your own sleep experiences. If you are lucky enough to have a great sleep pattern, you can ask one or more of your patients to complete a sleep diary.

> **Learning Exercise 10–1**   Using a Sleep Diary
>
> 1. Complete a sleep diary for 3 nights of your own sleep and/ or ask one of your patients to use the sleep log.
>
> 2. Review the results of recording sleep patterns. Consider these results in planning interventions based on the methods described in this chapter.

	Monday	Tuesday	Wednesday	Thursday	Friday	Saturday	Sunday
Bedtime							
Time fell asleep							
Hours asleep							
Sleep breaks							
Wake-up time							
Naps?							
Quality of sleep							
Alcohol/ medications?							

Figure 10–2.   Sleep diary.

Note.   This sleep diary is also provided in Appendix 1, "Worksheets and Checklists."

	Monday	Tuesday	Wednesday	Thursday	Friday	Saturday	Sunday
Bedtime	10:30 P.M.	10:49 P.M.				12:30 A.M.	11:30 P.M.
Time fell asleep	11 P.M.	11 P.M.				1 A.M.	1 A.M.
Hours asleep	6	5.5				6.5	5
Sleep breaks	3	4				2	4
Wake-up time	6:30 A.M.	6 A.M.				9 A.M.	7 A.M.
Naps?	No	No				Yes	Yes
Quality of sleep	Fair	Poor				Fair	Poor
Alcohol/ medications?	No	No				No	No

Figure 10–3. Grace's sleep diary.

Table 10–2. Psychoeducational resources for improving sleep

Books

Edinger J, Carney C: Overcoming Insomnia: A Cognitive Behavioral
  Approach—Therapist Guide. New York, Oxford University Press,
  2008

Hauri P, Linde S: No More Sleepless Nights. Hoboken, NJ, Wiley, 1996

Jacobs G, Benson H: Say Good Night to Insomnia: The Six-Week, Drug-
  Free Program Developed at Harvard Medical School. New York, Owl
  Books, 1999

Morin CM: Relief From Insomnia: Getting the Sleep of Your Dreams.
  New York, Doubleday, 1996

Web sites

www.cbtforinsomnia.com (interactive CBT Web-based program)

www.helpguide.org/life/insomnia_treatment.htm (psychoeducation
  about insomnia, cognitive-behavior therapy and relaxation tips, sleep
  diary, links to other sites)

www.sleepfoundation.org (podcasts, videos, print materials about
  different types of sleep disorders, online sleep store)

Note.   These resources are also listed in Appendix 2, "CBT Resources for
Patients and Families."

Psychoeducation

Educating patients about normal sleep and about maladaptive habits that
subvert sleep is a key element of CBT for insomnia. Psychoeducation can
be efficiently accomplished via assigned readings, handouts, and online
resources (see suggestions in Table 10–2). When patients find parts of the
treatment (e.g., sleep restriction) hard to accept, educational resources
can help validate the evidence base for these procedures.

Sleep Hygiene and Lifestyle Modification

Sleep hygiene recommendations and lifestyle management are used to
change habits that sabotage good sleep. Poor sleep habits include sleeping
with the television on all night or keeping work in the bedroom. The assessment of insomnia should include a careful behavioral analysis of the patient's
habits that may influence sleep. How much caffeine does the patient ingest
each day? When is the caffeine consumed? What is the bedroom environment? Does the patient have a routine to wind down at the end of the day?
What does the patient do if she wakes up during the night? After obtaining

---

Table 10–3. Good sleep practices

Have regular bedtimes and awakening times.

Have a wake-up routine that increases exposure to bright light as early as possible after waking.

Use caffeine sparingly, if at all, and always before noon.

Minimize alcohol use because it frequently causes rebound insomnia.

Avoid nicotine.

Avoid eating heavily close to bedtime. A light snack can be OK for some people.

Make certain that your bedroom is dark and quiet, and the temperature is comfortable.

Eliminate noise with earplugs or use a sound machine.

Try to establish a bedtime ritual and "wind down" as bedtime approaches—a bath, herbal tea, prayer, or meditation can be very helpful in calming you after the stimulation of the day. Leave worries out of bed.

Develop an exercise routine and complete it before 5 P.M.

---

this information, the therapist and patient can problem-solve obstacles to making changes in habits that would promote improved sleep. Patients are often unaware of basic steps they can take to improve the quality of their sleep. Table 10–3 lists some common elements of healthy sleep hygiene.

Stimulus Control

Stimulus control methods are an extension of the sleep hygiene recommendations described in the previous subsection. A somewhat more detailed plan is constructed to help patients 1) reduce exposure to stimuli that may interrupt sleep and 2) set up a healthy routine for promoting good sleep. Cognitive restructuring may be needed to convince patients to implement stimulus control, because they can have beliefs about sleep that perpetuate the habits that worsen insomnia (i.e., "I must have the TV on to fall asleep," "If I don't get enough sleep at night, I should take an afternoon nap"). Table 10–4 lists some useful stimulus control methods for improving sleep.

Sleep Restriction

Sleep restriction is a powerful technique that can help patients with chronic insomnia. This method is not typically used for sleep disruption

---

Table 10–4. Stimulus control methods for improving sleep

Use your bed only for sleep or sexual activity. Sleep is a habit, and the more you associate the bed with sleep, the better. Do not pay bills, eat, work on your computer, watch TV, argue, or talk on the phone in bed.

Remove distractions such as exercise equipment, hobby and craft supplies, or unopened mail from the bedroom.

Improve the comfort of your bed. Consider new, more comfortable pillows and sheets; rearrange the bedroom furniture; or get a new mattress if needed.

If you are unable to sleep after 15 minutes, do not stay in bed; instead, sit up and do a monotonous and/or soothing activity in a dimly lighted room. When you feel sleepy again, return to bed. Do not watch the clock but estimate the 15 minutes. Repeat this as often as needed.

---

associated with acute episodes of depression, mania, or psychosis. The purpose of sleep restriction is to consolidate and increase the efficiency of sleep. This technique can restore the normal homeostatic rhythm to patients' sleep cycles. To employ sleep restriction, the clinician requests that the patient decrease the amount of time spent in bed by a modest amount (e.g., to 85% of his average total sleep time) and to take no naps during the day. If the patient usually spends 7 hours per night in bed, the clinician might suggest that the patient set an alarm and get up after 6 hours.

When sleep restriction is employed, the natural drive to sleep will usually increase. The patient is then asked to gradually increase sleep by a small increment (15 minutes) each night, as long as he sleeps without interruption. Patients often need significant amounts of education to motivate them to engage in this strategy, and some spontaneously reveal beliefs they have about sleep that compound their insomnia (i.e., "I cannot function with fewer than 8 hours of sleep"). Clinicians need to be mindful of preexisting conditions (e.g., bipolar disorder, seizure disorder) that can be made worse by deliberately decreasing sleep time; sleep restriction should be avoided in these situations.

Relaxation Training

Relaxation training is another component of CBT for insomnia. This technique is described in detail in Chapter 9, "Behavioral Methods for Anxiety." Relaxation training can be taught by the clinician in a session with live practice, and a recording can be made of the in-therapy instructions. Also, several excellent relaxation training CDs are commercially available (see "Resources for Relaxation Training and Practice" in Appendix 2, "CBT Resources for Patients and Families"). We usually suggest that patients build their skills in relaxation training by practicing this technique during the day when they are not especially anxious and are not trying to get to sleep. This practice can help the patient to implement the method with less effort at bedtime or during periods of wakefulness.

Positive Imagery

An additional CBT method for anxiety described in Chapter 9, "Behavioral Methods for Anxiety," can be used to reduce or shift away from worrisome thoughts, tension, or other problems that are interfering with sleep. Positive imagery and related methods such as mindfulness can help people focus their attention on calming mental images that can help induce sleep. Examples of positive imagery include focusing on pleasant memories of walking along a beach or sitting beside a mountain stream on a fine day in early summer, or imaging the casting stroke of an accomplished fly fisherman. Positive imagery is the favorite technique for personal use by one of the authors, who experiences middle-of-the-night awakenings.

Cognitive Restructuring

Cognitive restructuring can be employed to decrease automatic thoughts and beliefs that are serving as powerful maintenance factors for insomnia. Harvey (2005) described a series of sleep-related beliefs that occur both at night and in the daytime that can perpetuate insomnia. These can include beliefs about the daytime effects of poor sleep and misattributions about the deleterious effects of poor sleep (e.g., "I performed poorly at work today because I slept poorly"), dysfunctional and unrealistic beliefs about sleep itself (e.g., "If I don't get 8 hours of sleep, I will be a total mess"), and beliefs about what one should do to make certain that sleep occurs in a particular way (e.g., "If I don't sleep for 8 hours, I should stay in bed as long as I need to make up for it"). Individuals with insomnia are more prone to worry and to have anticipatory anxiety about being able to sleep. They also automatically scan for sleep-related threats (e.g., "If the room is too cool, I will never get to sleep"). Selective attention to these threats can aggravate dysfunctional sleeping patterns. Table 10–5 displays some common automatic thoughts about sleep that can be targets for CBT interventions.

 All of the methods described in Chapter 7, "Targeting Maladaptive Thinking" (see Table 7–9), can be used to modify dysfunctional cognitions about sleep. For example, Socratic questions can help determine the

Table 10–5. Typical automatic thoughts that interfere with sleep

I will have a terrible day if I don't sleep well.

People must sleep 8 hours per night to function.

If I sleep poorly, I must take a nap to make up for it.

I can't function without a good night's sleep.

I will never be able to get back to sleep.

I cannot go back to sleep if a noise awakens me.

If I wake up and I don't feel rested, I know it will be a bad day.

Worrying in bed at night helps me sort things out.

accuracy and utility of a patient's thoughts about sleep. Thought records, sleep/wake logs, and behavioral experiments for restricting sleep can be employed to help a patient develop new and more accurate perspectives about sleep. The goal of these interventions is also to decrease the cognitive arousal often associated with poor sleep. Figure 10–4 shows a sequence of cognitive restructuring that led a patient to a less rigid and more adaptive belief about need for sleep.

Video Illustration 11 highlights the practical CBT methods for treating sleep problems that are described in this chapter. This segment shows Dr. Sudak working with Grace after she has started her new job.

Dr. Sudak quickly assesses Grace's sleep habits and finds that Grace is carrying lots of worries and pressures from the day into the time when she is trying to fall asleep. Also, her bedroom environment is less than ideal. She keeps leftover work from her job and various assignments from her children's classes next to her bed so that she can deal with them when time is available.

Another of Grace's problems is falling asleep with the TV on and then waking up to turn it off. She explains that after her husband's death, she began to keep the TV on because "It is company" and she "likes the noise." Still another problem is her irregular sleep and wake times. On weekends she stays up late, sleeps in, and takes naps.

▶ **Video Illustration 11.** CBT for Insomnia: Dr. Sudak and Grace

In this video, Dr. Sudak uses several of the CBT methods from Table 10–1 to help Grace improve her sleep. A major initiative in this brief session is to use stimulus control procedures to improve Grace's sleeping environment. They work collaboratively to design a plan to 1) keep the TV off, 2) get all of the work stuff out of the bedroom, and 3) substitute a sound generator with soothing audio instead of the TV.

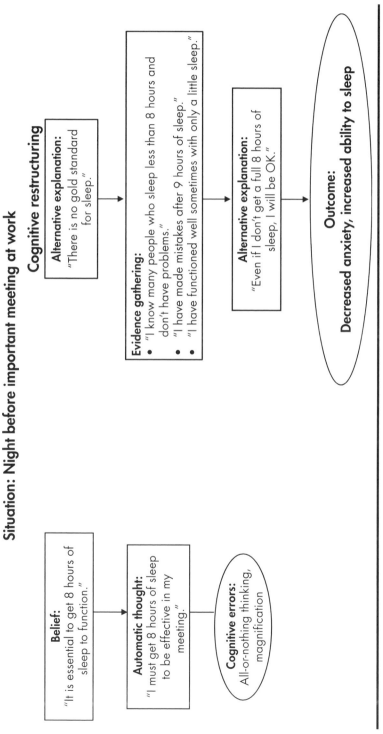

Figure 10–4. A cognitive restructuring sequence leading to a more adaptive belief about sleep.

Dr. Sudak and Grace also decide that Grace will set aside a time and place (not the bedroom) for completing tasks and addressing worries earlier in the evening, and she will work toward making sleep and wake times more routine on all days of the week. All of these changes are part of a behavioral experiment in which Grace is asked to modify her routine and then observe the effects on her sleep. This type of behavioral experiment demonstrates a fundamental principle of CBT—partnering with the patient to try new behaviors, collecting data about the project, and evaluating the outcome in an empirical style.

Summary

Key Points for Clinicians

- Dysfunctional cognitions about sleep, emotional and physiological arousal, maladaptive sleep behaviors, and the daytime consequences of poor sleep can become part of a vicious cycle that maintains and/ or deepens problems with insomnia.
- CBT methods for insomnia are typically directed at 1) modifying or building coping skills for worries or other cognitions that interfere with sleep and 2) promoting healthy sleep behaviors.
- CBT interventions are highly effective for insomnia.
- A mini-formulation of the patient's sleep-related thoughts, emotions, and behaviors will help in providing targeted treatment.
- Sleep diaries can be very useful tools for assessing sleep problems and planning interventions.
- Sleep hygiene and lifestyle modification are highly important components of the CBT approach to insomnia.
- Many useful educational tools can help patients develop better sleep habits. Books and Internet-delivered programs can help clinicians provide efficient psychoeducation in brief sessions.
- Some of the specific methods that are used for promoting good sleep are stimulus control, relaxation training, positive imagery, sleep restriction, and cognitive restructuring.

Concepts and Skills for Patients to Learn

- If you have insomnia, your sleeping habits or lifestyle patterns may be a big part of the problem. Some of the habits that can interfere with getting a good night's sleep are drinking beverages with caffeine, having irregular sleep and wake times, lack of exercise, use of alcohol or drugs, and having a bedroom environment that distracts you from sleep.

- Changing habits and lifestyle can be the key ingredient in an effective plan to improve sleep.
- People also can have trouble shutting off worries at bedtime, or they can have beliefs about sleep that can sabotage the ability to sleep well. CBT can help you learn to reduce or better cope with worries and to develop sleep-promoting beliefs.
- A number of different CBT techniques can help people get restful sleep. Some of these methods include 1) teaching you to relax your mind, muscles, and emotions; 2) building skills in using positive images to calm yourself; and 3) experimenting with restricting your time in bed to help you sleep better.

References

Bastien CH, Morin CM, Ouellet MC, et al: Cognitive-behavioral therapy for insomnia: comparison of individual therapy, group therapy, and telephone consultations. J Consult Clin Psychol 72:653–659, 2004

Cho HJ, Lavretsky H, Olmstead R, et al: Sleep disturbance and depression recurrence in community-dwelling older adults: prospective study. Am J Psychiatry 165:1543–1550, 2008

Currie SR, Clark S, Hodgins DC, et al: Randomized controlled trial of brief cognitive-behavioural interventions for insomnia in recovering alcoholics. Addiction 99:1121–1132, 2004

Edinger JD, Mears MK: Cognitive-behavioral therapy for primary insomnia. Clin Psychol Rev 25:539–558, 2005

Espie CA, Inglis SJ, Tessier S, et al: The clinical effectiveness of cognitive behaviour therapy for chronic insomnia: implementation and evaluation of a sleep clinic in general medical practice. Behav Res Ther 39:45–60, 2001

Ford DE, Kamerow DB: Epidemiologic study of sleep disturbances and psychiatric disorders: an opportunity for prevention? JAMA 262:1479–1484, 1989

Harvey AG: A cognitive theory and therapy for chronic insomnia. J Cogn Psychother 19:41–59, 2005

Morin CM: Cognitive-behavioral approaches to the treatment of insomnia. J Clin Psychiatry 65 (suppl 16):33–40, 2004

Morin CM, Espie CA: Insomnia: A Clinical Guide to Assessment and Treatment. New York, Springer, 2004

Morin CM, Culbert JP, Schwartz SM: Nonpharmacological interventions for insomnia: a meta-analysis of treatment efficacy. Am J Psychiatry 151:1172–1180, 1994

Morin CM, Colecchi CA, Stone J, et al: Behavioral and pharmacological therapies for late-life insomnia: a randomized clinical trial. JAMA 281:991–999, 1999

Morin CM, Bastien C, Guay B, et al: Randomized clinical trial of supervised tapering and cognitive behavior therapy to facilitate benzodiazepine discontinuation in older adults with chronic insomnia. Am J Psychiatry 161:332–342, 2004

Murtagh DRR, Greenwood KM: Identifying effective psychological treatments for insomnia: a meta-analysis. J Consult Clin Psychol 63:79–89, 1995

National Sleep Foundation: 2008 Sleep in America poll. Available at: www.sleepfoundation.org. Accessed December 25, 2009.

Newman AB, Enright PL, Manolio TA, et al: Sleep disturbance, psychosocial correlates, and cardiovascular disease in 5201 older adults: the Cardiovascular Health Study. J Am Geriatr Soc 45:1–7, 1997

Pollak CP, Perlick D, Linsner JP, et al: Sleep problems in the community elderly as predictors of death and nursing home placement. J Community Health 15:123–135, 1990

Simon GE, Von Korff M: Prevalence, burden and treatment of insomnia in primary care. Am J Psychiatry 154:1417–1423, 1997

Smith MT, Huang MI, Manber R: Cognitive behavior therapy for chronic insomnia occurring within the context of medical and psychiatric disorders. Clin Psychol Rev 25:559–592, 2005

Zavesicka L, Brunovsky M, Matousek M, et al: Discontinuation of hypnotics during cognitive behavioral therapy for insomnia. BMC Psychiatry 8:80, 2008

CHAPTER 11

Modifying Delusions

```
┌─────────────────────────────────────────────┐
│              LEARNING MAP                     │
│                                               │
│          Overview of CBT for delusions        │
│                                               │
│                      ⇩                        │
│                                               │
│        Fifteen brief CBT methods for delusions│
│                                               │
│                      ⇩                        │
│                                               │
│      Case example of CBT for delusions: Helen │
│                                               │
│                      ⇩                        │
│                                               │
│      Practice case: planning a CBT intervention for │
│                     delusions                 │
└─────────────────────────────────────────────┘
```

Psychiatric treatment of patients with psychotic symptoms is commonly conducted in sessions that are briefer than 50-minute hours (Kingdon and Turkington 1991; Tarrier et al. 1993; Turkington and Kingdon 2000). Brief sessions are used because these patients have 1) problems with concentration and attention that are aggravated by active delusions and/or hallucinations; 2) thought disorder; 3) negative symptoms such as apathy or social withdrawal; and 4) low motivation for lengthy, cognitively taxing treatment appointments. Despite these potential impediments to the psychotherapeutic process, an extensive research effort has supported the value of using cognitive-behavior therapy (CBT) methods to augment pharmacotherapy for patients with schizophrenia and other psychoses (National Institute for Clinical Excellence 2009).

Interested readers can find comprehensive descriptions of CBT methods for psychosis in several texts (Kingdon and Turkington 2005; Morrison et al. 2004; Wright et al. 2009). In this chapter, we briefly outline the core CBT strategies for working with delusions and then offer suggestions for 15 valuable interventions that can be used in brief sessions. Case examples are included to illustrate use of CBT methods for psychoses and to provide opportunities for building skills in this approach.

Overview of CBT for Delusions

General procedures for using CBT for delusions are listed in Table 11–1. These fundamental methods are used for working with delusions in a variety of psychiatric disorders, including schizophrenia, schizoaffective disorder, and major depression with psychotic features.

Delusions Are Viewed as Misperceptions That Can Be Modified With CBT Methods

Because delusions have classically been seen as all-or-nothing phenomena that are not amenable to reason (Jaspers 1913), clinicians have not usually been taught to directly question or attempt to modify delusions or other psychotic symptoms with psychotherapeutic methods. In fact, working with delusional content has been actively discouraged (Fish 1962). The reasoning for this "hands-off" approach has been a concern that delusions might be exacerbated due to the mechanism of reinforcement—the more you discuss delusions, the worse they get.

The idea that direct therapeutic interventions for treating delusions might be possible was first explored in an early case study by Aaron Beck (1952). The work of Strauss (1969) was also influential in the development of the CBT approach to psychosis because it showed that delusions and hallucinations could be viewed as points on a continuum. Thereafter, a number of case studies (e.g., Hole et al. 1979; Kingdon and Turkington 1991) and randomized controlled trials (e.g., Sensky et al. 2000; Tarrier et al. 1993; Turkington et al. 2002) showed that patients did not become more deluded or more behaviorally disturbed when psychiatrists focused on their delusions; in fact, they often improved.

Table 11–1. General features of cognitive-behavior therapy (CBT) for delusions

Delusions are viewed as misperceptions that can be modified with CBT methods.

A comprehensive cognitive-behavioral-biological-sociocultural model guides treatment.

A collaborative therapeutic relationship is required for effective use of CBT for delusions.

Normalizing and educating are fundamental methods in the CBT approach to psychotic symptoms.

A Comprehensive Cognitive-Behavioral-Biological-Sociocultural Model Guides Treatment

The comprehensive and integrative model described in Chapter 1, "Introduction," can be used to formulate and plan CBT interventions for psychotic symptoms (Wright et al. 2009). Psychoses are considered to be illnesses that have very strong genetic and biological roots. As with many other complex disorders, however, environmental factors are thought to play a highly significant role in disease expression and in amelioration or maintenance of symptoms. Thus, in planning treatment interventions, clinicians may consider developmental influences such as early traumas, bullying, or other stressful events that may have played a role in triggering the patient's symptoms; comorbid problems such as substance use or abuse or anxiety disorders; and the patient's strengths and supports. The case illustrations detailed later in this chapter show the use of a comprehensive, integrative formulation in planning CBT interventions for psychotic symptoms.

A Collaborative Therapeutic Relationship Is Required for Effective Use of CBT for Delusions

Developing a collaborative-empirical therapeutic relationship, as described in Chapter 3, "Enhancing the Impact of Brief Sessions," is a crucial step in implementing CBT methods for psychotic symptoms. Clinicians may need to adapt their clinical style to begin to work in this way. For example, special efforts may be required in the beginning of treatment to put patients at ease. Depending on the severity and phase of illness (e.g., amount of hypervigilance and paranoia), clinicians may need to start the engagement with discussions about nonthreatening or neutral topics, such as news items or the weather. Then, after a greater degree of comfort is evident in the relationship, clinicians can start to direct their questioning toward delusional content or other psychotic symptoms.

As demonstrated in the video illustrations that we discuss later in this chapter, clinicians who are using CBT should show an attitude of respect for patients' delusional perceptions. Instead of being dismissive of the possible validity of the cognition, clinicians should use an empirical approach and express genuine interest in understanding the delusional belief. Rather than being collusive or humoring, the clinician should take the stance that the belief is a hypothesis that can be checked out and tested through questioning and behavioral experiments. Part of this process involves *examining the evidence*—a standard CBT technique that allows the patient and clinician to determine the validity, if any, of parts of the delusional belief.

Being open to confirming at least some components of the delusional belief can often help the clinician to engage patients in productive CBT work. For example, in Chapter 5, "Promoting Adherence," we described Glenn, a patient with schizophrenia who was refusing treatment with clozapine because he believed it was an experimental drug. When Glenn participated in a collaborative exploration of this belief with Dr. Wright, one of the pieces of evidence that was uncovered was that a research study was being conducted at the facility. By validating this finding, and then explaining that the research study had nothing to do with clozapine, which was already approved by the U.S. Food and Drug Administration, Dr. Wright helped the patient to change his delusional belief and then accept treatment with this medication.

Normalizing and Educating are Fundamental Methods in the CBT Approach to Psychotic Symptoms

The term *normalizing* in this context refers to the process of destigmatizing psychosis by helping patients to see that symptoms such as delusions and hallucinations are very common and that they can be stimulated by stress, grief, sleep deprivation, and other life events that many people experience. An important observation that can be shared with patients is that persons from normal community samples frequently report paranoia and delusions (Johns and van Os 2001). The prevalence of delusions has been shown to be between 6% and 9% (Freeman 2006).

Normalizing and educating go hand in hand. After making some normalizing comments, clinicians can educate patients further using guided discovery and mini-lessons (as described in Chapter 3, "Enhancing the

Impact of Brief Sessions"). Handouts, readings, or Web sites can also be used to help the patient learn about psychosis and its treatment. The Web site www.paranoidthoughts.com and a linked self-help book by Freeman et al. (2006) provide excellent information that normalizes delusions and helps people learn to cope better with these experiences. Table 11–2 has a list of valuable books, handouts, and Web sites that can be recommended to patients with psychotic symptoms.

Fifteen Brief CBT Methods for Delusions

We have found that a large number of CBT methods are useful for treating patients with delusions in brief sessions. The selection of methods is based on the case formulation. Two or more of these methods are often combined in a session. For example, Socratic questioning and examining the evidence might set the stage for developing a coping card, or a behavioral experiment might be used to help generate alternative explanations and to build coping skills for managing delusions. We offer the following menu of choices for clinicians who want to augment pharmacotherapy for psychosis by adding targeted CBT methods in brief visits.

1. **Explore the delusion using Socratic questioning.** Patients with delusions typically jump to conclusions and form strong beliefs without considering enough evidence. Illogical conclusions can be explored sensitively with a series of questions that encourage patients to look at a broader range of evidence and to take a fresh perspective on the situation.

   Patient: I believe that at times I must be screaming and shouting in public.
   Clinician: (doubts that patient is actually exhibiting this behavior because history and family report suggest no evidence of screaming or shouting in public) That's a frightening idea. Has somebody told you that you were screaming and shouting? How would you know if this was actually happening?
   Patient: I don't know. It just seems that people are looking at me all the time like I have done something wrong.
   Clinician: Maybe we could think together about your fears. How would people typically react if somebody suddenly started screaming in public?
   Patient: I guess they would get real upset. They might run away or call the police.
   Clinician: OK. Let's check what happens when you are out in public. Has anyone ever run away or called the police on you, or reacted in any other strong manner?
   Patient: No, nothing like that.

Table 11–2. Resources for patients with psychosis

Books

Freeman D, Freeman J, Garety P: Overcoming Paranoid and Suspicious Thoughts. London, Robinson, 2006

Mueser KT, Gingerich S: The Complete Family Guide to Schizophrenia. New York, Guilford, 2006

Romme M, Escher S: Understanding Voices: Coping with Auditory Hallucinations and Confusing Realities. London, Handsell, 1996

Turkington D, Kingdon D, Rathod S, et al: Back to Life, Back to Normality: Cognitive Therapy, Recovery and Psychosis. Cambridge, UK, Cambridge University Press, 2009

Handouts

Kingdon DG, Turkington D: Understanding what others think, in Cognitive Therapy of Schizophrenia. New York, Guilford, 2005

Kingdon D, Turkington D: What's happening to me? A voice hearing pamphlet, in Cognitive Therapy of Schizophrenia. New York, Guilford, 2005

Web sites with educational information

Hearing Voices Network
www.hearing-voices.org
Provides practical advice for understanding voice hearing.

National Alliance on Mental Illness
www.nami.org
Provides education on severe mental disorders, support for patients and families, advocacy.

National Institute of Mental Health
www.nimh.nih.gov
Provides general information on research and treatment of severe mental disorders.

Gloucestershire Hearing Voices & Recovery Groups
www.hearingvoices.org.uk/info_resources11.htm
Provides examples of coping skills for voice hearing.

Paranoid Thoughts
www.paranoidthoughts.com
Gives helpful advice on coping with paranoia.

Belief: TV shows are sending me messages. They know all about me.

Evidence for	Evidence against
Content of show often has same themes as problems in my life.	*Filmed in other cities, often weeks or months before being shown.*
Characters can be angry or can seem to tease me.	*Why would writers of the show have any interest in my life here in Kentucky?*
They are always going on about sex, and I don't get any.	*My sister and mother tell me that there is no chance that the TV is sending me special messages.*
	My illness makes me overly sensitive to things.
	I am paying too much attention to TV instead of other things in my life.

Figure 11–1. Examining the evidence for a delusion: Rhonda's example.

Source. From Wright JH, Turkington D, Kingdon DG, et al: *Cognitive-Behavior Therapy for Severe Mental Illness: An Illustrated Guide.* Washington, DC, American Psychiatric Publishing, 2009, p. 109. Used with permission. Copyright © 2009 American Psychiatric Publishing.

They go on to discuss the subtle signals that the patient thinks might mean that he has caused some major social gaffe (such as screaming in public) and conclude with the explanation that his illness makes him very sensitive to social cues but that he has not behaved inappropriately.

2. **Write out the evidence for and against a belief.** A two-column worksheet can be used to write down evidence for and against a belief and to work toward generating alternative beliefs. Writing down the evidence can encourage patients to pay attention to the findings and to recall work done in the session. This method can also be used for homework if the patient is able to benefit from homework exercises. Figure 11–1 shows an example of a written exercise in examining the evidence.

3. **Explore the antecedents of a delusion.** Ask the patient when this belief first became apparent and what was happening in his life at that time. The purpose is to show the patient that perhaps he jumped to a conclusion when under stress and that other explanations are possible.

Clinician: How did this belief about the Mafia first start?
Patient: I was in an Italian restaurant and the waiter gave me a knowing
     look.
Clinician: What were you doing before the meal?
Patient: I had been at the job center, but they didn't have any work that
     day.
Clinician: How did you lose your previous job?
Patient: I had a little business cleaning houses, but I lost some customers,
     and I had a bank overdraft. Then everything fell apart. (tears
     and anger)
Clinician: I'm really sorry to hear about all of your troubles. It sounds like
     you were under great pressure at that time. Sometimes when
     we are really stressed, it can color how we see things. I wonder
     if all of the stress could have played a part in causing you to
     start worrying about the Mafia being after you.

4. **Identify the fine details of the delusional belief.** It is not enough to
   know that a person believes that the police have her under surveillance. Clinicians who are providing CBT need to seek details about
   the mechanisms that the patient believes are being employed. This
   information can then be used to help revise the patient's thinking.
   Some mechanisms that might be reported include computers, satellites, phone lines, or tiny cameras. Psychoeducation and reality testing
   can then be directed at the specific reasons that the delusion seems
   believable.

5. **Develop coping strategies or rational responses for emotions (e.g.,
   shame, anxiety, sadness, or anger) linked to delusions.** Intense mood
   states that are reinforcing delusional beliefs can be recognized through
   direct questioning, imagery exercises to recreate stressful situations, review of thought records, or a variety of other standard CBT methods.

   Clinician: When you dwell on your belief that you are John the Baptist,
        and it is your mission to rid the world of pornography, how do
        you usually feel?
   Patient: Frustrated and angry with people who deal in such filth.

   This expression of emotion gives the clinician a possible way to work
   on the delusion. Perhaps the anger could be reduced by considering
   the evidence that if the news agent did not sell those magazines, he
   would become bankrupt. The anger could also be reduced by guiding
   the patient to consider that the pornography on sale is not illegal. Additionally, behavioral methods such as exercise or relaxation training
   might be considered to lower the level of anger and tension.

6. **Ask peripheral questions.** Peripheral questions are practical inquiries
   about the mechanisms by which a psychotic belief might function in

the real world. They are less probing than Socratic questions. Because peripheral questions are usually not threatening, they may be particularly useful for patients who hold rigid delusional beliefs. For example, if a patient reported, "A satellite is draining my thoughts and moving my genitals," the clinician might ask questions such as these: "How much does it cost to put up a satellite? Who might have paid such a sum? Where might the satellite be operated from? What is the lifetime of a satellite before it falls from its orbit?" These types of questions might stimulate the patient's curiosity about the validity of the delusional belief. They also could eventually lead to some helpful educational homework to check out the capacity of satellites to perform functions such as "draining thoughts" or "moving genitals."

7. **Work on helping the patient give up safety behaviors.** Patients often employ safety behaviors, which are maladaptive coping strategies that play into and reinforce delusions. Examples include placing tape over heating ducts (to counter the belief that neighbors can spy through the ducts), imagining a crucifix (to ward off the sense that an evil spirit is able to torment), or pasting aluminum foil on windows (to block out signals from a ray gun that the person believes is being used against her). In general, we do not address safety behaviors until we are making progress on testing out the delusion with other CBT methods. If the collaboration is strong and some headway is being made on modifying the delusion, patients can be asked to gradually reduce their involvement in safety behaviors and to monitor the effects of this plan. Work on safety behaviors for delusions uses the same basic principles as reduction in safety behaviors for anxiety disorders explained in Chapter 9, "Behavioral Methods for Anxiety."

8. **Develop and practice coping strategies.** Patients with delusions typically do not have well-developed coping strategies that give them rational ways of managing the distress associated with these symptoms. In Chapter 12, "Coping with Hallucinations," we explain how patients can use distraction, focusing, and metapsychological techniques for managing hallucinations. These methods can also be used effectively for delusions. Distraction techniques can include listening to music, practicing a hobby, cooking, or a variety of other healthy behaviors. Focusing techniques involve a shift of cognitive style from painful preoccupation with a delusion or hallucination to active methods of disputing or countering the symptom (e.g., rational responding with the statement "nobody has ever harmed me" in the case of a patient who believes he is the victim of a persecutory conspiracy, or use of positive imagery to focus on a more affirming or relaxing set of cognitions than the upsetting cognitions associated with

delusional thinking). Metacognitive techniques such as practicing mindfulness or working on accepting the presence of delusions as a part of everyday life (and not responding to them) can also help patients cope with paranoid thoughts.

9. **Devise a behavioral experiment to test the reality of the delusion.** Behavioral experiments usually involve a homework assignment to check out a delusional belief or to try acting in a different manner. The experiments need to be graded so only moderate levels of anxiety are generated and so the patient has a reasonable likelihood of being able to follow through with the assignment. The experiments can be *exploratory* (to find new information about the delusion), *confirmatory* (to actually test out the delusion), or *retrospective* (to review the information from a partially completed experiment).

   The following is an example of a behavioral experiment:

   - The next time you are walking toward the subway and you have the sense that you are being followed, try to identify the person or persons who seem to be involved.
   - Walk the same route at least five times. Check to see if you observe the same person or persons repeatedly.
   - Try to come up with a reasonable explanation of what it would mean if you do not see the same people more than once. If you do see the same person or persons more than once, could it be due to any other reasons than that the person or persons are following you?
   - Bring these ideas to the next session so we can discuss them together.

10. **Discover if a seed of truth exists within the delusion.** Many delusions contain a seed of either historical or current truth. If the clinician and patient can reach some agreement on valid points about the delusional belief, a collaborative platform can be established for testing and modifying delusions.

   Patient: Some terrorists have my house under surveillance all the time.
   Clinician: It's certainly true that since 9/11 there is a general fear in the community about terrorists, but I wonder how active they have been in downtown San Antonio. Could we try to check this out?

11. **Keep an open mind.** It is important for collaborative work to be anchored in mutual respect and open-mindedness. Trust will develop more quickly when the patient sees the clinician as being open to

new ideas—for example, by the clinician giving full consideration to the possible validity or partial validity of delusional beliefs. An attitude of openness can encourage patients to disclose aspects of the delusional experience not previously shared with anyone.

12. **Generate alternative hypotheses.** When trust has developed and effective questioning has stimulated a degree of doubt, then it is time to generate some alternative explanations. The following are commonly asked questions: "Can you think of any other way to see this situation than [describe delusion]? If you asked someone you really trusted for his view of the situation, what might the person say? If you were a scientist who was trying to get to the truth about this situation, what questions might you ask?"

    Patients often have great difficulty generating alternative explanations. When the patient appears to be at a roadblock in finding alternatives, the clinician can tentatively suggest some possibilities. Even if the suggested alternatives are rejected, a percentage-of-belief score can be given for each alternative explanation, and the patient can be encouraged to continue to develop different ways of seeing the situation.

13. **Construct a pie chart.** Using a flipchart, a whiteboard, or a piece of paper, the clinician and patient can develop a pie chart that gives percentages of belief to various alternative explanations. It is important not to start by rating the delusion itself because it might be awarded the whole pie. Typically, more rational explanations are given low levels of belief when this method is first introduced. However, the pie-chart method can stimulate a sense of inquiry, and the clinician can work with the patient to gradually give rational explanations more credence.

14. **Perform an Internet search for the delusion.** Interesting information concerning the delusion can be perused if Internet access is available (e.g., using Google). This method can provide useful subject matter to discuss during the brief session. For example, one patient who was terrified that chimeras would invade the city became more settled when the Internet information revealed that chimeras are fictional creatures that are reported to have a very brief life span.

15. **Clinician does homework on the delusion.** A patient with very strong conviction in a delusion may not be responsive to Socratic questioning, examining the evidence, or completing homework. In such instances, it can be helpful for the clinician to offer to learn more about the belief. The patient might suggest where information could be found, and the clinician could then bring the findings back to the next session for discussion.

Case Example of CBT for Delusions: Helen

Helen is a 30-year-old woman with a history of schizophrenia who was introduced in Chapter 5, "Promoting Adherence," and was featured in Video Illustration 4, "CBT for Adherence II."

Helen's principal symptoms include delusions of being possessed by shadows that can possibly act through other persons (e.g., boyfriend, family, friends) to harm her or make her do things that she would never want to do. In addition to having delusions, Helen hears voices that are very mean and derogatory. The voices cause great distress. Behavioral responses include isolation, shuttering herself in a dark house, and even avoiding watching TV or listening to music. She has stopped previous activities such as drawing or painting, but has a previous track record of creativity.

Helen experienced traumas and strains when she was growing up. Her father worked out of the home as a salesperson and was gone for long periods of time. Her mother also worked and was preoccupied with ill parents. Helen fell out of a moving car at about age 10. The mild concussion had no lasting effects, but the event rattled her psychologically and added to her sense of vulnerability and lack of protection from family. She was abused by a step-uncle but hasn't yet been able to talk much about this in therapy sessions.

Although she was a good student, she had lots of trouble in her first year at college. It appeared that a vulnerability to psychosis (aunt and grandmother were hospitalized for psychosis, and Helen had early trauma), coupled with the unsettling freedoms of being away at school (e.g., increased sexual experiences, lack of structure, sleep disruption, and especially cannabis abuse) tipped her into an acute episode of hallucinations and delusions. She received treatment with medication and had substantial improvement (without full return to baseline) but needed to leave school. After a period of recovery at home, she started work in an office as a clerical assistant. This went fairly well for about a year, but she then began to slip back into paranoia. There was a good deal of suspiciousness about coworkers, and she had to quit this job. Subsequently, she has not worked and has become dependent on a boyfriend, John.

Helen's relationship with John has some positives: She really does care about him, he has been reasonably supportive, and he has a good job as a construction worker. However, she is stressed by his long absences from home (he must go to other cities for periods of weeks for construction jobs), and she often thinks that the shadows can control him and change his eyes. Also, they live in a basement apartment that is dark and isolating.

Helen's current relationships with her family of origin are distant. Her parents and a brother and sister live quite far away. Thus, she gets little or no support from them. She did have some friends in the past—Joanna was a special friend. However, Helen sees little of them now.

Helen was hospitalized once at about age 19. Subsequently, she has had intermittent treatment with medications. However, she has never been very consistent with taking antipsychotics and has often stopped medications because of weight gain or other side effects. She has recently started treatment with Dr. Turkington. At the point of Video Illustration 12, she has had five previous sessions, which focused on assessment, initial engagement, normalizing, educating, and adherence.

▶ **Video Illustration 12.** Working With Delusions I: Dr. Turkington and Helen

Video Illustration 12 shows how several methods for delusions can be interwoven in a successful, brief CBT session. The segment begins with a discussion about a homework assignment to log some examples of incidents related to delusions about being controlled by the eyes of other people. Helen describes one particular example of perceiving that the eyes of her boyfriend John and others can "turn pale" and "pinpoint." Then she cannot look at their eyes because the "shadows" would know how she feels inside and could take her over. She also describes safety behaviors, including pretending that she is looking at other people but avoiding eye contact, pinching herself "till it really hurts," and wearing tight bands around her wrists that push energy out of her. Dr. Turkington then begins to ask Socratic questions and to look for alternative explanations.

> Dr. Turkington: It sounds like you believe this thing about the shadows and the possession through the eyes very strongly…How much do you actually believe it?
> Helen: 100% I believe it.
> Dr. Turkington: OK…Are there any other possible explanations for this experience?
> Helen: For why their eyes are going funny?
> Dr. Turkington: Yes.
> (Because Helen isn't able to generate an alternate view by herself at this point, Dr. Turkington draws from Helen's homework to help her see that other explanations might be possible.)
> Dr. Turkington: But what about your log from the previous week? In the first example, you showed me that John said he was going away and you felt quite stressed about that.
> Helen: Yes.

Dr. Turkington then goes on to explain that Helen had been nervous, her boyfriend was likely to have been concerned about her, and he may have looked at her in a concerning way. They work on an alternate explanation that she is reading too much into the look in his eyes because of her suspiciousness. After Dr. Turkington asks again for alternate explanations, Helen says that John could have been annoyed and squinted at her. Another idea is that people having an irritant in one of their eyes, such as a bothersome contact lens, could be a factor.

The next step in the intervention was to make a pie chart. These elements were identified and rated for degree of belief:

- John is concerned, and there is stress in our relationship (15%)
- I'm paranoid—taking things too personally (10%)
- John is annoyed with me (20%)
- Somebody could have something in her eye (15%)
- Shadows (50%)

As you can see, the total percentage was 110%. Although the video does not show Dr. Turkington asking Helen to rerate the items to yield a total of 100%, this strategy could have been used at this session or a later visit. Nevertheless, the pie-chart method appeared to help Helen consider alternative explanations.

Because Helen was still giving the delusional explanation the greatest value, Dr. Turkington follows up with an additional intervention designed to reduce safety behaviors. He suggests a homework assignment of watching a film (Helen chooses *Breakfast at Tiffany's*) and looking at people's eyes. Helen reports that she knows that people's eyes in movies cannot actually possess her, but she still averts her eyes and pinches herself. The vignette ends with her agreeing to an assignment of looking into the eyes of the performers without pinching herself.

▶ **Video Illustration 13.** Working With Delusions II: Dr. Turkington and Helen

Video Illustration 13 begins with a review of one homework assignment in which Helen was asked to watch the actors' eyes in a movie. Dr. Turkington then asks Helen to build on her success in doing this assignment by asking her boyfriend to attend a treatment session and to watch his eyes during the session. This suggestion causes too much anxiety (Helen rates the anxiety at 95%), so they collaboratively decide to engage in a behavioral experiment to watch the eyes of staff persons in the outpatient clinic.

To help prepare Helen for the experiment, Dr. Turkington outlines some specific objectives, such as watching a person's eyes for at least 10 seconds without using safety behaviors. They also work on a coping strategy of using positive, relaxing imagery to reduce anxiety. The last part of the vignette shows Dr. Turkington asking a series of questions to help Helen check out her thinking if she does begin to perceive some variation in the eyes of the staff members.

These two video illustrations of Dr. Turkington and Helen demonstrate a number of CBT methods for delusions, including basic procedures such as developing a well-functioning, collaborative relationship; normalizing symptoms; and providing psychoeducation. Additionally, Dr. Turkington uses Socratic questioning, examining the evidence, behavioral experiments, coping strategy development, a pie chart, and other techniques from the 15 brief CBT methods for delusions listed earlier in the chapter.

Practice Case: Planning a CBT Intervention for Delusions

In the following exercise, you are asked to devise a CBT strategy for a person with delusions. The exercise involves planning treatment interventions for Anna Maria, a 46-year-old woman with a long history of schizophrenia.

> **Learning Exercise 11–1** Planning a CBT Intervention for Delusions
>
> 1. During an early session, you attempt to ask Anna Maria about her delusions that other people can read her thoughts, but she isn't very responsive. She seems guarded and hesitant to talk about these concerns. You decide that asking some peripheral questions might put her at ease. Anna Maria has previously told you that she has enjoyed reading, she looks forward to visits with a niece and a nephew, and she attends a day program where she eats both breakfast and lunch. Write a few peripheral questions that you might consider using.
>
> 2. At a later session, you ask Anna Maria about her anxiety and safety behaviors linked to her delusion of telepathy. She replies with an example. When she tries to go to public places, such as malls or grocery stores, she gets the sense that people are looking at her—they can see right through her and know exactly what she is thinking. Then she becomes extremely anxious, gets sweaty palms, and has a sick feeling in her stomach. She usually tries to stop all of her thoughts (to "go blank"), and she pulls up her collar and hunches her shoulders to try to protect herself. But this doesn't help much, so she runs home as quickly as possible. Construct a mini-formulation. Try to identify some points in the mini-formulation where you might use CBT methods to help Anna Maria with her delusions.
>
> 3. You are starting to make some progress with Anna Maria. She is now interested in learning more about telepathy.

What is it? Has it been tested scientifically? How many people might have experiences like hers? List some homework assignments that might help educate her on telepathy and related experiences.

4. The next time you see Anna Maria, she has read a handout about delusions ("Understanding What Others Think" [Kingdon and Turkington 2005]) and she has brought in a diary of evidence for her telepathy. You examine the diary and use Socratic questioning to generate other possible explanations of why people may give her "funny looks." Try to imagine your work with Anna Maria unfolding, and write down some of the possible alternative explanations that you are able to identify.

5. In the next brief session with Anna Maria, you put the alternative explanations on a pie chart to give her a visual illustration of the possible alternatives. Draw out a pie chart with the ideas that you identified in step 4 of this exercise.

6. Anna Maria is now reporting that she is less convinced that people can read her thoughts. Design a behavioral experiment to test this out in the outpatient clinic.

Summary

Key Points for Clinicians

- For patients with psychotic symptoms, CBT is often conducted in brief sessions. Long, intensive sessions may be too taxing for some patients with psychotic illnesses.
- Delusions are viewed as misperceptions or cognitive distortions that can be modified with CBT methods.
- A collaborative-empirical therapeutic relationship is a basic requirement for effective CBT with patients who have delusions.
- A comprehensive cognitive-behavioral-biological-sociocultural model is used to direct treatment.
- CBT for delusions relies heavily on the processes of normalizing and educating.
- Standard CBT methods such as Socratic questioning, examining the evidence, developing alternative explanations, doing behavioral experiments, and building coping strategies can be modified for treatment of delusions.

Concepts and Skills for Patients to Learn

- Paranoid thoughts and delusions are very common experiences. Many people report that they have these types of thoughts.
- Delusional thinking can be triggered by a variety of stresses, including sleep deprivation, grief, trauma, and illegal drug use.
- Most people who have delusional thinking have an underlying biological vulnerability (i.e., a "chemical imbalance" in the brain). Medications are a very important part of therapy because they treat this vulnerability.
- People with delusional thinking can also benefit from visits with a doctor and/or therapist who can suggest ways to cope with delusions and anxiety.
- By working together with a doctor and/or therapist, you can learn specific ways to manage fears more effectively.
- If you are receiving psychotherapy or counseling for delusions, try to tell your doctor and/or therapist the details about your fears and be open to looking at other ways of explaining situations.

References

Beck AT: Successful outpatient psychotherapy of a chronic schizophrenic with a delusion based on borrowed guilt. Psychiatry 15:305–312, 1952

Fish FJ: Schizophrenia. Bristol, UK, Wright, 1962

Freeman D: Delusions in the nonclinical population. Curr Psychiatry Rep 8:191–204, 2006

Freeman D, Freeman J, Garety P: Overcoming Paranoid and Suspicious Thoughts. London, Robinson, 2006

Hole RW, Rush AJ, Beck AT: A cognitive investigation of schizophrenic delusions. Psychiatry 42:312–319, 1979

Jaspers K: General Psychopathology (1913). Translated by Hoenig J, Hamilton MW. Manchester, UK, Manchester University Press, 1963

Johns LC, van Os J: The continuity of psychotic experiences in the general population. Clin Psychol Rev 21:1125–1141, 2001

Kingdon DG, Turkington D: Preliminary report: the use of cognitive behavior therapy with a normalizing rationale in schizophrenia. J Nerv Ment Dis 179:207–211, 1991

Kingdon DG, Turkington D: Cognitive Therapy of Schizophrenia. New York, Guilford, 2005

Morrison AP, Renton JC, Dunn H, et al: Cognitive Therapy for Psychosis: A Formulation-Based Approach. New York, Brunner-Routledge, 2004

National Institute for Clinical Excellence: Guideline Update 1: Schizophrenia. London, National Institute for Clinical Excellence, 2009

Sensky T, Turkington D, Kingdon D, et al: A randomized controlled trial of cognitive-behavioral therapy for persistent symptoms in schizophrenia resistant to medication. Arch Gen Psychiatry 57:165–172, 2000

Strauss JS: Hallucinations and delusions as points on continua function: rating scale evidence. Arch Gen Psychiatry 21:581–586, 1969

Tarrier N, Beckett R, Harwoods S, et al: A trial of two cognitive-behavioral methods of treating drug-resistant residual psychotic symptoms in schizophrenic patients, I: outcome. Br J Psychiatry 162:524–532, 1993

Turkington D, Kingdon D: Cognitive-behavioral techniques for general psychiatrists in the management of patients with psychosis. Br J Psychiatry 177:101–106, 2000

Turkington D, Kingdon DG, Turner T: Effectiveness of a brief cognitive-behavioral therapy intervention in the treatment of schizophrenia. Br J Psychiatry 180:523–527, 2002

Wright JH, Turkington D, Kingdon DG, et al: Cognitive-Behavior Therapy for Severe Mental Illness: An Illustrated Guide. Washington, DC, American Psychiatric Publishing, 2009

CHAPTER 12

Coping With Hallucinations

Overview of CBT for Hallucinations

The general cognitive-behavior therapy (CBT) methods described in Chapter 11, "Modifying Delusions," are also applied in teaching patients how to cope better with hallucinations: a comprehensive cognitive-behavioral-biological-sociocultural model is used for understanding hallucinations; a highly collaborative therapeutic relationship needs to be developed to allow productive CBT work; and normalizing and educating are essential basic procedures. Readers are referred to Chapter 4, "Case Formulation and Treatment Planning," for guidelines on performing integrative case conceptualizations and to Chapter 11 for details on developing effective therapeutic relationships and performing normalizing and educating activities with patients with psychotic symptoms.

In the treatment of hallucinations, as in the treatment of delusions, CBT is viewed as adjunctive therapy to antipsychotic medication. The goals of adding CBT to pharmacotherapy are to 1) help people develop adaptive beliefs or meanings about the experience of hearing voices or other hallucinations; 2) build skills for coping with hallucinations; 3) reduce the distress associated with hallucinations; 4) if possible, reduce the intensity of symptoms; and 5) enhance adherence to pharmacotherapy. The list of 20 CBT methods provided in the next section is drawn from our clinical work in treating hallucinations in brief sessions with combined CBT and pharmacotherapy and is consistent with the strategies used in empirical research on CBT for schizophrenia (Sensky et al. 2000; Turkington et al. 2006; Wright et al. 2009).

Twenty Brief CBT Methods for Hallucinations

1. **Inquire about patients' explanations for their hallucinations.** Patients often keep their explanations of the voices hidden, yet these explanations can have a profound effect on their behavior. For example, a patient who believes that the secret police are talking to him and that he must take all steps possible to prevent them from finding him would likely be very guarded and evasive. In contrast, a patient who is hearing a voice say, "You're stupid...You deserve to die," but believes "I have an illness—a chemical imbalance—and I don't need to pay attention to the voices" might be calm and function reasonably well even in the face of having persistent hallucinations.

   We suggest that clinicians directly ask patients for their opinion on the causation of the voices. After these ideas are elicited, educational and cognitive restructuring methods can be used to develop more adaptive explanations. Table 12–1 shows some changes in explanations that have been made in some of our patients who experience hallucinations.

2. **Use a voice diary.** Voice hearers often derive benefit by considering how voice severity fluctuates in different circumstances (Turkington et al.

Table 12–1. Modified explanations for hallucinations

Dysfunctional explanations	Functional explanations
"It is a bug in my ear/brain planted by the CIA/police."	"It is my schizophrenia acting up."
"It is radio waves from terrorists."	"It is due to stress."
"It is an evil spirit talking to me."	"Maybe my medications need to be adjusted."
"Aliens are communicating with me."	"Maybe the problem is that I am not getting enough sleep."
"It's all caused by witchcraft."	"These voices are a special gift."

Source. From Wright JH, Turkington D, Kingdon DG, et al: *Cognitive-Behavior Therapy for Severe Mental Illness: An Illustrated Guide.* Washington, DC, American Psychiatric Publishing, 2009, p. 132. Used with permission. Copyright © 2009 American Psychiatric Publishing.

2009). A simple voice diary can be constructed in a small notebook that the patient can carry for recording experiences. These data can then be reviewed in subsequent treatment sessions. Figure 12–1 shows some entries from a voice diary that demonstrate variations over a 2-day period.

Voice diaries can be used to plan activities that may be associated with a reduced intensity of hallucinations, or they can be used to spot activities for which better coping strategies may be needed. For example, the patient who completed the diary shown in Figure 12–1 might 1) plan to spend more time quietly reading and listening to music, 2) work on ways to reduce exposure to parental arguments, or 3) experiment with using distracting or focusing strategies (described later in the chapter) to manage the experience of taking a bus to the day center program.

3. **Write down the voice content on paper or on a whiteboard.** Writing down the voice content can provide an excellent opportunity for patients to examine their hallucinations in the cold light of day in the presence of a clinician. The patient's degree of belief (expressed as a percentage), the perceived power of the voices, and possible distortions in thinking (cognitive errors) can be discussed. Some of us keep a whiteboard in our offices so that the writing can be displayed in large, easily seen print. If a whiteboard is not available, a sheet of paper and some pens will suffice.

4. **Explore the link between sleep habits and voices.** Discussing the influence of sleep on hallucinations offers an opportunity for normaliz-

Day and time	Activity	Voice loudness (Scale: 0–10)
Monday 9 A.M.	In kitchen with parents— they are arguing and criticizing me	9
Monday Noon	Lunch at day center	2
Monday 1 P.M.	Art therapy	3
Monday 4 P.M.	Home, quietly reading and listening to music	1
Tuesday 10 A.M.	Taking bus to day center—people seem to be staring at me	8
Tuesday 3 P.M.	Playing pool with friends at center	3

Figure 12–1. Example of a voice diary.

ing the voice-hearing experience. Clinicians can 1) point out that poor sleep often makes voices worse and 2) explain how sleep deprivation can cause this problem in many people. Also, efforts can be made to use the treatment interventions for sleeping problems described in Chapter 10, "CBT Methods for Insomnia," to improve sleeping habits. When needed, appropriate pharmacotherapy can be prescribed for sleep disruption.

5. **Find out where the voices come from (geographical localization).** The clinician can ask the patient, "Do they get louder in any particular area as you walk around the consulting room?" If not, the clinician can engage the patient in attempts to explain this phenomenon. For example, Janelle believed that her voices were coming from electrical outlets and that everyone else could hear them. Having agreed that

her psychiatrist's voice became louder as she walked toward him, she then experimented by starting in a far corner of the room and walking toward an electrical outlet. The voices did not get louder. This exercise was an important step in bringing her to the realization that the voices were coming from her own brain.

6. **Record the voices (reality testing).** When patients say they are hearing voices, the clinician can turn on a tape or digital recording device in the consulting room to attempt to record the voices. Patients should write down what their voices were saying at the time of the recording and then listen to the playback. They are often gratified to hear no evidence of the hallucinations and can subsequently enter social arenas with more confidence that others cannot hear these voices.

7. **Ask about typical emotional reactions to hearing voices.** Usual reactions can include shame, anger, anxiety, and sadness. Because these emotions can worsen the intensity of hallucinations, a good target for therapeutic interventions can be a reduction of feelings that surround the voice-hearing experience. Some of the methods that might be used for this purpose are developing rational responses for automatic thoughts, positive imagery, and relaxation training.

8. **Ask about typical behavioral reactions to hearing voices.** Some of the most common behaviors are hiding away, withdrawal, and reduced socialization. These safety behaviors can act to exacerbate and maintain hallucinations. The clinician can suggest that the patient try some other activities to see how the voices might change. A graded exposure plan might be useful.

> Theo, a 38-year-old man with schizophrenia, had been a fairly accomplished piano player before he became ill. He had even performed in college recitals. However, he had been hearing voices telling him, "You're no good…Who are you kidding?…You'll make a fool of yourself if you ever let anyone hear you play." As might be expected, he had given up the piano entirely, and he largely stayed to himself. Part of the CBT strategy for Theo was to gradually try a behavioral experiment to start practicing the piano on his own, and then to play the piano for a few old friends. He was eventually able to perform with a small group at a church. As he progressed through this graded task assignment, he gained an increased sense of mastery over the hallucinations.

9. **Ask other people if they can hear the voice (reality testing).** Patients usually believe at some level that others can probably hear the voices, especially when the hallucinations are perceived as being loud, clear, and in the real world. When they have not asked a parent, close friend, or mental health professional whether they too can hear the

Table 12–2. Short list of distraction techniques for hallucinations

Humming

Listening to music

Praying

Painting

Walking in the fresh air

Phoning a friend

Exercising

Yoga

Taking a warm bath

Watching TV

Doing a crossword or other puzzle

Playing a computer game

voices, this reality testing exercise can make a good homework assignment. Clinicians can help patients select an appropriate person who can be taken into their confidence in this way.

10. **Practice a distraction technique (e.g., listen to music, exercise, try to read a magazine).** The clinician should first ask if the patient has tried anything before that seemed to help. After writing a short list of distracting coping strategies, the patient can select one or more ideas to implement for homework and use a voice diary to record any benefits. If a patient cannot identify any possibilities for distracting activities, the clinician can ask about previous hobbies, interests, or skills that might be tried. Alternatively, the "List of 60 Coping Strategies for Hallucinations" (provided in Appendix 1, "Worksheets and Checklists," and available for download from www.appi.org/pdf/62362) can be reviewed in a brief session. We recommend that clinicians copy and place this list of 60 coping strategies in a file so that it can be accessed easily when needed in treatment sessions. Table 12–2 includes an abbreviated list of distraction techniques for hallucinations.

11. **Practice a focusing technique (e.g., using rational responses).** This method involves asking patients to focus their attention on the voice-hearing experience and attempt to reduce distress by taking direct action. If the voices are self-condemning, then the patient can try to respond rationally—perhaps by talking into a cell phone with thoughts that counter the overly critical messages from the hallucinations. For example, Theo, the patient with schizophrenia who had stopped playing the piano, responded to his voices with these thoughts: "I actually

am a good person…I've never hurt anyone…I studied piano a long time and can still play pretty well. People at church say they'd like to hear me play again."

Another focusing technique is subvocalization. The patient is asked to try a competing activity, such as reading out loud, when the voices are active. The words are whispered under the breath, rather than spoken out loud. This technique needs to be modeled and practiced in session to help patients learn to subvocalize in a socially acceptable way and to avoid verbalizing more and more loudly. The clinician can explain that the speech areas of the brain are active during the voice-hearing experience and that engaging in another activity that uses this part of the brain can reduce the intensity of the hallucinations.

Positive imagery can also be a useful focusing technique. Mental images can be simple distractions (e.g., imagining oneself on a beach) or active methods of focusing on and refuting hallucinations (e.g., "I image the voice being locked in a closet, and then a blanket being placed over it…The voice gets softer and softer as these things are done"). Patients should be warned that focusing techniques can sometimes make voices louder before they start to improve. However, learning to use focusing methods can have many positive benefits.

12. **Practice a metacognitive technique.** Some of the most useful coping methods require taking a completely different attitude toward the voice-hearing experience. Instead of being troubled by the voices or struggling to make them go away, the patient accepts that voices will occur but gives them little or no power. The voices may then end up as background noise of no significant consequence. Mindfulness is a good example of a metacognitive technique (Bach and Hayes 2002). The voices are perceived in a neutral mindset; the patient simply observes the voice activity without trying to force the voices away or being too distressed about them. Some of our patients who have had the best adjustment to persistent hallucinations have become mindful of their voices but get on with life despite them.

13. **Bring the voices on (to reduce the omnipotence of the voices).** Patients can often feel even more in charge if they can bring on and switch off the voices. The following are examples of control strategies: 1) listening to rap music (makes the voices worse), and then changing to mellow jazz (calms the voices); 2) staying up late at night to the point of mild sleep deprivation (makes voices more frequent and louder) versus avoiding caffeine, winding down, and getting to sleep by 11 P.M. (minimizes voices); and 3) staying in the kitchen when parents are arguing (makes the voices very intense) compared

with leaving the room and going to a quiet spot to do some light reading (softens the voices).

14. **Work on schemas (to bolster self-esteem).** One reason that patients may believe the messages that very negative voices are giving to them is that the hallucinations are resonating with an underlying maladaptive schema (e.g., "I'm a loser," "I'm stupid," "I'm unlovable"). If the clinician suspects that the patient has a negative core belief, Socratic questions can be used to uncover the schema and test it for accuracy. The clinician might ask the voice hearer, "Do you really believe that you are such a loser as the voices say?" Further steps could include examining the evidence for the belief, trying to develop a more reasonable and self-affirming belief, and developing a homework assignment to practice behaving in a manner consistent with the revised belief.

15. **Put the voices "on trial."** To use this method, patients are asked to act like a lawyer in a courtroom. They can cross-examine the voices using the empty chair technique, questioning how the voices have come to a particular conclusion and what evidence supports this conclusion. The clinician can help the patient realize that perhaps the voices do not have all the answers.

16. **Build trust using self-disclosure.** If the clinician has had a hypnagogic or other hallucinatory experience, this could be disclosed to the patient. Hallucinations are a normal component of the grieving process, and many people have experienced this phenomenon.

17. **Discuss a famous voice hearer.** Actor Anthony Hopkins, Brian Wilson of the Beach Boys, and John Frusciante of the Red Hot Chili Peppers are all voice hearers. They are highly competent and creative individuals despite their voices. Telling patients about these public figures can help them accept their own symptoms and work to develop effective coping skills to manage hallucinations.

18. **Discuss the link between illegal substances and hallucinations.** Patients are often aware that certain drugs make them paranoid; however, they may be less aware of the association between drugs and hallucinations. A mini-lesson in a brief session or a handout describing the link between certain substances and various mental states can help patients begin to take steps to change drug-taking behavior. Methods from Chapter 13, "CBT for Substance Misuse and Abuse," can then be used to tackle substance abuse or misuse problems.

19. **Go to the Gloucestershire Hearing Voices & Recovery Groups Web site (www.hearingvoices.org/uk).** This Web site can provide many helpful hints. Patients often believe that no one else can understand their symptoms. It can be a great relief to find that voice hearers around the world are meeting regularly and supporting each other.

Problem

> *Voices criticize me. They tell me that I'm no good and that I shouldn't play the piano.*

Coping strategies

- *Review my list of strengths:*
  - *— I never hurt people, I'm kind, and I help others when I can.*
  - *— I did well in school till I got sick.*
  - *— I had lots of training in piano and can still play pretty well.*
  - *— People seem to like to hear me play.*
- *Listen to recordings of concert music.*
- *Keep busy with working in the yard, going to a movie, or doing other things that stop me from dwelling on the voices.*
- *Follow my step-by-step plan to gradually build back my confidence and skill in playing the piano.*
- *Use a pill box to remember to take medications. They do help when I take them.*

Figure 12–2. Theo's coping card.

20. **Write a coping card.** The coping card technique, which is used in many other applications in brief CBT sessions, is also a core method for working with hallucinations. The key points of strategies developed in treatment sessions can be summarized on the card, which the patient then uses as a reminder to put these ideas into practice in daily life. A coping card written with Theo, the man with schizophrenia described earlier in this chapter, is shown in Figure 12–2.

Case Example of Improving Coping Skills for Hallucinations: Helen

Helen's history was described in some detail in Chapter 11, "Modifying Delusions." In addition to her problems with delusions, she was hearing voices that were very mean and derogatory (e.g., "You're crap…It's your fault…You don't do anything…You are useless"). The voices caused great distress and at times were associated with despair and hopelessness. Helen's unhelpful behavioral responses to the voices included isolation, shuttering herself in a dark house, and even avoiding watching TV or listening to music. She had stopped formerly enjoyable activities, such as drawing or painting, but had a previous track record of creativity.

▶ **Video Illustration 14.** Coping With Hallucinations: Dr. Turkington and Helen

In the beginning of the brief session shown in Video Illustration 14, Dr. Turkington reviews Helen's voice diary and finds that her demeaning voices are clearly more troublesome in the evening. The voices are upsetting her terribly and are stimulating considerable sadness. After Dr. Turkington makes some empathic comments, he asks if these messages are similar to some of her own thoughts of self-criticism. Helen confirms that this is true. They then test whether the voices are giving a true account of her self-worth.

The next part of the intervention is geared toward building Helen's self-image by helping her counter the voices with accurate statements about herself (e.g., "I'm trying…I'm doing my best…I have been ill…In the past I have been creative and hard working…I have friends…Despite our problems, John still likes me"). These positive features are to be recorded on a cell phone for Helen to play back frequently when the voices are tormenting her. Dr. Turkington and Helen also work on a distracting activity of drawing in the park. Helen had been interested in artwork previously and seems motivated to give this activity a try. A specific goal is set for her to draw in the park twice in the coming week for 30 minutes on each occasion.

Practice Case:
Planning a CBT Intervention for Hallucinations

The following practice case provides the opportunity for you to consider which of the 20 brief CBT techniques presented earlier in this chapter you would use to treat Nanda, a 26-year-old man with a history of chronic schizophrenia, cannabis abuse, and trauma in childhood.

> **Learning Exercise 12–1** Planning a CBT Intervention for Hallucinations
>
> 1. Nanda had no family history of major mental illness and had a reasonably normal childhood except that his father was a truck driver who was often away from home. Unfortunately, Nanda was physically beaten by a babysitter at age 7 years and then bullied by an employer at age 16 years. At about that time, he began smoking cannabis and became increasingly withdrawn and self-absorbed. Nanda subsequently developed paranoid delusions that police cars were following him and that he could feel satellites burning his skin and genital area with lasers. He also had persistent severe auditory hallucinations of critical voices telling him

he "deserved to get hurt," he was a "loser," and other very negative messages. Nanda believed that the voices were coming from the satellites and could be heard by his neighbors.

Can you think of at least two ways to work with Nanda's hallucinations in brief sessions? Can you help him develop any other explanations for the hallucinations? Write a brief plan to help Nanda begin to develop some degree of doubt about the certainty that the voices are coming from satellites. If you have a colleague who can role-play Nanda, try out these methods in a simulated brief session.

2. As you work with Nanda, you find that he is very ashamed of having a psychiatric illness and feels alienated from others. He has a very isolated and lonely lifestyle. You conclude that the stigma of mental illness is weighing heavily on Nanda and that efforts to normalize his experiences may help him to engage better in therapy and have more success in coping with hallucinations. Write a brief plan for using at least two strategies for helping reduce the stigma that Nanda is feeling. If possible, role-play using these methods with an associate.

3. Nanda is trusting you more, and the collaborative nature of the therapeutic relationship is improving. He is more forthcoming about his cannabis use and admits that he is using this drug fairly heavily. Although the cannabis initially gives him a feeling of relaxation and reduced anxiety, it appears to worsen his hallucinations. Write a discussion that you might have with Nanda about the link between cannabis use and his voice hearing. Try to practice this discussion in a role-play with a colleague. You will learn about CBT methods for substance abuse in the next chapter.

4. As the therapy in brief sessions proceeds, you are able to have more extensive discussions with Nanda about his explanation for having hallucinations. He surprises you by saying that he thought the hallucinations might have something to do with being physically abused as a child and then being bullied as a teenager. You ask him how these incidents could have possibly influenced his beliefs that he is being persecuted by the police and that voices are being projected from satellites. He tells you that the whole thing is a punishment.

Next you write down this explanation for the hallucinations on paper or a whiteboard and begin to work with Nanda on developing a more functional and less self-condemning explanation. Think of some Socratic questions or other cognitive restructuring methods that you might use to help him revise this maladaptive belief. Then try to practice using these techniques in a role-play exercise.

Summary

Key Points for Clinicians

- In treating hallucinations, CBT is often conducted in brief sessions. Long, intensive sessions may be too exhausting for many patients with intrusive distressing hallucinations.
- To plan effective CBT interventions, clinicians need to develop a case formulation that assesses the significance of current and past stresses, exacerbating influences, automatic thoughts and core beliefs, typical behavioral responses to hallucinations, biological and medical contributors, and patient strengths.
- Standard cognitive restructuring techniques, such as Socratic questioning, examining the evidence, and developing rational explanations, can be modified for treatment of hallucinations.
- CBT for hallucinations relies heavily on the process of generating new and more effective coping strategies.

Concepts and Skills for Patients to Learn

- Hallucinations are commonly experienced by many different people.
- Hallucinations can be triggered by a variety of stressors, including lack of sleep, sensory deprivation, intense grief, illegal drugs, and traumas of various types.
- Try not to be ashamed of what your voices are saying. Voices often say unpleasant things. Your doctor or therapist will be able to help you feel more comfortable about having hallucinations if you are able to tell her about them.
- Antipsychotic medications can reduce or eliminate hallucinations.
- CBT can be very helpful in learning to cope with hallucinations. The goals of this treatment are to assist you in understanding hallucinations and finding specific ways to control them.

References

Bach P, Hayes SC: The use of acceptance and commitment therapy to prevent the rehospitalization of psychotic patients: a randomized controlled trial. J Consult Clin Psychol 70:1129–1139, 2002

Sensky T, Turkington D, Kingdon D, et al: A randomized controlled trial of cognitive-behavioral therapy for persistent symptoms in schizophrenia resistant to medication. Arch Gen Psychiatry 57:165–172, 2000

Turkington D, Kingdon D, Weiden PJ: Cognitive behavior therapy for schizophrenia. Am J Psychiatry 163:365–373, 2006

Turkington D, Kingdon D, Rathod S, et al: Back to Life, Back to Normality: Cognitive Therapy, Recovery and Psychosis. Cambridge, UK, Cambridge University Press, 2009

Wright JH, Turkington D, Kingdon DG, et al: Cognitive-Behavior Therapy for Severe Mental Illness: An Illustrated Guide. Washington, DC, American Psychiatric Publishing, 2009

CHAPTER 13

CBT for Substance Misuse and Abuse

LEARNING MAP

Understanding cognitive processes in substance abuse

Readiness for change: motivational enhancement

Gaining stimulus control: identifying persons, places, and things

Implementing a sobriety plan

Self-monitoring and dealing with negative cognitions

Relapse prevention

Misuse and abuse of alcohol and psychoactive drugs commonly complicate the lives of people with psychiatric disorders. The high rate of co-occurrence is in part the result of the ubiquity of substance abuse and addiction. Excluding nicotine dependence, most systematic surveys (e.g., Kessler et al. 2005) indicate that rates of substance abuse and dependence are 15%–20% in the U.S. adult population, with men having higher rates of most substance-related disorders than women. Problems with substance abuse and dependence are even more frequent among people with psychiatric disorders such as schizophrenia and the mood and anxiety disorders. Lifetime rates for alcohol and substance abuse for persons with these conditions have been reported to be up to three times those of the general public (Daley and Thase 2000).

Such high rates of co-occurrence reflect both the importance of shared causal factors and the likelihood that at least some vulnerable individuals gravitate toward the problematic use of alcohol and other substances as a means of self-medication (Khantzian 1985). Even when the problematic substance use begins as self-medication, treatment of the primary psychiatric disorder often is not sufficient, and specific treatment for substance misuse or abuse is warranted. Just as it is misguided to ignore the non–substance abuse disorder in a treatment plan for an individual with alcoholism or another substance abuse disorder, it is similarly a mistake to try to treat a mood, anxiety, or psychotic disorder in an individual with problematic substance use without implementing a sobriety plan (Daley and Thase 2000). In this chapter, we focus on the use of cognitive-behavior therapy (CBT) strategies within brief sessions to address problematic use of alcohol, marijuana, sedative-hypnotics, and other substances of abuse. These brief methods are not intended for use with individuals who have severe addictions and for whom inpatient or ambulatory detoxification programs are clinically indicated.

Understanding Cognitive Processes in Substance Abuse

Problematic use of and addiction to alcohol and other substances are the result of complex, interdependent biopsychosocial processes that involve genetic vulnerabilities, experiential and contextual factors, and conditioning of the neural circuitry that mediate appetitive and hedonic behaviors (Baler and Volkow 2006). What typically begins as a series of purely voluntary or volitional acts may slowly (in the case of alcohol or marijuana) or rapidly (with crack cocaine) segue into a self-perpetuating, cyclical process in which conditioned stimuli (i.e., persons, places, things,

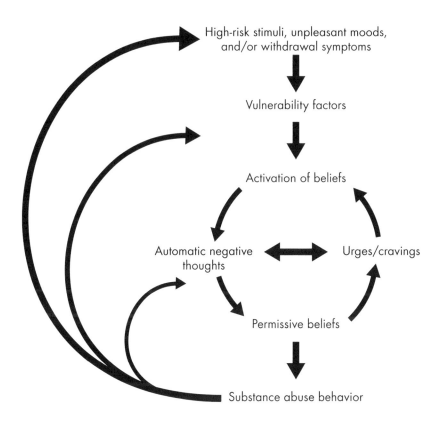

Figure 13–1. Cognitive-behavioral model of substance abuse.

Source. Reprinted from Thase ME: Cognitive behavior therapy for substance abuse disorders, in *American Psychiatric Press Review of Psychiatry*, Vol. 16. Edited by Dickstein LJ, Riba MB, Oldham JM. Washington, DC, American Psychiatric Press, 1997, p. 50. Used with permission. Copyright © 1997 American Psychiatric Press.

or thoughts and feelings) trigger urges and cravings, which in turn motivate the instrumental behaviors that result in alcohol or drug use (Thase 1997; Figure 13–1). For heuristic reasons, an *urge* is described as the behavioral inclination or response predisposition to use drugs or alcohol in certain contexts, and the term *craving* is used to describe the state characterized by an admixture of dysphoric cognitions, affects, and physiological arousal that are provoked by conditioned cues.

Beyond the thoughts that may serve as the stimuli that elicit urges and cravings, other cognitions, including automatic negative thoughts and beliefs about substance abuse, may increase the likelihood that the urge or craving will result in substance abuse (Thase 1997). For example, an automatic thought such as "my life is already in shambles—I might as well go ahead and get high" or a belief such as "cravings are irresistible" can facilitate the dysfunctional behaviors associated with drug or alcohol use by undermining the individual's attempts to exercise volitional control to cope with the craving or urge. Other cognitions can promote drug or alcohol use by enabling the individual to engage in self-deception or minimize the perceived consequences of getting high. "I'll get drunk this one last time and will start a sobriety plan tomorrow" is one example of such a permissive cognition.

Cognitive-behavioral approaches are among the best studied psychosocial interventions for alcohol and other substance abuse and dependence disorders and have been shown to increase the likelihood of abstinence and reduce the subsequent risk of relapse (Dutra et al. 2008; Kadden 2003). Virtually all members of this relatively broad class of interventions begin with recognition of the stimuli that elicit urges and cravings and the patterns of cognition that accompany these states. Cognitive restructuring techniques and behavioral rehearsal strategies are then used to practice healthier alternatives to coping without drinking or using drugs. Imagery techniques can be used to elicit urges or cravings to facilitate in vivo practice with newly learned coping behaviors.

Traditional 12-step approaches to treatment of problematic alcohol and drug use also emphasize recognition of the persons, places, and things that serve as stimuli to provoke urges and cravings, as well as the importance of negative cognitions (e.g., the Alcoholics Anonymous [AA] adage that "stinking thinking leads to drinking"). Unlike CBT, 12-step methods suggest dealing with self-deceptive or permissive cognitions with the tenet that the addicted individual is powerless over the addiction and that control must be ceded to a higher power. Although these particular beliefs are not consistent with the collaborative and constructivist roots of CBT, few other inherent incompatibilities exist between the treatment models. Thus, most cognitive-behavior therapists encourage their patients also to attend self-help programs such as AA or Narcotics Anonymous (Thase 1997). The CBT approach is, after all, rooted in empiricism, and clinicians are encouraged to draw upon and incorporate all strategies that work. In fact, in one clinical trial comparing treatments for cocaine dependence funded by the National Institute on Drug Abuse, participants who were randomly assigned to receive the combination of individual and group sessions of drug counseling following the traditional 12-step methods were significantly more likely to become abstinent than were those randomly assigned to receive a course of individual CBT without 12-step groups (Crits-Christoph et al. 1999). For individuals with more severe addictions, a more efficient way to facilitate abstinence might be an early emphasis on relatively simple methods that emphasize complete avoidance of the persons, places, and things associated with alcohol or drug use and "giving up" the illusion of self-directed control over coping with urges or cravings.

Readiness for Change: Motivational Enhancement

It is not uncommon for people seeking treatment for a psychiatric disorder to initially minimize or deny problematic alcohol or drug use. If the substance use is indeed clinically problematic, there will likely be other opportunities to make the diagnosis. For example, the magnitude and extent of alcohol or drug use should always be reassessed when treatment of the presenting problem is not achieving the desired effect. On other occasions, significant others may express their concerns to the mental health professional, or some pivotal life event may propel problematic substance abuse into the therapeutic spotlight. Before launching into a series of interventions, however, the clinician needs to understand the individual's readiness to recognize or deal with a substance abuse problem. For this purpose, methods drawn from the motivational interviewing approach are appropriate, relatively easy to learn, and particularly well suited for use in brief sessions (Hettema et al. 2005; Madson et al. 2009; Sobel and Sobel 2003).

With Darrell, whose treatment for depression was described earlier in Chapter 6, "Behavioral Methods for Depression," and Chapter 8, "Treating Hopelessness and Suicidality," the life event that forced dealing with a drinking problem was an arrest for driving under the influence (DUI). In the initial interview, Darrell denied problems with alcohol or substance abuse and reported that he drank a few beers with his friends "several times a month." However, later in treatment, Darrell was pulled over on the way home from a bar and cited for DUI.

▸ **Video Illustration 15.** CBT for Substance Abuse I: Dr. Thase and Darrell

The session shown in Video Illustration 15 opens with Dr. Thase suggesting that they go right to the agenda item of the DUI citation. Darrell initially minimizes the event and says that he is not proud of it. He explains that he "had a few" when he was out with friends and happened to get pulled over at the wrong time, as though the incident was simply a matter of bad luck.

Dr. Thase notes that Darrell's mother called to express her concern that her son has a drinking problem. Then Dr. Thase gently confronts Darrell by noting that two of the criteria for a diagnosis of alcohol abuse are a DUI and the concern of a family member. Next he asks Darrell how much he had to drink that night. Darrell says that he had only a few beers. However, he could not really remember the number, and he drank the beers relatively quickly. His blood alcohol level was 0.09. As the session proceeds, Dr. Thase lets Darrell know that his mother has provided additional information that Darrell is drinking alone at home in the evenings. Darrell admits that he drinks 3 beers 5 nights a week and that when he is out with friends he can consume up to 8 beers during the course of 3–4 hours. Yet, he again downplays the significance of his drinking behavior when he says, "I never wanted to think that it is such a big problem…such a big deal."

Because Darrell clearly has a problem with alcohol but still does not appear to be solidly committed to tackling the issue, Dr. Thase asks a series of questions designed to enhance motivation. First, he asks Darrell about the impact that the DUI arrest may have on his life. After Darrell says it is a "big deal" and that he is worried about it, he agrees to work with Dr. Thase on finding other motivators for change.

Dr. Thase: Can you think of other motivating factors to change your drinking behavior?

Darrell: I really don't want to worry my mom anymore…With her being sick and everything, she's got enough to worry about. I don't want to put her through that.

Dr. Thase: That's a good one. I guess it's also true that some of these nights that you are reaching a level of intoxication, you may not be able to help her the way you want to help her if there was an emergency.

Darrell: Yeah, I hadn't thought about it that way…But I definitely need to be there for her…especially when things are real bad.

Dr. Thase: So we have the legal troubles, we have to be of more help and less worry to your mom. Can you think of other motivators?

Darrell: You know…I think work is getting to be an issue now…Some mornings I will come in and either I didn't sleep too well because I've been drinking, or every once in a while I will have kind of like a hangover…It's kind of got me late to work, and you know I've missed a couple meetings.

Dr. Thase: Those are three good reasons. Can you think of any others?

Darrell: One of the big things is really trying to not be like my dad…He was a pretty bad drinker, and I just don't want to end up a loser like him…He's lost all of us and everything, and I don't want to go down that road.

This motivator is very emotionally resonant for Darrell, so Dr. Thase underscores the importance of this factor before continuing to build the list

Motivators for change	Demotivators
• *Arrest for driving under the influence—legal problems, jeopardy for jail time.*	• *I enjoy drinking beer.*
• *I don't want to worry or stress my mother.*	• *I get relief from stress when I drink beer.*
• *I need to be there for my mother.*	• *Many family members and friends are "social drinkers."*
• *Negative impact of alcohol on work performance.*	• *If I admit I have a drinking problem, then I have "joined the club" with my father.*
• *I don't want to be a loser like my father.*	
• *My physical health would improve.*	
• *Alcohol use can interfere with recovery from depression.*	

Figure 13–2. Motivational enhancement: Darrell's example.

of motivating factors. Although Darrell cannot think of any other items to add, Dr. Thase uses the clinician's prerogative to discuss two additional items: his overall health would improve (his blood pressure has been up and alcohol abuse could be a factor in this), and alcohol can interfere with the effectiveness of CBT and antidepressant medication and counteract his efforts to recover from depression.

Next, Dr. Thase turns to the possible demotivators. Darrell notes that he likes drinking beer, because it both tastes good and makes him feel good. Also, Darrell relates that when so much is going on in his life, he feels some relief when he drinks. Although Darrell's mother doesn't approve of his drinking, a lot of others in his family are heavy "social" drinkers; drinking appears to be a normal part of their lives. Dr. Thase suggests or "wonders aloud" that if Darrell admits that he has a drinking problem, then he is like his dad and has joined "the club."

In summing up, Darrell states that he wants to change: "I don't need anything else making my life worse right now." The key items identified through motivational enhancement methods with Darrell are summarized in Figure 13–2.

Gaining Stimulus Control: Identifying Persons, Places, and Things

Recognizing that urges and cravings to use alcohol or drugs are, in part, conditioned to occur in certain settings or in the company of particular people is an important step toward abstinence. Beginning to make life-style changes to minimize contact with the persons, places, and things associated with drinking or drug use is an important advantage in maintaining sobriety, particularly in the first weeks or months of abstinence. Potential lifestyle changes can include avoiding contact with people who are not respectful of the plan not to drink or use drugs, increasing time with people who are sober, and developing healthier leisure-time activities, including exercise. When a patient's social network is filled with friends and acquaintances who drink heavily or use drugs, making necessary changes with interpersonal contacts can be a daunting task, and the patient may need to reach out to peers met at AA or Narcotics Anonymous meetings or to try to reconnect with previously estranged family members or friends from the past.

Activity and pleasant events scheduling (see Chapter 6, "Behavioral Methods for Depression"), a CBT method suitable for brief sessions, may be a useful technique for helping patients organize their efforts to change. Also, the cognitive restructuring methods described in Chapter 7, "Targeting Maladaptive Thinking," can be used to modify dysfunctional thoughts, such as "Nobody would want to be around me if I am not drinking—I'd be a bore" or "Alcohol and drugs have been my best friends—I've forgotten how to make a real friend." In some cases, the abuse may have been associated with erosion or loss of social skills, and efforts to rebuild these skills may be needed.

A 45-year-old man with alcohol and cocaine abuse and major depression who was treated in brief sessions by Dr. Sudak provides an interesting example of problems in changing contacts with persons, places, and things. Paul had been a restaurant manager who really enjoyed "partying" with the staff after closing the restaurant each night. He had many contacts in the restaurant business, many of whom also had problems with substance abuse. He was around alcohol all the time when he was at work and had an extensive wine collection at home. Cocaine was readily available among his associates at the restaurant.

By the time Paul entered treatment, he had lost his job managing a restaurant but was still spending a lot of time with his old "friends" in the business. Part of Paul's treatment involved breaking off these contacts, at least for the first 6 months of therapy; looking for a new job that would not involve serving alcohol or bring him into routine contact with persons who used cocaine; divesting himself of his wine collection and other stores of alcohol; and developing a healthier schedule of activities. Figure 13–3 lists some of the specific activities that Paul built into his weekly schedule.

Another example of gaining stimulus control comes from the treatment of Miranda, a 35-year-old woman who initially sought therapy for

- *Drive 5-year-old son to and from school every day. Spend at least 4 hours a day watching him and/or playing with him so that wife can focus on her job.*
- *Exercise at gym for 1 hour four or five times a week.*
- *Attend Alcoholics Anonymous five times a week.*
- *Spend at least 2 hours each weekday in job search activities.*
- *Attend church every Sunday and once more during the week.*
- *Meet with three friends from high school who have a jam session playing bluegrass music twice a week. Explain to them that I have an alcohol and drug problem and need their help to not consume substances when we play music.*
- *Go to coffee shop with brother (a nondrinker) to sit and talk two or three times a week.*
- *Attend farmer's market every Tuesday afternoon and Saturday morning with family.*

Figure 13–3. Planned activities to promote sobriety: Paul's example.

an anxiety disorder but soon revealed a significant problem with alcohol dependence. She worked as a paralegal in a law firm that had a strong tradition of the "team" going to a bar after work twice a week for "happy hour." They also celebrated legal victories with long "alcohol-soaked" dinners. In her therapeutic work with Dr. Wright, Miranda decided to tell her boss and coworkers that she had an alcohol problem and would not be attending the social events after work. She also committed to stop going on cruises—one of her favorite vacation activities—because the free-flowing alcohol available on the boats might trigger a relapse.

About 3 months into her treatment, Miranda was able to resume going out after work with her coworkers and to drink nonalcoholic beverages when others were consuming alcohol. An especially challenging part of coping with the stimuli of these occasions was the criticism and undermining that she experienced from one of the other office staff members. This woman repeatedly said things such as, "I hate for you to have to give up something you love so much…You really don't need to do this." Fortunately, Miranda was able to spot that her coworker also had a problem with substance abuse. When Miranda checked this person's Facebook page, she found that many of the entries had references to alcohol use.

Later in treatment, after 2 years of sobriety and many brief CBT sessions, Miranda was ready to take a cruise with her husband. She reported, "I love taking cruises, and I have been around alcohol enough that I can resist the urges…I'm 'allergic' to alcohol…I can't touch it, and I know I will be OK." This case demonstrates the gradual reintroduction of exposure to people, places, and things associated with substance misuse and abuse.

- *Review list of motivators daily.*
- *Talk to my best friend about my alcohol problem and ask him to help.*
- *Remove all beer and alcohol from apartment.*
- *Attend Alcoholics Anonymous as agreed with Dr. Thase.*
- *Use activity schedule to plan ways to reduce risk for drinking.*
- *Have weekly sessions with Dr. Thase.*

Figure 13–4. A sobriety plan: Darrell's example.

Much like the graded exposure to anxiety stimuli described in Chapter 9, "Behavioral Methods for Anxiety," the CBT approach for substance abuse helps people build confidence and skills in effectively managing stimuli that have previously led to dysfunctional behavior. Although some stimuli are best avoided on a long-term basis (e.g., "crack houses," other places where illegal drugs are easily acquired, liquor stores), most people with substance abuse histories will eventually need to learn ways to maintain sobriety when confronted with common stimuli, such as social occasions where alcohol is served.

Implementing a Sobriety Plan

When the patient agrees with the clinician that the use of alcohol or drugs is problematic and that it is possible to abstain, the next step is to develop a sobriety plan. In Darrell's case, the sobriety plan included frequently reviewing his list of motivators for sobriety, confiding to his most sympathetic friend that he needed to stop drinking because of the DUI, and asking for this friend's help to remove the beer and liquor from his apartment (Figure 13–4). In addition to rallying support from Darrell's social network, Dr. Thase encouraged Darrell to attend AA, noting that meetings are held in his office building on Mondays, Thursdays, and Saturdays. After Dr. Thase provided a brief explanation of why AA could help, Darrell said that he was willing to try attending meetings.

Because work had already been done in CBT on activity scheduling, Darrell was able to quickly draw on this method to reduce contact with stimuli that might increase his risk of drinking and to build up the number of positive activities that might help him to abstain from alcohol. Further CBT sessions were also an important part of the sobriety plan. Darrell and Dr. Thase agreed to meet for a weekly, brief session every Friday morning before Darrell started work. Fridays had been a day of heightened vulnerability to alcohol use because Darrell often went out to sports bars after work to celebrate the end of the workweek.

Self-Monitoring and Dealing
With Negative Cognitions

Another part of CBT for substance abuse involves dealing with the automatic negative thoughts and beliefs about drinking or drug use that will inevitably surface during the first days and weeks of abstinence. The brief session shown in Video Illustration 16 begins with Dr. Thase reviewing Darrell's self-rated depression score. Dr. Thase then asks Darrell how the sobriety plan is working. Darrell reports that the plan is going well and that he has not had any alcohol for the past 2 weeks. He has been attending one AA meeting each week, and he has been reviewing his list of motivators to change at least once daily. Thinking about being available to help his mother, the likely consequences of a second DUI, and not wanting to be like his father has been helping Darrell to maintain his motivation not to drink.

▶ **Video Illustration 16.** CBT for Substance Abuse II: Dr. Thase and Darrell

After reinforcing the good results and giving Darrell credit for these changes, Dr. Thase asks if Darrell has had any problems carrying out the plan. Darrell notes that he has been stressed when he goes out with friends or with women.

> Darrell: It is weird to not be drinking, I will say that…everybody expects you to have a drink.
> Dr. Thase: Has anyone actually said anything to you about this?
> Darrell: No, I can't say that anyone has said anything to me…I guess I wonder if they are kind of thinking about it.
> Dr. Thase: So what are you worried that they are thinking about?
> Darrell: I guess…"Is he some kind of nerd or a geek?…He doesn't drink. He doesn't fit in." And women…they want a guy who can handle himself…It just kind of looks bad if you don't have a drink.

When Dr. Thase points out that Darrell may be having automatic thoughts about the reactions of women to his not drinking, Darrell's first reaction is that the thought is a true statement. Therefore, Dr. Thase decides to use the downward arrow technique to unravel the meaning of the thought.

> Dr. Thase: If that is true, what does it mean about you?
> Darrell: You're a loser and a geek kind of guy, and they don't want to be with you.
> Dr. Thase: And if you're a loser and a geek and they don't want to be with you, what's the next step in your life?

> Darrell: You end up alone…and you can't get married…You really won't be with anybody.

Dr. Thase then shows Darrell how a worry can go through a downward spiral to the point of concluding that he will end up "alone, isolated, cut off, never married…basically failing."

They next begin to test the accuracy of the automatic thoughts and beliefs. Dr. Thase asks, "How certain are you of the fact that women want a guy who can handle his alcohol?" Darrell answers, "Fairly certain." Dr. Thase then asks if this applies to all women. Darrell notes that it may apply to 50% of women. They discuss some women who may not be bothered—those who attend AA and those with family histories of alcohol abuse. Then Dr. Thase asks the pivotal question:

> Dr. Thase: Do you have to drink to handle yourself?
> Darrell: I guess you don't have to drink to handle yourself…You could handle yourself in other ways.
> Dr. Thase: Or perhaps part of handling yourself is not drinking…knowing when it is best not to drink.
> Darrell: Yeah…Maybe that's kind of a thing that would make a woman feel better about you.

After making some progress on modifying automatic thoughts in the brief session, Dr. Thase suggests a homework assignment in which Darrell will keep track of his automatic thoughts about what people may be thinking about him, test the accuracy of the thoughts, and see if this makes him feel more comfortable about not drinking.

Relapse Prevention

Cognitive-behavioral approaches to substance abuse begin with the recognition that most individuals who have abused drugs or alcohol will, at some point, suffer a lapse or relapse (Marlatt and Gordon 1985; Thase 1997). Relapse prevention thus is viewed as a potential lifelong endeavor. For most patients, the relapse prevention plan includes ongoing awareness and management of high-risk situations; practice with coping with thoughts and feelings that have been associated with substance use; effectively using supports such as family, friends, and/or AA; making healthy lifestyle choices; and regular sessions with the clinician. A hallmark of CBT is that the skills learned during brief sessions and practiced via homework assignments can be used for a lifetime.

Learning Exercise 13–1   Using CBT for Substance Misuse or Abuse

1. The next time you have a brief session with a patient who reports problematic use of alcohol or another drug, explore the patient's readiness for change by asking about factors that might motivate against and for continued substance use.

2. If drinking or substance use appears to be interfering with treatment response, try to collaboratively develop a sobriety plan.

3. Use an activity schedule or other behavioral method to work on reducing contact with potential triggers for abuse and to enhance involvement in activities that may promote abstinence.

4. Use a thought change record to elicit and modify the patient's automatic negative thoughts and beliefs that are associated with urges or cravings to drink or use drugs.

5. Use guided imagery to elicit an urge or craving and a behavioral rehearsal exercise to practice successful coping.

Summary

Key Points for Clinicians

- Problematic use of alcohol and other substances frequently complicates other psychiatric disorders and, if not specifically addressed, can undermine treatment efforts. When substance abuse is present, it becomes a primary target for CBT interventions.
- A variety of CBT methods can be used in brief sessions to address problematic substance use. These methods include 1) providing psychoeducation about the impact of substance abuse on outcomes and overall health; 2) using motivational interviewing techniques to improve readiness for change; 3) identifying the persons, places, and things associated with substance use and using activity schedules or other behavioral methods to manage these influences; 4) recognizing and modifying permissive cognitions; 5) collaboratively developing and implementing a sobriety plan; and 6) encouraging attendance at self-help programs such as AA.

- More severe substance use disorders, including those that meet criteria for dependence, may warrant more intensive interventions, including ambulatory or inpatient detoxification. Clinicians working with these patients also can use CBT methods in combination with other treatment strategies, including pharmacotherapy.
- After initial treatment goals are achieved, ongoing cognitive-behavioral relapse prevention strategies are a useful approach to help the patient maintain sobriety and to reduce the potential for renewed problem substance use.

Concepts and Skills for Patients to Learn

- People with psychiatric illnesses have a high risk of problematic use of alcohol and other substances. Substance misuse, abuse, and dependence often have a negative effect on treatment outcomes.
- Problematic alcohol and drug use are treatable. When people are able to abstain from alcohol and drug use, the symptoms of their other psychiatric problems are more likely to improve.
- One way to increase the likelihood of abstaining from alcohol or drug use is to think about both the advantages of sobriety (i.e., motivators) and the likely disadvantages of abstaining (demotivators). People who are ready to change (i.e., those who have a clear sense that the advantages outweigh the disadvantages) have a better chance of achieving sobriety. Make a list of both the reasons for stopping alcohol or drug use as well as the likely problems and disadvantages that you will encounter if you try to implement a sobriety plan. Review this list frequently.
- CBT teaches people how to spot and reverse the negative thoughts and urges that promote alcohol or drug use. Learning and practicing these methods can help you achieve and maintain sobriety.
- If you are having significant withdrawal symptoms or are unable to abstain from substance use, make sure to tell your clinician. Also, ask for help from your family, friends, or anyone else who could give you support. Sometimes more intensive approaches to treatment are initially necessary to help people stop drinking or using drugs.
- People who attend self-help programs such as Alcoholics Anonymous have a better chance of achieving and maintaining sobriety.

References

Baler RD, Volkow ND: Drug addiction: the neurobiology of disrupted self-control. Trends Mol Med 12:559–566, 2006

Crits-Christoph P, Siqueland L, Blaine J, et al: Psychosocial treatments for cocaine dependence: National Institute on Drug Abuse Collaborative Cocaine Treatment Study. Arch Gen Psychiatry 56:493–502, 1999

Daley DC, Thase ME: Dual Disorders Recovery Counseling: Integrated Treatment for Substance Use and Mental Health Disorders, 2nd Edition. Independence, MO, Herald House/Independence Press, 2000

Dutra L, Stathopoulou G, Basden SL, et al: A meta-analytic review of psychosocial interventions for substance use disorders. Am J Psychiatry 165:179–187, 2008

Hettema J, Steele J, Miller WR: Motivational interviewing. Annu Rev Clin Psychol 1:91–111, 2005

Kadden RM: Behavioral and cognitive-behavioral treatments for alcoholism: research opportunities. Recent Dev Alcohol 16:165–182, 2003

Kessler C, Berglund P, Demler O, et al: Lifetime prevalence and age-of-onset distributions of DSM-IV disorders in the national comorbidity survey replication. Arch Gen Psychiatry 62:593–602, 2005

Khantzian EJ: The self-medication hypothesis of addictive disorders: focus on heroin and cocaine dependence. Am J Psychiatry 142:1259–1264, 1985

Madson MB, Loignon AC, Lane C: Training in motivational interviewing: a systematic review. J Subst Abuse Treat 36:101–109, 2009

Marlatt GA, Gordon JR: Relapse Prevention: Maintenance Strategies in the Treatment of Addictive Behaviors. New York, Guilford, 1985

Sobel LC, Sobel MB: Using motivational interviewing techniques to talk with clients about their alcohol use. Cogn Behav Pract 10:214–221, 2003

Thase ME: Cognitive-behavioral therapy for substance abuse, in American Psychiatric Press Review of Psychiatry, Vol. 16. Edited by Dickstein LJ, Riba MB, Oldham JM. Washington, DC, American Psychiatric Press, 1997, pp 45–71

CHAPTER 14

Lifestyle Change:
Building Healthy Habits

```
┌─────────────────────────────────────────────┐
│                                               │
│              LEARNING MAP                     │
│                                               │
│   CBT techniques that can facilitate habit change │
│                                               │
│                     ⇩                         │
│                                               │
│             Case example: Grace               │
│                                               │
│                     ⇩                         │
│                                               │
│      Practice case: developing a plan for     │
│                 habit change                  │
│                                               │
└─────────────────────────────────────────────┘
```

Many patients receiving psychotropic medications have achieved good symptom relief or remission, but have difficulty achieving some of their life goals. Others have habits that may impact the course of their psychiatric illness or a medical illness if not managed differently. This chapter details strategies that can be used in brief sessions to help patients change maladaptive habits and reach goals. Cognitive-behavior therapy (CBT) can be a practical and effective method for helping patients reach important milestones that lead to healthier, more balanced, and fulfilling lives.

Making life changes can be a challenge for anyone. Patients who want to form new habits frequently lack a systematic approach that works. When patients fail to make desired changes, they often blame themselves rather than acknowledge the significant obstacles that usually exist in acquiring new behaviors. Self-condemnation can reinforce maladaptive beliefs about the possibility of change and undermine efforts to reach goals. The problem with self-blame is compounded by a barrage of messages from popular magazines, Internet sites, and advertising about "quick-fix solutions" to complex life problems. The CBT approach to lifestyle change acknowledges and normalizes the difficulty in building healthier habits and tries to help people focus on solving problems instead of criticizing themselves.

CBT Techniques That Can Facilitate Habit Change

Research studies have supported the use of brief interventions to initiate and maintain habit change. For example, Grilo and Masheb (2005) and Carels et al. (2008) demonstrated that CBT techniques administered with guided self-help or in brief group treatment were successful for patients with binge eating disorder and in helping these patients maintain weight loss. In Table 14–1, we list some of the CBT methods commonly used to assist people in changing habits. Because basic procedures for using these techniques have been described previously in this book, the emphasis in this chapter is on their practical application for problems with procrastination or reaching goals.

Goal Setting

One way to achieve meaningful change is to help patients set clear, specific, and manageable goals. In Chapter 9, "Behavioral Methods for Anxiety," we demonstrated how useful goals can be developed in brief sessions for treating problems such as agoraphobia and obsessive-compulsive disorder (e.g., being able to go to malls, grocery stores, and other public places and stay with minimal anxiety [a rating of 10 or lower on a 100-point scale]; reducing time spent checking and counting to less than 5% of waking hours). Using the same collaborative process, goals can be set for altering patterns of procrastination or building new habits. The following are some examples from patients we have treated:

- Todd—a patient who is unemployed and is procrastinating about taking action to find a new job:
  1. Update résumé within 2 weeks.
  2. Spend at least 2 hours per day "working" on finding a job.
  3. Be back to work within 4 months—even if it is not my ideal job.

Table 14–1. Cognitive-behavior therapy techniques that can facilitate change

---

Goal setting

Motivational enhancement

Time management

Self-monitoring

Graded task assignments

Problem solving

Cognitive restructuring

Building coping skills for distressing emotions

- Judy—a patient with extreme obesity:
  1. Log food intake and limit calories to 1,600 or fewer calories per day.
  2. Walk on treadmill at least four times a week for at least 30 minutes. Log the exercise.
  3. Follow a medically supervised diet and exercise plan for 6 months to prepare for bariatric surgery.
  4. Lose at least 40 pounds before the surgery.

- Raphael—a patient with chronic pain who has been told by his doctor to exercise but has not yet been able to maintain an exercise program:
  1. Get a personal trainer who is experienced in working with chronic pain—commit to sticking with the program for at least a 6-week trial.
  2. Do the 6-week trial even if pain goes up temporarily.
  3. After the 6-week program, work with the trainer to develop a program for the long haul. Find an exercise program that will help manage my pain.

The goal-setting process with these three patients followed the principles shown in Table 14–2.

After reasonable goals have been set, clinicians need to help patients find solutions when they run into difficulties in staying the course. For example, a problem can arise when goal setting triggers automatic thoughts or beliefs about the expectations of other people. Sometimes these thoughts can sabotage attempts to do things differently. To illustrate, Dr. Sudak discovered that Grace had a belief that she should spend all her free time with her children. Because this belief was interfering with her getting

---

Table 14–2. Tips for goal setting in brief sessions

Use mini-lessons or other efficient psychoeducational methods to teach patients how to set effective goals.

Choose realistic goals that have a reasonable chance of being achieved with a brief session format for treatment. Avoid sweeping, overgeneralized goals that may make patients feel overwhelmed or hopeless about making progress.

Be specific.

Choose goals that lend themselves to practical CBT-oriented solutions.

Guide patients to select goals that are meaningful, and address significant concerns and problems.

Consider setting both short-term goals that could be attained in the near future and one or more longer-term goals that may require ongoing work in CBT.

Try to use terms that make goals measurable and will help gauge progress.

If patients have difficulty working toward goals, regroup and determine barriers to reaching goals. Develop plans for overcoming obstacles and/ or revise the goals.

Note.   CBT=cognitive-behavior therapy.
Source.   Adapted from Wright JH, Basco MR, Thase ME: *Learning Cognitive-Behavior Therapy: An Illustrated Guide.* Washington, DC, American Psychiatric Publishing, 2006. Used with permission. Copyright © 2006 American Psychiatric Publishing.

involved in an exercise plan, Dr. Sudak encouraged Grace to ask her kids how they would feel if she spent 2 hours each Saturday morning playing tennis with a friend. Grace was surprised to find that her children were enthusiastic about her plan and actually had some suggestions of ways they could help her—by making breakfast on Saturday, doing some laundry, and watching a favorite TV program together.

Motivational Enhancement

Once goals are defined, motivational enhancement can be a vital part of a brief intervention. Drawing from motivational interviewing techniques (see Chapter 5, "Promoting Adherence," and Chapter 13, "CBT for Substance Misuse and Abuse"; Miller and Rollnick 2002; Sobel and Sobel 2003), patients can be encouraged to identify and write down major motivating and demotivating influences. The motivators can then be highlighted, reinforced, and burnished to help patients stay on track. Interfering or demotivating factors can be understood and, if possible, countered with behavioral plans. Judy, the patient with extreme obesity, had a history of many failed diets and short-lived exercise programs. A key motivator now was her desire to have bariatric surgery. Dr. Wright used motivational methods to enhance the power of this influence and was also able to help Judy define and intensify the power of other motivators.

> Dr. Wright: I know that you need to stick with a medically supervised diet for 6 months to qualify for the bariatric surgery, but I am wondering what is motivating you to do all of this.
>
> Judy: Well, I went to that class that the bariatric surgeon gave, and he explained that people who have been severely overweight for a long time have a tiny chance of ever losing a whole lot of weight and keeping it off without surgery.
>
> Dr. Wright: OK, I understand that point, but what is making you want to go through the surgery and the lifestyle changes that need to go along with it? What things are making you want to take this path?
>
> Judy: Being overweight is slowly killing me. My joints are wearing out, I can hardly walk a block without getting tired, I have diabetes, and I had to stop gardening and doing any real work around the house. (They go on to list some of the other major downsides of Judy's obesity [see Figure 14–1]. Then Dr. Wright asks Judy to identify the possible advantages of the bariatric surgery and lifestyle change.)
>
> Dr. Wright: Let's look at the flip side of the coin. If you had success with the surgery and you were able to change your lifestyle with healthier eating and exercise habits, what would the benefits be? How would you see your life as being different? Try to be realistic with your expectations.
>
> Judy: I could get around so much better without all of this weight. I could work in the garden again and help out my mother—she isn't getting any younger. I'd live a lot longer and be able to see my grandchildren grow up.
>
> Dr. Wright: Sounds good. Anything else?
>
> Judy: Sure. I would feel so much better about myself. Also, I don't think that I would be as depressed.

(After detailing other items listed in Figure 14–1, Dr. Wright asks Judy about demotivators and then begins to work out a plan to cope with them.)

> Dr. Wright: You've been building a good case for sticking with your plan. Are there some things that could get in the way of success? Some things that could sap your motivation and make you want to go back to the old ways? Even with lap band surgery, people can still hang on to a lot of weight if they don't change their lifestyle.

Motivators

- *Be able to have bariatric surgery and to have the surgery be a success.*
- *My health—to avoid dying early, to get rid of diabetes if possible, to not wear out my joints.*
- *Be able to live a full life: gardening, taking care of my mother, going out with friends, walking without getting out of breath.*
- *Losing a lot of weight and getting into shape would be a huge boost to my self-esteem.*
- *Maybe start to date again, find a satisfying relationship.*
- *Wear clothes that fit well and look good on me.*
- *Be able to eat food without guilt.*

Demotivators

- *I have always needed to eat when I get nervous or sad and lonely. I couldn't keep doing this.*
- *My whole family loves to eat. They could get upset if I change, and they don't. They could pressure me to eat the food they prepare or bring home.*
- *I've been heavy for so long that I'm not sure how I would react if I lost a lot of weight and people looked at me in a different way.*

Figure 14–1. Judy's list of motivators and demotivators for a diet and exercise program.

Judy: Yeah, I realize that. You're wanting me to be honest about things that would make me want to cheat in following the plan or to give up?

Dr. Wright: Can you think of things that could undermine your motivation?

Judy: Yes, when I get nervous I want to eat. Anytime I feel sad or lonely, I seem to need to eat something.

Dr. Wright: One idea to help you with the plan might be to work on some alternate coping strategies instead of using food. Would that be OK?

Judy: Yes, I know I need to do that.

They then went on to identify other possible interfering influences or demotivators, and over the course of several visits worked out a comprehensive plan for achieving her goals. Judy's list of motivators and demotivators is shown in Figure 14–1. Judy's baseline weight was 336 when the intervention plan was started. At the time this book was written, she was 5 months into her plan and had 1 month to go before the bariatric surgery. She had seen Dr. Wright every 2 weeks for a brief visit in which she reviewed her diet and exercise logs, discussed progress and obstacles, and worked to improve the regularity of her meals and quality of her diet. Her weight at the end of 5 months was 274 pounds, a 62-pound weight loss. Judy was exercising at least 45 minutes five times daily and was looking forward to her surgery.

Although Judy's treatment seemed to be heading toward a good outcome, success was far from assured. She could easily stray from the course of developing a healthier lifestyle, or she could later foil the effects of the bariatric surgery by consuming large amounts of easily digestible food. Therefore, continued treatment was planned. Of course, many other patients with similar problems fail in their attempts to change unhealthy habits, even when they are receiving CBT. Our practices are full of people who would like to change habits but have not yet done so. Change is difficult and often requires many attempts to achieve even partial success. However, experiences such as seeing the hard work that Judy did with her plan inspire us to keep trying to meet the challenging tasks of habit change and to use some of the additional methods we describe in the following subsections.

Time Management

An effective plan for implementing and sustaining change usually takes time and sustained effort. Thus, time management is often a key component in attempts to break through procrastination or modify long-standing habits. Two principal questions need to be asked about time: "How much?" and "When?" Patients may not budget sufficient time for implementing a plan for change, or they fall into the trap of making an initial commitment for a behavioral change but then putting it off or finding that they get "too busy" or "run out of time."

Specificity and regularity are often highly important variables in sustaining a behavioral change plan. Contrast these two plans:

1. I'll start an exercise program sometime this month.
   Pitfalls: 1) amount of time required has not been specified or planned; 2) detailed schedule of when to exercise has not been developed; 3) plan does not indicate how exercise will fit into rest of patient's schedule.
2. I will go to the YMCA, which is only two blocks from my work, on Tuesdays and Thursdays for 1 hour after work. It will take about 15 minutes to walk there and put on gym clothes. I will work out for 1 hour. By the time I take a shower and drive home, it will be about 7 P.M. My wife supports this plan and doesn't mind if I come home later these nights. I will also walk in my neighborhood for at least

45 minutes on Saturday or Sunday afternoon before dinner. My wife wants to walk with me.

Strengths: 1) plan is highly specific; 2) regular times during week have been set aside for exercise; 3) patient has coordinated schedule with work and home commitments; 4) family is supportive of changes; 5) plan appears to be practical and achievable.

Activity scheduling, a technique described in Chapter 6, "Behavioral Methods for Depression," can help patients determine whether they can commit sufficient time to ensure that they can accomplish a project. This tool can help patients take control of their time as they identify which activities they may need to replace or modify to reach a goal. Activity scheduling can also be a great help in tracking progress and accountability toward goal attainment by recording time spent working on the task at hand.

Self-Monitoring

One of the most powerful methods that clinicians can use to help patients change is to teach them to monitor their own behavior. We have already given one example of self-monitoring in this chapter—the diet and exercise logs kept by Judy, the patient who was preparing for bariatric surgery. A multitude of other self-monitoring techniques can be applied, including sleep diaries; computerized exercise records that calculate and track repetitions, distances covered, and calories expended; work plans for completing projects; and activity schedules. In fact, we used self-monitoring to avoid procrastination and keep a steady course toward completion of this book. We developed a work plan, monitored our efforts to meet sequential goals in the timeline, and gave each other feedback about the progress we were making.

Table 14–3 lists advantages of self-monitoring. Self-monitoring can produce change by itself. It can focus and intensify the patient's attention on the problem area and help him identify particular triggers for problem behavior or the consequences of behavior. Patients can keep a journal of instances of desired behavior to increase accountability and to decrease selective memory for success or failure. Self-monitoring also can help identify obstacles that could hamper change efforts.

Self-monitoring can give the patient information about situations in which stimulus control can be a relevant tool to facilitate new habits. For example, someone who wants to exercise more regularly may be more successful if she has a gym bag packed and in the car rather than having to go home for clothes after work, because going home presents a greater

---

Table 14–3. Advantages of self-monitoring

Draws attention to the plan for change. Can encourage expenditure of effort on sticking with the plan.

Provides positive reinforcement for change.

Increases accountability.

Can help identify problems in following the plan.

May promote use of stimulus control methods to shape desired or undesired behavior.

Can help spot facilitating or sabotaging cognitions.

Provides realistic appraisal of progress.

---

potential for the patient to get derailed or distracted. Some patients may determine a need to remove "electronic distractions" (e.g., computer, instant messaging, video games, phone, TV, Facebook) to effectively work on a project. It can help to cue the start of a work period by discontinuing these activities and setting time limits for how long the activities will be put aside.

Another important function of self-monitoring is to help patients realistically appraise and reward successes appropriately. One of the positive rewards or reinforcers for taking steps toward change is the simple gratification of seeing progress. Self-monitoring with logs, diaries, or computerized measurement systems can solidify and amplify this form of positive reinforcement. Also, a self-monitoring system can be used to build in self-reinforcers. Small treats (e.g., buying a book, downloading music, having a special meal at a restaurant, getting a new piece of clothing) can serve as rewards for reaching a modest short-term goal. Bigger rewards (e.g., taking a trip, buying a bicycle, acquiring some new electronic gear) can be planned for making more extensive changes.

> **Learning Exercise 14–1**   Using Self-Monitoring as a Tool for Behavioral Change
>
> 1. Identify a behavior you wish to change or modify.
>
> 2. Design a plan to monitor the occurrence of the behavior with a log, diary, or other system in the next week.
>
> 3. Implement the self-monitoring plan and see what you learn about the behavior.

Graded Task Assignments

A classic way to tackle challenging goals and to change habits is to use the graded task assignment system described in Chapter 6, "Behavioral Methods for Depression." Most people are familiar with the idea that breaking down a large or daunting task into smaller pieces and then taking it a step at a time can produce results, yet many have trouble executing this type of step-by-step procedure. Thus, clinicians may need to coach patients on how to use this technique and help them overcome barriers that get in their way.

In the following example, Dr. Thase is working with Todd, a man who lost his job and has been struggling to put in any meaningful and productive time to find a new one. Most of the time when Todd tries to sit down to read the employment section of his newspaper or go online to check on possibilities, he gets overwhelmed and "finds something else to do." Then he feels guilty and defeated because he has not accomplished anything toward getting back to work. As stated in the "Goal Setting" section earlier in this chapter, Todd had set goals (update résumé within 2 weeks; spend at least 2 hours per day "working" on finding a job; be back to work within 4 months—even if it is not his ideal job), but he tells Dr. Thase that he has not been able to make any significant progress in reaching these objectives.

> Dr. Thase: I think you have set some realistic goals, but something seems to be getting in the way of your making progress. What happens when you try to work on your résumé or you try to spend the 2 hours on job-hunting activities?
>
> Todd: It just seems so overwhelming. The job market is so tough right now, and my confidence is so low. I guess I just have trouble facing all of the hurdles that I'll have to jump through to get a job.
>
> Dr. Thase: I know that losing the job has hit you pretty hard, and you need to build your self-confidence back up again. I think I have an idea for a system that can help you start to make some progress. Sometimes when tasks seem to be overwhelming and people are procrastinating, they can have a breakthrough by organizing a step-by-step plan.

(Dr. Thase explains the graded task assignment method and engages Todd in the process of designing a plan. They decide to break two of his goals—updating his résumé and spending 2 hours each day "working" on finding a job—into smaller pieces.)

> Todd: Well, getting the résumé updated is the first priority. I can't do much of anything until I shape up the résumé.

Goal   *Update and improve my résumé.*

Steps   *1.   Turn on computer. Review and print out current résumé.*

2.   Go to bookstore and buy recommended book on writing effective résumés.

3.   Spend 1 hour daily of my "work" time reading this book.

4.   As I read the book, make notes on my current résumé for ideas for improvement.

5.   Target problem areas on résumé (time between jobs) and get solution for handling this from the book.

6.   Write a first draft of a revised résumé.

7.   Ask Paul to review it and give me feedback.

8.   Finalize changes to résumé and have it ready to send to possible employers.

Figure 14–2.   A step-by-step plan: Todd's example.

Dr. Thase: So, following along with this idea about building a stepwise plan to accomplish tasks, what might be the first thing to consider doing?

Todd: Turn on my computer and actually look at the résumé—I've been avoiding doing this.

Dr. Thase: OK, and assuming that you look at the résumé, what next?

Todd: Take the advice of my friend, Phil, and get a book that gives instructions on how to write an effective résumé.

During the next few minutes of this brief session, Dr. Thase helped Todd develop the graded task assignment plan shown in Figure 14–2. The first two parts of the plan were assigned for homework. At the next session, they reviewed the homework, did troubleshooting on following the rest of the plan, and developed a graded task assignment for the goal of spending at least 2 hours daily "working" on finding a job.

Problem Solving

After the clinician and patient have set goals and have a clear description of the task at hand, problems can hinder change efforts. In brief sessions, psychiatrists and patients can develop mini-formulations to identify two categories of problems that frequently undermine attempts to change habits: practical problems and psychological problems. Once the type of difficulty is specified, brief cognitive-behavioral interventions can be used to overcome roadblocks that are interfering with attempts to reach goals. Problem-solving techniques are often helpful when practical issues are hindering progress. Psychological problems are addressed in the next section of this chapter, "Cognitive Restructuring."

The basic steps for problem solving are outlined in Table 14–4. First, the problem needs to be clearly defined and stated. Second, the patient and clinician brainstorm a variety of strategies that might be considered for attacking the problem. After evaluating the pros and cons of each idea, they can choose and commit to a strategy that may be most likely to work. The last step of the problem-solving procedure is to evaluate the effectiveness of the solution and rework the plan, if needed.

Before committing to a plan, patients may need to do some research about potential strategies, such as asking friends how they have approached similar situations. Socratic questions can be helpful in forming a plan and can empower patients to consider solutions that have a good likelihood of success. Once patients execute a productive plan, it is very important to keep a written record of what has happened. The written record can become a potent tool to use if setbacks occur in the future.

If patients have skill deficits that interfere with the process of change (e.g., lack of assertiveness, poor organizational abilities, insufficient knowledge, or limited experience), the clinician may need to add skills training exercises to the problem-solving plan. Judy, the patient with obesity described earlier in this chapter, had very poor skills in eating a healthy and balanced diet. When she brought her first diet log to brief sessions with Dr. Wright, it was readily apparent that her eating habits needed to be modified if she were to reach her goals.

Judy's family members were all obese, and they had perpetuated a family culture of "grazing" with high-calorie or "junk" foods. Her earliest logs showed that she was often consuming over 4,000 calories a day with "fast food" that could be eaten at virtually any time of the day. She also had frequent snacks of foods such as pizza rolls, ice cream, and potato chips. Judy had never cooked a balanced meal and had little knowledge of how to do so. Also, she had no significant experience with sitting down for a regularly scheduled meal and eating the food with a mindful presence.

During the 5 months that Judy had been treated by Dr. Wright at the time this book was written, they had worked together to build skills for 1) meal planning, 2) improving the balance and variety of meals, 3) preparing food, 4) eating on a regular schedule and avoiding frequent snacks, and 5) developing a mindful attitude when eating meals.

Cognitive Restructuring

The discomfort involved in breaking old habits can stimulate multiple thoughts and beliefs that short-circuit the change process. Thoughts such

---

Table 14–4. Problem-solving steps

---

1. Formulate the problem in a specific, clear way.
2. Brainstorm. List as many solutions as possible without editing.
3. Evaluate the pros and cons of each solution.
4. Choose a strategy and formulate a plan.
5. Implement the plan.
6. Evaluate the effectiveness and revise the plan if necessary.

---

as "It's not fair," "It's too hard," "I'm too upset," and "I don't feel like it" can lead patients to give themselves permission to break away from their efforts to change. Clinicians can help identify these types of thoughts in brief sessions by asking patients what went through their minds when they did not engage in the strategy that was planned. Then the cognitive-behavioral techniques previously detailed in this book, such as thought change records and examining the evidence (see Chapter 7, "Targeting Maladaptive Thinking"), can be used to deal with the dysfunctional cognitions.

Thoughts that disrupt change efforts often have common themes, such as failure, perfection, or the need to put off a task because of other concerns (Leahy 2001). Once therapists discover these themes, mini-formulations (see Chapter 4, "Case Formulation and Treatment Planning") can be developed in brief sessions to help patients see how their thinking process is affecting progress. An illustration of a mini-formulation drawn by Dr. Thase and Todd, the man who was working to find a new job, is shown in Figure 14–3.

Some thoughts about change (e.g., "It's hard to do this…It will take a lot of effort") may be accurate but not very helpful in supporting efforts to reach goals. The following are good questions to ask in such circumstances: "How useful is this thought to you?" "What will happen if you continue to have this thought?" A frequently neglected intervention to help patients achieve desired outcomes is to help them define and accept what the real consequences of certain behavior changes will be. This line of questioning can often elicit a number of thoughts about what is "fair." Although it may not be "fair" that I cannot eat ice cream every night, this fact will not help me get into my pants every day. We have often found that patients can benefit from collecting data about prior experiences when they have been able to complete tasks that they did not wish to do or endured something unpleasant (e.g., cleaning up a big mess, going to work when very tired, taking care of sick children in the middle of the night).

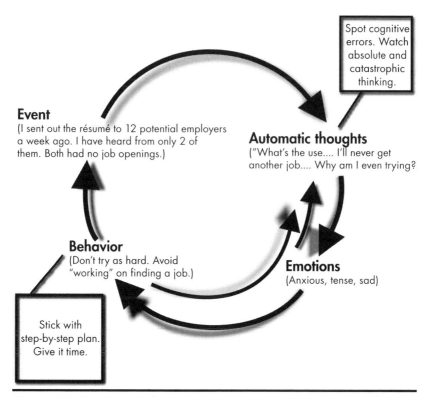

Figure 14–3.   A mini-formulation for procrastination: Todd's example.

A common trap that can subvert change is the need to do something perfectly to have it "count." Clinicians can help patients understand that if they wait for perfection, little may get done. They can use cognitive restructuring methods, such as exploring advantages and disadvantages, to modify perfectionistic beliefs. Behavioral experiments in which patients agree to purposely perform tasks at less than 100% effort or skill may help them relax rigid standards and try to make needed changes.

Building Coping Skills for Distressing Emotions

Many patients also avoid tasks in response to distressing emotions. They may have learned that procrastination can at least temporarily decrease an unpleasant emotion such as anxiety. When intense emotions are playing a role in avoidance, clinicians can use techniques described in Chapter 9, "Behavioral Methods for Anxiety," such as relaxation training and positive imagery, to assist patients in being more comfortable with altering their procrastinating behavior.

Exposure therapy is an additional technique that may be helpful in some cases. The patient can be asked to try to engage in the task that is feared for progressively longer periods of time until the anxiety diminishes. A bonus in using exposure methods is that they can help patients recognize maladaptive cognitions that are perpetuating the problem. And exposure therapy can promote testing of predictions about whether or not the distressing emotions are endurable.

Another way that painful emotions can interfere with reaching goals is when patients give themselves permission to engage in certain behaviors because of their emotional state (e.g., "I deserve ice cream because my boss yelled at me and I am upset"). In these types of situations, clinicians can help patients keep in mind the consequences of engaging in unwanted behavior ("gaining weight will not make my boss nicer to me") and employ healthier tactics to cope with upsetting emotions.

Case Example: Grace

A number of key CBT principles are at work in Video Illustration 17. Dr. Sudak quickly assesses Grace's prior experiences with exercise as they begin to conceptualize the problem. She asks Grace to consider her past and present motivators for exercise and identifies practical obstacles that could interfere with her becoming more physically active. Grace identifies a possible plan, and they work together to put that plan into action.

▶ **Video Illustration 17.** Breaking Through Procrastination: Dr. Sudak and Grace

This video also provides a demonstration of how automatic thoughts can contribute to procrastination. An important question that Dr. Sudak asks is whether thoughts about exercise influence Grace's level of motivation. Grace says, "If I don't do it every day, it doesn't count." Notice how Dr. Sudak examines this thought with Grace by asking questions such as, "You've got an idea that says that if you don't do it every day, it doesn't count…Do you know if it's true?" "What do you know about the health benefits of exercise?" "What's another way to think about exercise?" These Socratic inquiries help lead Grace to a different conclusion: "Exercising some is better than nothing." This alternative view may make it more likely that she will engage in physical activity.

One of the other methods shown in this video illustration is self-monitoring. Dr. Sudak recommends that Grace use an activity schedule to log the number of times she exercises in the week. Dr. Sudak then normalizes the need for self-monitoring by telling Grace, "Keeping a record is a help for all of us." Dr. Sudak hopes that the normalizing strategy can enhance Grace's self-regard and make it more likely that Grace might use self-monitoring in the future when faced with similar difficulties.

Practice Case: Developing a Plan for Habit Change

Almir is a 28-year-old man who is trying to complete a thesis for a master's degree in biology. He has depression but now only has low-grade symptoms of this disorder. Almir has been treated successfully by you with antidepressants and CBT for the depression. His self-rating of depressive symptoms on a 0- to 10-point scale (0=no depression; 10=the most severe depression anybody could have) has fallen to the 1–2 range. However, a remaining problem is his procrastination about finishing the work required for his advanced degree. He has completed all the other requirements except the thesis describing his research. Although Almir has landed a job working in a commercial lab, he would like to receive the degree and perhaps go on with further graduate training.

Almir has essentially stopped work on writing his dissertation. He describes himself as having "writer's block." Some of the problems that you identify are the following: 1) Almir has never had a disciplined schedule for completing writing; 2) he has his papers for the thesis spread out in a disorganized fashion throughout his apartment—most are "hidden away so they don't remind me of the problem," but others are scattered in places such as the kitchen counter or even in the trunk of his car; 3) when Almir tries to work on the thesis, he gets easily distracted by e-mails, twitter messages, and a multitude of other tasks that "seem to be important at the time"; and 4) he has a flood of automatic thoughts (e.g., "I've let it go on too long already…I'll never get this done…I waste all my time and never get anything accomplished…This is too much for me") that are dragging him down and contributing to a vicious cycle of avoidance, maladaptive thoughts, and distressing emotions.

> **Learning Exercise 14–2** Using CBT to Combat Procrastination
>
> 1. Your job is to help Almir combat his problem with procrastination. The first step is to develop a mini-formulation by filling in the blank spaces in Almir's example below.
>
> 2. In a subsequent brief session, you are pleased to hear that Almir has been getting good benefit from using a thought

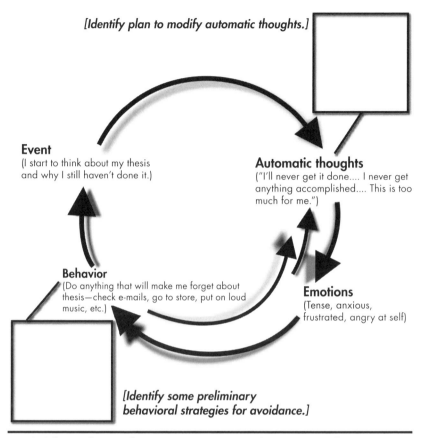

A mini-formulation for procrastination: Almir's example.

change record to develop more functional cognitions about completing the requirement for his degree. He now seems ready to work out a detailed step-by-step plan. Write out a graded task assignment for completing the thesis.

3. Your assessment revealed that Almir has a number of time management problems and distracting influences. Add to the plan some ideas for countering these issues.

4. To complete the plan, write your suggestions for using self-monitoring and self-reinforcement to assist Almir in meeting his goal.

Summary

Key Points for Clinicians

- Skillful use of goal setting can facilitate change. Targets should be specific and achievable.
- Motivational interviewing methods can be used to help people commit to and work toward change.
- Effective time management can be critical to the success of plans to modify habits.
- Self-monitoring tools can be used to track and reinforce progress. Written logs or diaries are often key elements of effective change plans.
- Graded task assignments help people use a stepwise approach to change instead of giving up in the face of challenging projects.
- Problem-solving methods may be needed to assist people in overcoming obstacles to change. Setbacks can provide an important opportunity for enhancing problem-solving skills.
- Core CBT methods for changing maladaptive cognitions can play an important role in helping people to modify self-defeating thoughts and to generate healthy attitudes about change.
- If distressing emotions are leading to avoidance, behavioral methods such as relaxation training, positive imagery, and exposure therapy may be needed to reduce the intensity of the emotion and promote efforts to change habits.

Concepts and Skills for Patients to Learn

- Changing habits is difficult for everybody. However, tools from CBT can help people change their lifestyle and reach their goals.
- Specific, manageable goals and a clear plan can help increase the chances for success.
- Try to build up the case for change. List the key motivators or advantages to doing things differently. Keeping the motivators at the top of your mind can be a big help when the going gets tough.
- One of the most useful methods for changing habits is to write down your efforts to change on a log and to review this with your doctor or therapist.
- Everyone needs rewards for effort. Try to build in some realistic rewards in your plan for change.
- Set aside enough time to work on change, and schedule routine times to engage in your new or revised habits.

- When a challenge seems big or a task seems overwhelming, break it down into smaller pieces that can be achieved step by step. With each step forward, you can build your confidence and skills.
- Most people run into problems in accomplishing plans for change. If this happens to you, your doctor or therapist can help you figure out solutions for the obstacles. Don't give up if problems arise—use them as learning opportunities.
- People can have a variety of self-defeating, self-critical thoughts when they try to change their habits. If you recognize these thoughts, you and your doctor or therapist can use CBT tools to help you develop a more positive attitude.
- If upsetting emotions, such as anxiety or anger, are getting in the way of building new habits, you can learn CBT methods to cope with these feelings and stay on track with your plan for change.

References

Carels RA, Konrad K, Young KM, et al: Taking control of your personal eating and exercise environment: a weight maintenance program. Eat Behav 9:228–237, 2008

Grilo CM, Masheb RM: A randomized controlled comparison of guided self-help cognitive behavioral therapy and behavioral weight loss for binge eating disorder. Behav Res Ther 43:1509–1525, 2005

Leahy R: Overcoming Resistance in Cognitive Therapy. New York, Guilford, 2001

Miller WR, Rollnick S: Motivational Interviewing: Preparing People for Change, 2nd Edition. New York, Guilford, 2002

Sobel LC, Sobel MB: Using motivational interviewing techniques to talk with clients about their alcohol use. Cogn Behav Pract 10:214–221, 2003

CHAPTER 15

CBT in Medical Patients

LEARNING MAP

Rationale for using CBT in medical illnesses

Empirical evidence for efficacy of CBT in medical illnesses

High-yield CBT interventions for patients with medical problems

---

A great deal of research and clinical work has been focused on the development of cognitive-behavior therapy (CBT) methods that can help patients with medical illnesses (Safran et al. 2008; Sensky 2004; Wright et al. 2008). Our goal in this chapter is to explain how some of the most practical and efficient CBT methods for patients with physical disorders can be implemented in brief sessions. Because CBT applications for medical illnesses may be unfamiliar to some readers, we outline a few of the important reasons for doing this type of work and provide a short tour through some of the empirical backing for this approach.

Rationale for Using CBT in Medical Illnesses

CBT, of course, is not used for treatment of the primary disease state in patients with medical disorders but is an adjunctive therapy that is targeted toward reducing symptom burden and helping people better accept and manage physical illnesses. Although many effective treatments are available for medical problems, a great number of patients have chronic diseases with residual problems such as pain, reduced mobility, weakness, or impaired daily functioning. Others are experiencing the onset of a severe illness and are struggling to come to grips with the diagnosis and engage in an effective treatment plan. Still others are grieving over loss of function or have problems adhering to needed treatments. CBT can be used to assist patients in coping with all of these situations.

An additional reason for using CBT is that patients with physical problems often have anxiety or depression that is sufficient to warrant referral to a mental health specialist for treatment. A variety of studies have found high rates of depression and anxiety in medical disorders such as heart disease (Januzzi et al. 2000; Lichtman et al. 2008), diabetes (Anderson et al. 2001), cancer (Spiegal and Giese-Davis 2003), and stroke (Morris et al. 1993). Depression is three times more common in patients following myocardial infarction than in the normal population (Lichtman et al. 2008) and is frequently observed in patients with positive human immunodeficiency virus (HIV) status (Dew et al. 1997).

Many patients who have mental illnesses such as bipolar disorder or schizophrenia and who are being followed with brief medication management develop physical illnesses over their lifetimes. Having a severe psychiatric disorder substantially increases morbidity and mortality from medical problems. Depression raises the risk of death in patients with cardiovascular disease (Focht et al. 2004; Lichtman et al. 2008; van Melle et al. 2004) and diabetes (Katon and Ciechanowski 2002) and decreases immune function in patients with positive HIV (Antoni et al. 2005). Another ominous finding is that patients with bipolar disorder and schizophrenia have shortened life spans because of increased rates of medical disorders, particularly cardiovascular disease (Newcomer and Hennekins 2007). Thus, clinicians who are providing combined CBT and pharmacotherapy for patients with psychiatric conditions also need to be on the lookout for medical problems in these patients, be advocates for their receiving high-level medical care, help them learn how to lead healthier lifestyles, and teach them coping skills for physical symptoms.

Empirical Evidence for Efficacy of CBT in Medical Illnesses

Numerous meta-analyses and reviews have found that CBT has benefits for patients with physical illnesses (Safran et al. 2008; Sensky 2004;

Wright et al. 2008). Positive results from adjunctive CBT include decreased distress and pain in patients with breast cancer (Tatrow and Montgomery 2006), better glycemic control in patients with diabetes (Lustman et al. 1998; Snoek et al. 2008), and decreased symptoms in a variety of patients with chronic pain (Linton and Nordin 2006; Linton and Ryberg 2001; Moore et al. 2000; Morley et al. 1999; Turner and Jensen 1993). Other studies have shown that treatment with CBT can help patients with multiple sclerosis to have improved psychological and physical functioning (Rodgers et al. 1996), enable people with hypertension to have decreased medication requirements (Shapiro et al. 1997), and benefit patients with fibromyalgia and chronic fatigue syndromes (Bennett and Nelson 2006; Deale et al. 2001; Stulemeijer et al. 2005).

The list of additional CBT applications in medical disorders is quite large and includes conditions such as asthma (Maes and Schlosser 1988), inflammatory and irritable bowel syndromes (Kennedy et al. 2006; Payne and Blanchard 1995), and temporomandibular joint syndrome (Mishra et al. 2000; Turner et al. 2006). Taken together, these studies suggest that CBT can be combined with indicated physical treatments to enhance quality of life and daily functioning in many patients with medical illnesses.

High-Yield CBT Interventions for Patients With Medical Problems

The CBT approach to treating people with medical disorders in brief sessions uses all of the general procedures outlined in Chapters 1, "Introduction"; 2, "Indications and Formats for Brief CBT Sessions"; 3, "Enhancing the Impact of Brief Sessions"; and 4, "Case Formulation and Treatment Planning." Special attention should be paid to understanding the meanings that patients attach to having a medical diagnosis and requiring treatment, screening for depression and anxiety that may have been triggered by the medical illness, and developing effective coping strategies for physical symptoms. Also, clinicians need to coordinate their work with the plans of other physicians who are treating the patients. Table 15–1 lists some of the high-yield CBT methods that we recommend for assisting people who have medical problems. These methods are discussed in the following subsections.

Identify Patient's Explanatory Model for the Illness

Psychological problems produced by medical illnesses are highly influenced by the personal meaning that a patient imparts to having the dis-

---

Table 15–1. Ten high-yield cognitive-behavior therapy
interventions for patients with medical problems

---

1. Identify patient's explanatory model for the illness.
2. Provide psychoeducation.
3. Employ motivational interviewing.
4. Use cognitive-behavior therapy tools to promote adherence.
5. Teach patients skills to facilitate communication with care providers.
6. Implement activity scheduling to enhance personal control.
7. Problem-solve when necessary.
8. Take steps to reduce arousal.
9. Correct misconceptions and distortions.
10. Facilitate grieving and acceptance of losses.

---

ease (Sensky 2004). Categories of dysfunctional thinking about illness include maladaptive thoughts and beliefs about the experience of being ill; about the consequences of a particular illness; about the type of illness itself; or about physicians, medications, or hospitals. Some of these ideas can be widely held in a patient's culture or subculture and may need thoughtful exploration to effect change. A few examples of meanings that might be attached to having an illness are noted in Table 15–2. CBT methods can be directed at modifying potentially deleterious meanings and developing and strengthening positive meanings.

An illustration of the way personal meaning can be addressed effectively in a brief session can be found in Dr. Sudak's treatment of Allan, a 53-year-old man who has been struggling since having a heart attack 6 months ago. He is a high school teacher who previously was an avid exerciser. He believed that his vigorous exercise program, which included running marathons, would "immunize" him against having an early heart attack. He had an uncle who died suddenly of a heart attack at age 54; however, Allan's father, who was a very active man, lived into his mid-80s until his death 2 years ago.

Now Allan seems adrift. He feels very vulnerable to sudden death and is avoiding any exercise, despite his doctor's report that his heart is much better and that moderate exercise is highly recommended. Allan also is avoiding having sex with his wife due to an intense fear that the exertions of sex will be too much for his heart. Before the heart attack, they had a "great" sex life.

The meanings that Allan has attached to having an unexpected heart attack appear to include a 180-degree switch from feeling fully protected by exercise to his current view of being totally vulnerable. Understanding

---

Table 15–2. Personal meanings that may be attached to having a medical illness

---

Meanings that could negatively impact adjustment

Having this condition means that I am weak.

This just proves that life is futile. Why try so hard?

It is shameful to have this problem.

Natural remedies are always better than chemicals that doctors push. I can do this better on my own.

Everything I did to live a healthy life was a waste.

You have to be careful about trusting doctors. They are in the pockets of the drug companies.

If I can't do everything I used to do, it isn't worth trying.

I deserved to get this illness.

Meanings that could positively impact adjustment

It is tough luck, but anybody can get this type of disease.

This disease will test me, but I can approach it like any other problem. Get as much information as possible—then figure out the best solution.

I've coped with lots of other problems; I can face this illness.

I've seen other people fight this disease; I can too.

This is a wake-up call to live a healthier life.

I need to live my life in a meaningful way with this illness.

I am not my disease; I am still myself.

My doctor, my family, and I can be an effective team to fight this problem. I need to make sure that we are on the same page with our plans.

---

this switch helped Dr. Sudak formulate a plan for helping Allan develop a more realistic view of his personal health, including risks involved in exercise and sex.

▶ **Video Illustration 18.** Helping a Patient With a Medical Disorder I: Dr. Sudak and Allan

In Video Illustration 18, Dr. Sudak uses Socratic questions to help Allan evaluate his predictions about physical activity and to uncover his explanatory model for his current physical state—a feeling of intense exhaustion. Allan reports that he believes heart disease is the cause of his severe tiredness ("I haven't recovered completely from the heart attack").

Because Dr. Sudak is aware of the cardiologist's report and recommendations, namely that he has had an excellent recovery from the heart attack and that a moderate exercise program is needed, she works with Allan to develop alternative explanations for his fatigue (e.g., stress, depression, deconditioning). This line of questioning leads to a conversation about his lack of confidence about his physical health and his fears that his heart condition is similar to that of his uncle who died at a young age. Dr. Sudak uses the following Socratic questions in asking Allan to discover information about himself and his heart:

- "What is different between you and your uncle?"
- "What did the doctors say about your heart after the heart attack?"
- "Why would they want you to exercise?"
- "What would it take to build your confidence?"

Dr. Sudak also uses capsule summaries to rapidly synthesize the data at hand and to emphasize key points to Allan (e.g., "In your head you know it might be a good thing to exercise, at least in a moderate way, but you're not feeling so confident about doing that"). They wrap up their work in this brief session by making a coping card with facts about the current state of Allan's heart (e.g., "My cardiologist says I'm recovering nicely") and his doctor's recommendations for physical exercise. Allan agrees to use the card as a reminder and confidence booster as he increases walking to five times a week and measures his fatigue before and after walking on a 0- to 100-point scale.

> **Learning Exercise 15–1**   Understanding the Meanings of Medical Illnesses
>
> 1. Think of a patient in your practice who has a chronic physical disorder. What meanings and beliefs about the problem could possibly interfere with the patient's managing the illness?
>
> 2. Write out a mini-formulation that shows how key maladaptive beliefs are influencing the patient's emotions and behavior.
>
> 3. Add a plan to work with these beliefs to the mini-formulation.

Provide Psychoeducation

Patients have access to a great variety of resources to help them learn about medical illnesses and partner with their doctors in effective disease management. This explosion of medical information has both positive and negative ramifications. Many patients get good information about their illnesses from Web sites and printed publications. Skilled use of these resources in briefer sessions can be a powerful tool to further patients' participation in their own care. Internet-based information can be a problem, however, because the quality of information available to patients is so variable and because the sheer amount of material can be overwhelming. Thus, clinicians need to become familiar with good resources and to determine the optimal amount of exposure that will promote effective learning. In brief sessions, clinicians can pinpoint the salient information that patients need to manage their conditions and can assist them in finding and understanding the most useful educational materials. Sometimes we go online in brief sessions to give patients a boost in locating valuable information.

> **Learning Exercise 15–2** Finding Educational Resources for Medical Problems
>
> 1. Choose two or three of the most common medical problems experienced by the patients in your practice.
>
> 2. Spend about 10–15 minutes looking online for resources that could help patients who are seeking information about these illnesses.

Employ Motivational Interviewing

The motivational interviewing techniques discussed in Chapter 14, "Lifestyle Change: Building Healthy Habits," can also be used to benefit patients with medical disorders who have been advised to stop smoking, reduce or discontinue alcohol use, lose weight, exercise regularly, or change other habits. Many of the other methods detailed in Chapter 14 for lifestyle change can be used as well.

One patient mentioned in Chapter 14 was Raphael, a man with chronic pain who had been told by his doctor that he should start an exercise program. Although Raphael had set reasonable goals for the program, he had not been able to get started. Therefore, Dr. Turkington used motivational interviewing as part of the treatment plan to help Raphael engage in exercise. Figure 15–1 shows the motivators and demotivators that they identified. Highlighting the motivators helped Raphael get going with the exercise program, and Dr. Turkington and Raphael were able to work on plans to cope with the demotivators. The most powerful demotivators were the expectations that pain could get worse or that he

Motivators

* *Sticking with a reasonable exercise program will build strength in my muscles, increase flexibility, and eventually help me cope with the pain.*
* *Exercise will help me be more functional around the house.*
* *My wife and kids really want me to get back in gear.*
* *I hope exercise will help me have sex more comfortably.*
* *A long-term motivator is to build myself up to the point that I could work again.*
* *Exercise can reduce depression.*

Demotivators

* *The pain could get worse, at least for a while. Exercise increased my pain in the past.*
* *I could get even less functional if I go into spasms and can't even sit in a chair.*
* *I'm so out of shape that I would be ashamed to go to a gym.*
* *The equipment and the facility cost money.*

Figure 15–1. Raphael's list of motivators and demotivators for an exercise program.

would actually be less functional for a while if his back hurt too much to drive or sit at his desk. The strategy that they decided on was for Raphael to begin a professionally supervised and very gradual exercise routine and to use a coping card that listed some of his positive motivators about the long-term value of exercise. When he looked at the costs of working with a trainer versus the costs of continued pain and disability, he decided the investment in the exercise plan would be a good one.

Use CBT Tools to Facilitate Adherence

The dozen CBT methods described in Chapter 5, "Promoting Adherence," can be quite useful in helping patients follow medication regimens for physical illnesses. Some of the most useful of these procedures are modifying automatic thoughts about having an illness or taking medication, pairing medication taking with another activity that is accomplished routinely, using reminder systems, identifying barriers to compliance, and developing a written adherence plan.

Teach Patients Skills to Facilitate Communication With Care Providers

Communicating with physicians and navigating the complexity of the medical care environment are daunting tasks when a person is healthy

---

Table 15–3. Skills to facilitate communication with care providers

---

Before the medical appointment, spend time organizing your questions.

Write down your questions in advance. This will help you remember to cover all important topics.

Keep a list of all your diagnoses, medications, and the doctors who have prescribed the medications. Update the list each time a change is made. This list can be particularly helpful when you are seeing multiple doctors from different practices. Do not assume that all your doctors know every medicine you are taking.

Keep a list of the names, phone numbers, and addresses of all your doctors. Take this list with you to each doctor's visit.

Do not be afraid to take notes during your appointment with your doctors. It is very easy to forget key information. Written notes will help you remember important facts.

Ask your doctor about policies and procedures for phone, e-mail, and written communications. It is good to know in advance how your doctor will handle phone calls or other communications.

Be assertive and persistent if needed. Because most doctors are very busy, they may not always be fully sensitive to your need for information. However, they will usually respond if you ask questions in a straightforward way.

It is OK to ask doctors questions about sensitive topics. It is much better to openly discuss these topics than to leave an appointment with important questions unanswered.

---

and well informed. Clinicians may have had this experience themselves with an illness. Imagine, then, what the experience could be like for a person with fewer resources and less information. Psychiatrists can be a great support in helping patients understand illnesses, communicate better with their care providers, and manage the challenges of the network of care. Table 15–3 lists some of the methods that our patients have found useful.

If communication problems with physicians are not resolved by following the general guidelines listed in Table 15–3, a clinician can use part of the brief session to help a patient examine automatic thoughts about her physicians (some of which may be true), role-play more assertive behavior, employ behavioral experiments, or use other CBT methods to try to resolve the problem.

In Video Illustration 19, Dr. Sudak demonstrates this type of work in a brief session when she helps Allan build his confidence for discussing a sensitive topic (i.e., his concerns about harming his heart if he has sex).

Table 15–4. Activity scheduling for patients with medical problems

---

Collect data about pain, medication side effects, energy, and other variables through the day.

Schedule activities that are important (pleasurable events, necessary tasks to deal with symptoms or side effects) during times of day that are best for the patient.

Use schedule as behavioral reminder for taking medications.

Plan behavioral experiments to test predictions about the illness.

Schedule relaxation or worry time.

Dr. Sudak identifies and lists Allan's concerns, explores his automatic thoughts about his cardiologist, and suggests that he write down his questions for his doctor before his next visit. Allan admits that his mind "goes blank" when he sees his cardiologist and that he remembers little of what is said. Therefore, he plans to take a pad with him so he can take notes and review them after the appointment.

▶ **Video Illustration 19.** Helping a Patient With a Medical Disorder II: Dr. Sudak and Allan

Implement Activity Scheduling to Enhance Personal Control

Behavioral skills learned in CBT (see Chapter 6, "Behavioral Methods for Depression," and Chapter 9, "Behavioral Methods for Anxiety") can help patients with practical problems that stem from physical illness. One of the most commonly used methods, activity scheduling, is shown in Video Illustration 18. Dr. Sudak uses an activity schedule in this video to help Allan plan physical activity and collect data by rating his level of fatigue before and after walking. The activity schedule helps to organize the information gathered during the behavioral experiment and provides a tool to remind Allan of the homework assignment. Table 15–4 lists some creative uses for activity schedules for patients with medical illnesses.

Activity schedules can help patients have a better sense of personal control when they use the schedules to better organize their time and take control of their days. They can also use activity schedules to determine whether the beliefs they have about symptoms are actually true. For example, patients with chronic pain, when asked, might say that their

Problem

- *Pain interferes with my doing chores (cooking, cleaning, painting, yardwork).*
- *Wife works all day and gets irritated when I don't help out.*
- *I end up feeling like I am lazy—that I don't contribute anything to the family.*

Plan

1. *Have full discussion with wife about my pain and my limitations. Negotiate a step-by-step plan for me to gradually increase responsibility for household chores.*
2. *Ask wife to try to hold the criticism for a while and give me support for trying to take on some responsibility. If this doesn't work, ask her to come to some of my sessions with Dr. Turkington.*
3. *Use relaxation and positive imagery to try to reduce pain while I am working on chores.*
4. *Continue with the exercise program to build my strength and to "harden" me for working while experiencing pain.*
5. *Recognize self-critical thoughts. Write them down on a thought change record and use this system to give myself credit for trying.*

Figure 15–2. Raphael's coping card.

pain is constantly severe and never remits. Such patients can use hourly observation with ratings of symptoms to see whether the pain varies with different activities (e.g., distracting or enjoyable tasks vs. times of boredom, loneliness, or tension). Another good application for activity schedules is planning the time necessary for effective disease management, such as exercise, medication, or rest. Also, scheduling techniques can help patients allocate time for implementing rewards to reinforce new habits that they must acquire to successfully manage their symptoms.

Problem-Solve When Necessary

When patients with medical disorders are confronted with practical problems, such as financial concerns, transportation issues, housing, and coping with the demands of managing their physical illnesses, clinicians can recommend the problem-solving methods that are outlined in Chapter 14, "Lifestyle Change: Building Healthy Habits." The ideas that are generated with problem-solving techniques can be summarized in a coping card, as shown in Figure 15–2. Dr. Turkington and Raphael, the man who was facing chronic pain, developed this card to help him manage a problem with functioning in the home setting.

Take Steps to Reduce Arousal

Raphael's problem-solving plan included the use of progressive relaxation and positive imagery to cope with pain. These techniques (detailed in Chapter 9, "Behavioral Methods for Anxiety") can also be applied in many other situations in which patients with medical disorders are experiencing excessive arousal or physical tension. Other methods that can be considered for this purpose are breathing retraining and mindfulness. Autonomic arousal and/or tension of the skeletal musculature can make the symptoms of a medical disorder more difficult to tolerate (e.g., in fibromyalgia, headache, or temporomandibular joint syndrome). Thus, efforts to use CBT to reduce excessive arousal may pay significant dividends.

Correct Misconceptions and Distortions

In Video Illustration 18, Dr. Sudak uses Socratic questioning to help Allan modify some of his dysfunctional thinking after a heart attack. Prior to the heart attack, Allan had a positively distorted view of the value of exercise (i.e., that exercise provides "immunization" against heart disease). Following the heart attack, he has excessive fear of exercise and exaggerates his vulnerability to bad outcomes that could be related to physical activity. Several thinking errors, including magnification, ignoring the evidence, and absolutistic thinking, are involved. By the end of this session, Allan appears to have a less distorted view of exercise and is able to commit to a plan of increased physical activity.

Cognitive restructuring is also used in Video Illustration 19 when Dr. Sudak helps Allan examine the evidence about the risks of sudden death from engaging in sex with his wife. Allan remembers a newspaper article that he read in the past about a man who died after having sex. This demonstrates that Allan has thinking errors that are promulgating a dysfunctional belief. This single incident is overgeneralized and magnified to the extent that he concludes that he will have a higher probability of having a heart attack if his heart rate goes up during sex. When Dr. Sudak points out that there probably have been many people who have had sex with their partners without any damage to their hearts and who were not written up in the newspaper, Allan chuckles and admits that his thinking has been skewed.

In working with patients with medical disorders, clinicians may have many opportunities to use the standard cognitive restructuring methods described in Chapter 7, "Targeting Maladaptive Thinking." The following are some examples of misconceptions and distortions about physical illnesses that our patients have reported.

- "I'm going straight downhill"—A patient with chronic obstructive pulmonary disease visualized herself racing down a snowy slope in a runaway sled with no control, yet much evidence indicated that her symptoms could be managed effectively.
- "The pain has robbed me of everything I ever wanted"—A patient with chronic pain had indeed lost much function and was unable to work, but she still had loving family relationships, interests that could be used as opportunities for growth, and the capability to learn new skills.
- "I will lose control and totally embarrass myself...I need to stay by myself and avoid all social activities"—A patient with irritable bowel syndrome who once had an "accident in public" magnified the risk of having bowel problems in public, minimized his capacity to cope with this problem if it did occur, and exaggerated the reactions that others might have.

Facilitate Grieving and Acceptance of Losses

Another way for practitioners to help medical patients in brief sessions is to provide opportunities for them to express appropriate grief, anxiety, and anger about the illness and the issues they face as a result of the physical problems. The therapist often provides one of the only "safe havens" for such work; family and friends may wish to reassure the patient or express that the patient should be grateful for her current treatment. Sometimes loved ones may be too overwhelmed with their own sense of anxiety and loss to be able to assist patients in discussing reactions to illness and coming to a new level of acceptance.

Our discussions with medical patients about grief and loss often turn to existential themes. We use methods described by Frankl (1992) to help people find meaning and purpose in the face of serious illness (or impending death if the illness is terminal or likely to be so). We also may discuss patients' spiritual beliefs and assist them with engaging with spiritual counselors and using spiritual resources in managing loss and moving toward acceptance. In addition, classic CBT methods such as cognitive restructuring and behavioral activation can be useful with many patients who are grieving the losses associated with having a medical illness. Clinicians can help patients recognize and change cognitive distortions (e.g., "No woman would want to date a man who had prostate cancer surgery"; "I'll have to give up all the things I really enjoy"; "I'll just be a drag on my family") that may be aggravating or accelerating a sense of loss. Also, activity scheduling and graded task assignments can help reactivate patients as a part of working through grief. Becoming active again, at least in a partial way, can give patients with medical disorders hope that they can begin to cope with their grief and have a meaningful life.

Summary

Key Points for Clinicians

- CBT is used adjunctively in the treatment of medical disorders to reduce symptom burden and to help build coping skills.
- CBT methods have been shown to be useful for a wide range of medical disorders.
- The meanings that patients attach to having medical illnesses can have a major influence on their coping styles.
- As with other CBT applications in brief sessions, psychoeducation is a core component of treatment. Efficient educational methods, including mini-lessons, handouts, and Internet searches, can be tailored to the brief session format.
- A number of high-yield CBT methods can be used to help patients with medical disorders. These include motivational interviewing, adherence interventions, enhancement of communication with health care providers, activity scheduling, problem solving, relaxation training, positive imagery, cognitive restructuring, and efforts to facilitate grieving.

Concepts and Skills for Patients to Learn

- If you are having problems coping with a medical illness, it can help to discuss these difficulties with a clinician who has been trained in CBT.
- People can have beliefs and attitudes about medical illnesses that can undermine their attempts to effectively manage their problems.
- Lots of information about medical illnesses is available in books and on the Internet. Although it is usually helpful to gain knowledge about physical illnesses that you may have, discussions with your doctor or therapist are an important part of the learning process. Your doctor or therapist can help you cull out the most important and accurate information about medical illnesses.
- CBT can provide many useful tools to cope with physical illnesses. These methods can help people reduce tension and anxiety, make lifestyle changes if needed, build problem-solving skills, and communicate more effectively with their doctors or therapists.

References

Anderson RJ, Freedland KE, Crouse RE, et al: The prevalence of comorbid depression in adults with diabetes: a meta-analysis. Diabetes Care 24:1069–1078, 2001

Antoni MH, Cruess DG, Klimas N, et al: Increases in a marker of immune system reconstitution are predated by decreases in 24-h urinary cortisol output and depressed mood during a 10-week stress management intervention in symptomatic HIV-infected men. J Psychosom Res 58:3–13, 2005

Bennett R, Nelson D: Cognitive behavioral therapy for fibromyalgia. Nat Clin Pract Rheumatol 2:416–424, 2006

Deale A, Husain K, Chalder T, et al: Long-term outcome of cognitive behavior therapy versus relaxation therapy for chronic fatigue syndrome: a 5-year follow-up study. Am J Psychiatry 158:2038–2042, 2001

Dew MA, Becker JT, Sanchez J, et al: Prevalence and predictors of depressive, anxiety and substance use disorders in HIV-infected and uninfected men: a longitudinal evaluation. Psychol Med 27:395–409, 1997

Focht BC, Brawley LR, Rejeski WJ, et al: Group-mediated activity counseling and traditional exercise programs: effects on health-related quality of life among older adults in cardiac rehabilitation. Ann Behav Med 28:52–61, 2004

Frankl VE: Man's Search for Meaning: An Introduction to Logotherapy, 4th Edition. Boston, MA, Beacon Press, 1992

Januzzi JL, Stein TA, Pasternak RC, et al: The influence of anxiety and depression on outcomes of patients with coronary artery disease. Arch Intern Med 160:1913–1921, 2000

Katon WJ, Ciechanowski P: Impact of major depression on chronic medical illness. J Psychosom Res 53:859–863, 2002

Kennedy TM, Chalder T, McCrone P, et al: Cognitive behavioural therapy in addition to antispasmodic therapy for irritable bowel syndrome in primary care: randomized controlled trial. Health Technol Assess 10(19):1–84, 2006

Lichtman JH, Bigger JT, Blumenthal JA, et al: Depression and coronary heart disease. Circulation 118:1–8, 2008

Linton SJ, Nordin E: A 5-year follow-up evaluation of the health and economic consequences of an early cognitive behavioral intervention for back pain: a randomized, controlled trial. Spine 31:853–858, 2006

Linton SJ, Ryberg M: A cognitive-behavioral group intervention as prevention for persistent neck and back pain in a non-patient population: a randomized controlled trial. Pain 90:83–90, 2001

Lustman PJ, Griffith LS, Freedland KE, et al: Cognitive behavior therapy for depression in type 2 diabetes mellitus: a randomized, controlled trial. Ann Intern Med 129:613–621, 1998

Maes S, Schlosser M: Changing health behavior outcomes in asthmatic patients: a pilot study. Soc Sci Med 26:359–364, 1988

Mishra KD, Gatchel RJ, Gardea MA: The relative efficacy of three cognitive-behavioral treatment approaches to temporomandibular disorders. J Behav Med 23:293–309, 2000

Moore JE, Von Korff M, Cherkin D, et al: A randomized trial of a cognitive-behavioral program for enhancing back pain self care in a primary care setting. Pain 88:145–153, 2000

Morley S, Eccleston C, Williams A: Systematic review and meta-analysis of randomized controlled trials of cognitive behavior therapy and behavior therapy for chronic pain in adults, excluding headache. Pain 80:1–13, 1999

Morris PL, Robinson RG, Andrzejewski P, et al: Association of depression in 10-year poststroke mortality. Am J Psychiatry 150:124–129, 1993

Newcomer JW, Hennekins CH: Severe mental illness and cardiovascular disease. JAMA 298:1794–1796, 2007

Payne A, Blanchard EB: A controlled comparison of cognitive therapy and self-help support groups in the treatment of irritable bowel syndrome. J Consult Clin Psychol 63:779–786, 1995

Rodgers D, Khoo K, MacEachen M, et al: Cognitive therapy for multiple sclerosis: a preliminary study. Altern Ther Health Med 2:70–74, 1996

Safran SA, Gonzalez JS, Soroudi N: Coping with Chronic Illness. New York, Oxford University Press, 2008

Sensky T: Cognitive behavioral therapy for patients with physical illness, in Cognitive-Behavior Therapy. Edited by Wright JH (Review of Psychiatry Series, Vol 23; Oldman JM and Riba MB, series eds). Washington, DC, American Psychiatric Publishing, 2004, pp 83–121

Shapiro D, Hui KK, Oakley ME, et al: Reduction in drug requirements for hypertension by means of a cognitive-behavioral intervention. Am J Hypertens 10:9–17, 1997

Snoek FJ, van der Ven NC, Twisk JW, et al: Cognitive behavioural therapy (CBT) compared with blood glucose awareness training (BGAT) in poorly controlled Type 1 diabetic patients: long-term effects on HbA moderated by depression: a randomized controlled trial. Diabet Med 25:1337–1342, 2008

Spiegal D, Giese-Davis J: Depression and cancer: mechanisms and disease progression. Biol Psychiatry 54:269-282, 2003

Stulemeijer M, de Jong LW, Fiselier TJ, et al: Cognitive behaviour therapy for adolescents with chronic fatigue syndrome: randomised controlled trial. BMJ 330:14, 2005

Tatrow K, Montgomery GH: Cognitive behavioral therapy techniques for distress and pain in breast cancer patients: a meta-analysis. J Behav Med 29:17–27, 2006

Turner JA, Jensen MP: Efficacy of cognitive therapy for chronic low back pain. Pain 52:169–177, 1993

Turner JA, Manci L, Aaron LA: Short- and long-term efficacy of brief cognitive-behavioral therapy for patients with chronic temporomandibular disorder pain: a randomized, controlled trial. Pain 121:181–194, 2006 van Melle JP, de Jonge P, Spijkerman TA, et al: Prognostic association of depression following myocardial infarction and cardiovascular events: a meta-analysis. Psychosom Med 66:814–822, 2004

Wright JH, Beck AT, Thase ME: Cognitive therapy, in The American Psychiatric Publishing Textbook of Psychiatry, 5th Edition. Edited by Hales RE, Yudofsky SC, Gabbard GO. Washington, DC, American Psychiatric Publishing, 2008, pp 1211–1256

CHAPTER 16

Relapse Prevention

LEARNING MAP

CBT model of relapse prevention

⇩

Educating about the risk for relapse

⇩

Recognizing and treating residual symptoms

⇩

Identifying triggers or early warning signs for relapse

⇩

Developing relapse prevention plans

⇩

Involving significant others in relapse prevention plans

Although the short-term goal of cognitive-behavior therapy (CBT) is symptom relief, the ultimate measure of treatment success is maintaining and maximizing those gains over the long term, including the prevention of relapse or recurrence of major episodes of illness. The aims of successful therapy go far beyond those of acute phase therapy and include the ongoing use of self-directed interventions that are intended to reduce vulnerability and promote lifestyle changes.

Another fundamental tenet of CBT is that the recommended strategies for relapse prevention should be tested scientifically. In this regard, studies of CBT for major depressive disorder (Blackburn and Moore 1997; Bockting et al. 2005; Hollon et al. 1992, 2005; Kovacs et al. 1981; Paykel et al. 1999), bipolar affective disorder (Ball et al. 2006; Fava et al. 2001; Lam et al. 2001, 2003; Scott et al. 2001), panic disorder (Barlow et al. 2000), insomnia (Morin et al. 2009), and schizophrenia (Grawe et al. 2006; Gumley et al. 2003; Turkington et al. 2006, 2008) have demonstrated that CBT can have enduring benefit. Although not all studies are in agreement (e.g., see Scott et al. 2006) and the effects may diminish over a number of years (Paykel et al. 2005), the overall weight of the evidence supports the view that CBT significantly improves longer-term outcomes and reduces the risk of relapse across a broad range of disorders.

Many prescribing clinicians see patients for brief visits for long periods of time after an acute episode of illness has resolved or attenuated, especially when the patient has a history of previous recurrences of an Axis I disorder. Thus, these clinicians are well positioned to monitor for signs of potential relapse and to continue to work with patients to put CBT relapse prevention strategies into action. In this chapter, we discuss methods that are used to promote use of self-help strategies that can help patients become their "own therapists" as sessions are tapered or possibly discontinued. We view these self-help methods as a means to achieve enduring cognitive and behavioral changes and relapse prevention. We also provide practical illustrations on how to incorporate these strategies within longer-term treatment plans that emphasize maintenance pharmacotherapy.

CBT Model of Relapse Prevention

A relapse prevention component is built into CBT from the outset of therapy because this treatment emphasizes building skills to manage symptoms. During the course of treatment, patients are encouraged to use homework assignments to practice using these skills every day. As patients gain greater confidence in using the CBT methods that are the most helpful in managing symptoms, they are encouraged to apply these principles to a broader array of difficulties outside of specific homework assignments. At a core belief level, such confidence reflects an increasing sense of self-efficacy, with more functional attitudes and beliefs about coping with adversity (i.e., "I can deal with life's problems and, when necessary, can adapt and improvise new solutions"). This new approach to problem solving not only promotes greater self-reliance but also helps patients to better recognize when to ask others for help. The effective clinician shapes and reinforces these attitudes, beliefs, and behaviors and is able to convey to the patient the notion that ultimately the patient, rather than the person who delivered the therapy, is the primary agent of change.

Educating About the Risk for Relapse

The old saying that "forewarned is forearmed" is especially pertinent to the treatment of individuals with psychiatric disorders because relatively few will have only a single episode of illness during their lifetime. Although a certain amount of the "rose-colored glasses" optimism of well-being is likely to return as a patient recovers from an episode of psychiatric illness, he should be aware that additional troubles may lie ahead. The therapeutic approach to relapse prevention therefore begins with providing accurate information about the natural history of the disorder that is being treated and about what can be done to maximize the chances for sustained benefit.

People who are receiving this information often have a negative emotional response, with sadness or apprehension accompanying a wave of pessimistic automatic negative thoughts. The skilled clinician provides psychoeducation with an "open eye" to observing the changes in affect or behavior that may reveal such negative thoughts and capitalizes on the opportunity to help the patient verbalize the cognitions and address them in treatment sessions. Even when a patient shows no visible cues of an emotional response, the clinician should end a psychoeducational interchange by asking if the patient has any questions or any unspoken concerns or thoughts or feelings about the implications of what was discussed. Another beneficial practice is to suggest a homework assignment to monitor the patient's thoughts and feelings about the visit, in case the emotional response is delayed.

Recognizing and Treating Residual Symptoms

Complete symptom remission is the desired goal for the acute phase of treatment of all mental disorders for many reasons, including the fact that longitudinal studies of both major depressive disorder and bipolar disorder have documented that fully remitted patients have a lower risk of relapse (Jarrett et al. 2001; Perlis et al. 2006; Thase et al. 1992). Nevertheless, full remission may not always be possible. A significant minority of people who respond to 12–16 sessions of CBT for depression continue to manifest one or more persistent symptoms. As such, an important component of a relapse prevention plan is to identify these symptoms, review relevant CBT strategies that may help reduce these symptoms, and implement a plan to address them on an ongoing basis.

The process of crafting a longer-term plan often begins with an open-ended question such as, "As we approach the end of our regularly planned sessions, I've been wondering if you've identified particular symptoms or problems that are still a source of concern" or "In what ways are you still not feeling or functioning at your best?" Self-report assessment scales, such as the Patient Health Questionnaire–9 (Kroenke et al. 2001), the Quick Inventory of Depressive Symptomatology Self-Report Version–16 (Rush et al. 2003), or other instruments listed in Table 3–2 in Chapter 3, "Enhancing the Impact of Brief Sessions," also can used to identify residual symptoms. If one of these rating scales has been administered periodically during the acute phase of treatment as a means of objectifying progress, the particular pattern of symptom change and persistence should be readily discerned. On other occasions, new symptoms emerge during the course of treatment, or other problems that were not identified as particularly troublesome earlier in the course of treatment (e.g., social anxiety) become more prominent as other symptoms improve. In such cases, the clinician and patient might devote portions of one or two sessions to collaboratively mapping out the best approach to managing these problems.

Identifying Triggers or Early Warning Signs for Relapse

Because most psychiatric disorders run an episodic course, only a fortunate minority of individuals who seek treatment will have only a single episode of illness and remain well thereafter. More often than not, the individual will have some firsthand experience with relapse and recurrence and can provide some personally relevant details about the types of stresses or situations that are likely to provoke a relapse or symptomatic exacerbation. Some patients have a vulnerability to stressors in key domains, such as setbacks in interpersonal relationships or in careers, which can be inferred from their past history and their core beliefs. For other patients, particularly those who have already had a number of relapses and recurrences, the episodes may seem to occur "out of the blue," without provocation. However, even in these cases, patients can usually identify prodromal symptoms that serve as early warning signs of impending bouts of illness. For example, many people with recurrent mood disorders report that changes in their sleep-wake cycle, either insomnia or an increased need for sleep, can herald the onset of a depressive episode. In a similar manner, decreased need for sleep or an increased libido can precede the onset of an episode of hypomania or mania.

A specific method of using a symptom summary worksheet for identifying early signs of mood swings in bipolar disorder and designing strategies to interrupt escalations into mania or depression was described in Chapter 2, "Indications and Formats for Brief CBT Sessions." This type of written exercise could be used for any patient who has a condition with significant risk for relapse. Barbara's symptom summary worksheet from Chapter 2 is repeated in Figure 16–1. Individualized records such as these can encourage patients to monitor for early warning signs of relapse and to prepare in advance to use CBT strategies to stay well.

> **Learning Exercise 16–1**   Identifying Triggers or Early Warning Signs for Relapse
>
> 1. Select two or more patients from your practice whom you think have a significant risk for relapse.
>
> 2. Ask the patients questions to attempt to identify possible triggers for relapse. Examples: "Can you think of anything that might cause a setback? What kinds of stresses might increase the chances that the symptoms will come back?"
>
> 3. Use a symptom summary worksheet or a similar written exercise with these patients to develop customized lists of early warning signs for relapse.

Developing Relapse Prevention Plans

In the brief session format, relapse prevention plans are typically built over a series of visits and are strengthened incrementally as the patient moves from acute phase treatment to maintenance therapy. The plans can incorporate a variety of cognitive-behavioral and psychopharmacological methods that are customized to match the diagnoses, vulnerabilities, and strengths of each patient (Table 16–1).

Symptom	Mild	Moderate	Severe
Irritability	Edgy, quick to criticize others, voice may have a sharp tone.	May throw dishes or other things, yell at kids; show little concern for others' problems.	Scream and rant and rave. Have trouble sitting still —others better stay out of my way. Always on edge—work, home, everywhere.
Thinking I can do more than is realistic—not paying attention to real concerns.	Minimize real problems in my life—pay less attention to genuine worries like bills or work responsibilities.	Starting to get pumped up about special projects—taking on way more than I can actually handle. I push my way into positions where I am overcommitted.	Grandiosity out of control. I think I am the best in everything I do. I push others out of the way. don't listen to them—do it my way.
Sleeping too little	Stay up about 1 hour extra most nights because I am really enjoying myself or am involved in a special project.	Staying up 2 or more hours extra most nights. I am on a roll. I have lots of trouble shutting off my mind to go to sleep. Don't really want to sleep.	I am going a mile a minute—don't want to sleep at all. I could stay up for 3 or 4 nights before crashing.
Mind racing	Thoughts begin to pick up speed. This is subtle, but I start to feel more creative and full of life.	Thoughts definitely are speeding along. I don't pay much attention to what others are saying.	Thoughts are jumping around so fast that sometimes I don't make a lot of sense.
Getting into trouble	A bit of extra risk taking. I might drive 5–10 miles faster, and I might flirt more with men.	I say things that I shouldn't —off-color jokes. I wear more provocative clothes. I'm spending more than I should.	I am really in trouble now—spending more money than I have, racking up credit card debt, getting involved with the wrong kind of men.

Figure 16–1. Symptom summary worksheet for hypomanic and manic symptoms: Barbara's example.

Table 16–1. Building blocks for relapse prevention plans

Review and rehearse basic cognitive-behavior therapy skills.

Make lifestyle changes.

Develop coping strategies to prevent symptom escalation.

Use cognitive-behavioral rehearsal.

Optimize pharmacological regimen.

Promote adherence.

Review and Rehearse Basic CBT Skills

The methods that will ultimately be helpful for sustaining recovery and preventing relapse or recurrence are basically the same strategies and techniques that proved to be useful for treating the symptoms during the acute phase of therapy (e.g., recognizing and changing automatic thoughts, examining the evidence, behavioral activation and activity scheduling, exposure, using coping cards). Helping patients to practice and master these skills and encouraging them to use these methods to forestall symptom flurries can significantly enhance their abilities to effectively manage future stressors. Although research has not yet confirmed that the ongoing use of CBT strategies after completion of therapy is a critical element of successful prophylaxis—a definitive study of this hypothesis is ongoing at the University of Pennsylvania and the University of Texas Southwestern Medical Center—there is good reason to believe on clinical grounds that patients who adopt the CBT model and continue to practice coping strategies have the best chances for enduring benefit.

Written materials that summarize the procedures for cognitive and behavioral interventions may be particularly useful for helping patients to maintain their skills in CBT (see Chapter 3, "Enhancing the Impact of Brief Sessions"). These materials might include a therapy notebook, a folder with handouts used during CBT sessions, or index cards that summarize main points. Patients can refer back to this information when sessions have stopped or are reduced in frequency. For a patient who has difficulty with reading or writing, the therapist should inquire about strategies the patient used in the past to recall other important information and then develop appropriate materials. For example, an audio recording made by the clinician and patient might help with retention of key concepts and methods.

Patients should be encouraged to keep the materials they have collected during the acute course of therapy as a library or tool kit for subsequent self-directed work. An option that can be explored for effective cataloguing and retrieval of these resources is to store them electronically on a computer. Some of our more successful recent treatment experiences have involved individuals who used computerized versions of homework assignments, such as exposure logs or thought change records, which they review to track progress and to reinforce learning.

Whether pen-and-pencil or computerized storage methods are used, clinicians should create the expectation that therapy will work better and have more enduring value if CBT tools are saved and can be drawn upon later when needed. For example, a therapist might suggest something like this: "We've found that people who do homework assignments have a much better chance of benefiting from therapy. If you keep a record of our work in therapy, you can use this knowledge later in your life to help cope with new problems—like a gift that keeps on giving. Can we take a few moments to come up with a plan to ensure that you have a record of our work together so that you can easily find these tools if you need to use them?"

Make Lifestyle Changes

For patients with recurrent mood disorders and schizophrenia, certain lifestyle changes can play an important role in reducing the risk of relapse. For example, an individual with bipolar disorder may decide to adhere to a regular sleep and activities schedule, minimize caffeine intake, avoid "stimulating" activities in the evening, and work on improving stress management skills. A patient with a history of recurrent depression might opt to schedule a regular time for aerobic exercise every morning. Methods described in this book for insomnia (Chapter 10, "CBT Methods for Insomnia") and building healthy habits (Chapter 14, "Lifestyle Change: Building Healthy Habits") can be used in brief sessions to help patients make positive lifestyle changes that can be important parts of relapse prevention plans.

Develop Coping Strategies to Prevent Symptom Escalation

Barbara's symptom summary worksheet (Figure 16–1) had several early warning signs that could be valuable targets for a relapse prevention plan. In Video Illustration 1, we showed a demonstration of CBT directed at irritability, the first item on her list. Barbara had noted during her hospitalization that one of the important signs of an impending switch into mania was irritability. Dr. Wright worked with her to spot automatic thoughts and cognitive errors that were firing up her anger toward her

---

Problem: Anger and irritability with son

1. *When I start to get angry or irritable, stop to spot my automatic thoughts and check them out to see how accurate they are.*

2. *Try to take a balanced look at the situation.*

3. *Do something to step away from the situation...like take a walk or a "timeout."*

4. *Try talking with my son and work out a solution for the problem.*

Figure 16–2. Barbara's coping card.

son. They also developed a behavioral strategy to calm her emotions and to help her manage the situation more rationally.

Barbara's coping card, previously shown in Chapter 2, "Indications and Formats for Brief CBT Sessions," is repeated here (Figure 16–2) as an example of a CBT method that can be employed in a brief session to train patients in relapse prevention skills. The intervention started with Barbara learning to cope better with anger and irritability toward her son, but as therapy proceeded, Dr. Wright and Barbara worked on generalizing these same methods to other situations that could trigger similar reactions. They also developed coping methods for other warning signs on her symptom summary worksheet.

The next learning exercise asks you to plan some interventions for deescalating symptoms that may lead Barbara to a full relapse. You can pick standard CBT methods, or you can brainstorm and come up with other approaches that you think might work. For example, a plan for helping Barbara reduce risk-taking behavior could include straightforward methods, such as recognizing cognitive errors (e.g., minimizing or ignoring the evidence of the downside of her risk taking), but it could also involve an analysis of advantages and disadvantages. The latter technique could reveal some of the "positives" in feeling attractive to men, getting initial interest from others, having a temporary surge in pleasurable emotions, and so forth, that she would need to consider in building a workable plan.

Learning Exercise 16–2 Developing Coping Strategies to Prevent Symptom Escalation

1. Review Barbara's symptom summary worksheet. Choose two or more of the items (other than irritability).

> 2. Write a treatment plan for CBT methods that you could use for each of these items in brief sessions. Your goal is to help Barbara learn ways to interrupt the upswing into mania.

An additional example of the development of coping strategies that can be part of relapse prevention plans comes from the treatment of Brenda, a patient of Dr. Turkington with a diagnosis of schizophrenia. Although Brenda had learned to diminish the impact of auditory hallucinations in acute therapy, she continued to hear voices from time to time, and it seemed likely that they might worsen at some point in the future. In preparing for the future, Brenda and Dr. Turkington collaboratively developed a detailed list, recording symptoms or problems in one column and plans for coping with each of these possible problems in the other column (see Figure 16–3).

Use Cognitive-Behavioral Rehearsal

Elements of a relapse prevention plan that may involve responding to a very challenging life event or applying a CBT skill that has not been fully mastered can be strengthened by the use of rehearsal exercises. These exercises can follow a what-if or worst-case scenario. For example, if a patient's anxiety is often heightened in the context of marital discord, the patient may benefit from rehearsing strategies for coping with criticism from her spouse. If a patient is fearing some extremely stressful event (e.g., loss of a job, breakup of a marriage, ominous diagnosis of a medical problem), the clinician can help the patient think through how he might use personal strengths to face these situations.

When implemented skillfully, the worst-case scenario technique is done with great sensitivity and empathy. Clinicians assess patients' capacity to use this method productively, prepare them for the emotional arousal that may be engendered, and give them good CBT coaching on coping methods. An illustration of this type of work comes from Dr. Thase's treatment of Darrell. As introduced in Chapter 6, "Behavioral Methods for Depression," Darrell was struggling with the terminal illness of his mother. In a later session not shown in the video illustrations, Dr. Thase gently broached the topic of how Darrell might react when his mother did pass away. In his formulation of Darrell's problems, Dr. Thase had a concern that Darrell might become more depressed and resume alcohol abuse when his mother's illness reached a fatal conclusion.

> Dr. Thase: We've been making good progress on getting the depression under control and stopping drinking, but one thing that we haven't

Symptom or problem	Coping plan
• *If I sleep very poorly for 4 or 5 nights, the voices will get much worse.*	• *Stay away from caffeine. Call the doctor to ask for sleeping medication if this problem goes on for more than 2 nights.*
• *I could get caught up with worrying all the time and stop seeing friends.*	• *Allow myself no more than 1 hour of worry a day (usually from 4 P.M. to 5 P.M.). Do at least two enjoyable things a day to take my mind off my worries.*
• *I could start thinking that the devil is trying to tell me something.*	• *Remember what my pastor said about the devil. Remind myself that the devil in the Bible doesn't talk like the voice I sometimes hear.*
• *I could start dwelling on the past and thinking of all the problems I had as a young mother.*	• *Look at the coping card I wrote with my doctor. Tell myself, "I did the best I could. I am a good person and a good mother."*

Figure 16–3. Brenda's coping plan.

Source. Adapted from Wright JH, Turkington D, Kingdon DG, et al: *Cognitive-Behavior Therapy for Severe Mental Illness: An Illustrated Guide.* Washington, DC, American Psychiatric Publishing, 2009, p. 299. Used with permission. Copyright © 2009 American Psychiatric Publishing.

talked about much is how things might go for you when your mother does pass away. I've been thinking that it could help you to do some forecasting about how you might react and to do some work now to prepare yourself. What do you think about that idea?

Darrell: I try to avoid thinking about that as much as I can, but she probably only has another 3–6 months to live. It's going to be pretty rough on me.

Dr. Thase: I know that it will be an enormous hurt, and that you'll feel a lot of grief.

Darrell: Yeah, I'm really going to miss her.

Dr. Thase: Could we think ahead a little to see if there are some coping strategies that might work better than others when you do have to face this problem?

Darrell: That's probably a good idea. I guess I could slip back and lose a lot of the ground I've been gaining the last couple months.

Dr. Thase: So to start, could we make a brief list of some positive and negative coping methods?

Darrell: Sure. I guess the worst thing I could do would be to start drinking again.

They went on to generate the list in Figure 16–4, and in future sessions they came back to this topic several times to flesh out more details of effective coping methods and healthy grieving.

Optimize Pharmacological Regimen

For most of our patients with recurrent mood disorders and psychoses, long-term pharmacotherapy is a cornerstone of the relapse prevention plan. Because the focus of this book is on CBT methods, not psychopharmacology, we do not detail current methods of maintenance pharmacotherapy here. However, we want to emphasize the importance of appropriate, ongoing pharmacotherapy. The various practice guidelines published by the American Psychiatric Association provide good overviews of the methods of maintenance treatment with medication (e.g., see American Psychiatric Association 2000, 2002; Lehman et al. 2004).

Promote Adherence

Another important element of relapse prevention plans for people who are taking long-term medications is to use the CBT methods described in Chapter 5, "Promoting Adherence." Not uncommonly, clinicians assume that their patients are taking medication as prescribed when in fact they are not. By forgetting to ask about medication adherence, a clinician may inadvertently reinforce a patient's belief that taking the medication is no longer very important.

The following example is illustrative. Stan had a well-established diagnosis of bipolar disorder and had been doing well on lithium for more than 4 years following the successful treatment of a relatively severe episode of mania. During this time, he had been able to successfully taper and discontinue two adjunctive therapies (olanzapine and clonazepam), which were used during the height of the manic episode. Also, for the past 2 years, the frequency of his visits to his psychiatrist had been reduced to one brief visit every 3 months.

Stan's psychiatrist had not asked about medication adherence for the past year. Because Stan was always upbeat and complimentary about his treatment, the psychiatrist did not realize that for several years Stan had been thinking, "I'm sick and tired of taking medication all the time. I'll bet that I don't even need to take this drug anymore." As his doctor might have predicted had he known what Stan was thinking, Stan stopped the medication about 2 months before his most recent visit. Stan's wife had

How I could react after my mother dies

Unhealthy behaviors	Healthy behaviors
— *Resume drinking beer or other alcohol*	— *Attend AA meetings; get support*
— *Isolate myself; dwell on my emotional*	*from this group*
pain	— *Keep full schedule of activities*
— *Just go to work and come home and*	*with friends and family*
stare at TV	— *Exercise regularly; have at least one*
— *Get down on myself for not doing*	*positive thing to look forward to*
more for mother in her final years	*each day*
— *Try to suppress all my feelings;*	— *Avoid excessive blame for the past;*
act like I'm not hurt by her passing	*give myself some credit for being a*
— *Get more discouraged about life*	*good son*
and pull back from interests	— *Talk about my feelings when it is*
	safe—with my family, with Dr. Thase
	— *After the acute pain passes, try to*
	find some new hobby, work, or other
	interest where I can invest my energies

Figure 16–4. CBT rehearsal for relapse prevention: Darrell's list of unhealthy and healthy coping methods.

contacted the clinician to request an urgent appointment for her husband because he seemed much more irritable and was sleeping only about 4 hours each night. Unfortunately, Stan suffered a full relapse of mania before he was restabilized on lithium and other medications.

To help patients stick with longer-term pharmacotherapy regimens, we recommend that the principles outlined in Chapter 5, "Promoting Adherence," be followed even when symptoms seem to have been under control for long periods of time. Some of the key methods used in CBT for adherence include 1) fostering a highly collaborative therapeutic relationship with open dialogue about the pros and cons of medications; 2) simplifying medication regimens where possible; 3) minimizing side effects; 4) normalizing problems with compliance; 5) analyzing behavioral patterns associated with medication taking—and coaching patients on ways of incorporating medication into their daily routine; and 6) eliciting and modifying dysfunctional automatic thoughts and beliefs about pharmacotherapy.

Involving Significant Others in Relapse Prevention Plans

Research on schizophrenia, bipolar disorder, and depression has shown that people who have the benefit of an involved, supportive (i.e., not critical) family have a lower risk of relapse or recurrence (see, e.g., Butzlaf and Hooley 1998). Therefore, it can be useful to bring family members or other significant others into the process of developing and implementing a relapse prevention plan. Conversely, because self-monitoring or ongoing use of particular coping strategies may necessarily interfere with family time, it is wise to ensure that important people in the patient's life do not inadvertently undermine the coping plan (e.g., by saying, "I just don't understand why you still have to do those stupid assignments. Didn't you complete that therapy months ago?"). We often recommend that our patients invite family members or significant others to attend at least one of the acute phase treatment sessions. In addition to fostering a helping alliance with the loved ones, this visit also is useful to obtain additional information about how the patient is functioning and, on occasion, can reveal that a significant other also may need treatment. A successful visit with family or significant others can end with an open invitation for attending additional sessions in the future should the need arise.

> **Learning Exercise 16–3**   Developing a Relapse Prevention Plan
>
> 1. Select one or more patients from your practice for whom you would like to develop a CBT-oriented relapse prevention plan.
>
> 2. Collaboratively build a relapse prevention plan with each patient that contains at least three of these elements:
>
>   - A list of early warning signs for relapse
>
>   - Lifestyle changes that could possibly reduce the risk for relapse
>
>   - CBT methods for stopping the escalation of symptoms
>
>   - CBT rehearsal
>
>   - Methods for enhancing adherence
>
>   - Involvement of significant others

Summary

Key Points for Clinicians

- Extensive empirical evidence indicates that CBT has a long-term effect in reducing the risk for relapse.
- Educating patients about the risk for relapse is a wise practice.
- If significant residual symptoms remain after acute treatment for mood disorders, the longer-term outcome may be compromised. Thus, the clinician and patient should make an effort to recognize and reduce residual symptoms.
- The CBT model for relapse prevention empowers patients by teaching them the skills to become their "own therapists."
- Developing an early warning system for signs of impending relapse is a core element of the CBT approach.
- Relapse prevention plans can be developed in brief sessions in a variety of ways. The following are some commonly used methods:

  1. Reviewing and rehearsing basic CBT skills
  2. Making lifestyle changes
  3. Developing coping strategies to prevent symptom escalation
  4. Using cognitive-behavioral rehearsal

- The psychopharmacological components of the relapse prevention plan are often essential for good long-term outcome. CBT methods for adherence can be used to help patients use medications to stay well.

Concepts and Skills for Patients to Learn

- Unfortunately, many psychiatric illnesses can be recurrent; however, much can be done with medication and CBT to reduce the risk for relapse.
- One of the helpful features of CBT is that it teaches practical skills that can be used in two major ways: 1) to reduce or eliminate symptoms and 2) to stay well once an illness is in check.
- Successful treatment with CBT prepares you to use self-help skills throughout your lifetime to promote wellness.
- A particularly useful part of CBT for relapse prevention is developing a customized list of early warning signs that symptoms may be returning. If you can spot these signs, you can try to nip them in the bud before they become larger problems.
- Your doctor or therapist may suggest that you consider changes in lifestyle habits, such as sleeping and exercise, that could help you continue to make progress.

• Sometimes it can be useful to look ahead to try to identify possible stresses that could set you up for a return of symptoms. Even if you must confront tough challenges, you can work out a plan in advance for coping and staying healthy.

References

American Psychiatric Association: Practice guideline for the treatment of patients with major depressive disorder (revision). Am J Psychiatry 157(suppl):1–45, 2000

American Psychiatric Association: Practice guideline for the treatment of patients with bipolar disorder (revision). Am J Psychiatry 159(suppl):1–50, 2002

Ball JR, Mitchell PB, Corry JC, et al: A randomized controlled trial of cognitive therapy for bipolar disorder: focus on long-term change. J Clin Psychiatry 67:277–286, 2006

Barlow DH, Gorman JM, Shear MK, et al: Cognitive-behavioral therapy, imipramine, or their combination for panic disorder: a randomized controlled trial. JAMA 283:2529–2536, 2000

Blackburn, IM, Moore RG: Controlled acute and follow-up trial of cognitive therapy and pharmacotherapy in outpatients with recurrent depression. Br J Psychiatry 171:328–334, 1997

Bockting CL, Schene AH, Spinhoven P, et al: Preventing relapse/recurrence in recurrent depression with cognitive therapy: a randomized controlled trial. J Consult Clin Psychol 73:647–657, 2005

Butzlaf RL, Hooley JM: Expressed emotion and psychiatric relapse: a meta-analysis. Arch Gen Psychiatry 55:547–552, 1998

Fava GA, Bartolucci G, Rafanelli C, et al: Cognitive-behavioral management of patients with bipolar disorder who relapsed while on lithium prophylaxis. J Clin Psychiatry 62:556–559, 2001

Grawe RW, Falloon IR, Widen JH, et al: Two years of continued early treatment for recent-onset schizophrenia: a randomised controlled study. Acta Psychiatr Scand 114:328–336, 2006

Gumley A, O'Grady M, McNay L, et al: Early intervention for relapse in schizophrenia: results of a 12-month randomized controlled trial of cognitive behavioural therapy. Psychol Med 33:419–431, 2003

Hollon SD, DeRubeis RJ, Seligman ME: Cognitive therapy and the prevention of depression. Appl Prev Psychol 1:89–95, 1992

Hollon SD, DeRubeis RJ, Shelton RC, et al: Prevention of relapse following cognitive therapy vs. medications in moderate to severe depression. Arch Gen Psychiatry 62:417–422, 2005

Jarrett RB, Kraft D, Doyle J, et al: Preventing recurrent depression using cognitive therapy with and without a continuation phase: a randomized clinical trial. Arch Gen Psychiatry 58:381–388, 2001

Kovacs M, Rush AJ, Beck AT, et al: Depressed outpatients treated with cognitive therapy or pharmacotherapy. Arch Gen Psychiatry 38:33–39, 1981

Kroenke K, Spitzer RL, Williams JB: The PHQ-9: validity of a brief depression severity measure. J Gen Intern Med 16:606–613, 2001

Lam DH, Bright J, Jones S, et al: Cognitive therapy for bipolar illness: a pilot study of relapse prevention. Cognit Ther Res 24:503–520, 2001

Lam DH, Watkins ER, Hayward P, et al: A randomized controlled study of cognitive therapy for relapse prevention for bipolar affective disorder: outcome of the first year. Arch Gen Psychiatry 60:145–152, 2003

Lehman AF, Lieberman JA, Dixon LB, et al; American Psychiatric Association; Steering Committee on Practice Guidelines: Practice guideline for the treatment of patients with schizophrenia, 2nd edition. Am J Psychiatry 161 (suppl):1–56, 2004

Morin CM, Vallières A, Guay B, et al: Cognitive behavioral therapy, singly and combined with medication, for persistent insomnia: a randomized controlled trial. JAMA 301:2005–2015, 2009

Paykel ES, Scott J, Teasdale JD, et al: Prevention of relapse in residual depression by cognitive therapy: a controlled trial. Arch Gen Psychiatry 56:829–835, 1999

Paykel ES, Scott J, Cornwall PL, et al: Duration of relapse prevention after cognitive therapy in residual depression: follow-up of controlled trial. Psychol Med 35:59–68, 2005

Perlis RH, Ostacher MJ, Patel JK, et al: Predictors of recurrence in bipolar disorder: primary outcomes from the Systematic Treatment Enhancement Program for Bipolar Disorder (STEP-BD). Am J Psychiatry 163:217–224, 2006

Rush AJ, Trivedi MH, Ibrahim HM, et al: The 16-item Quick Inventory of Depressive Symptomatology (QIDS) Clinician Rating (QIDS-C) and Self-Report (QIDS-SR): a psychometric evaluation in patients with chronic major depression. Biol Psychiatry 54:573–583, 2003

Scott J, Garland A, Moorhead S: A pilot study of cognitive therapy in bipolar disorders. Psychol Med 31:459–467, 2001

Scott J, Paykel E, Morriss R, et al: Cognitive-behavioural therapy for severe and recurrent bipolar disorders: randomized controlled trial. Br J Psychiatry 188:313–320, 2006

Thase ME, Simons AD, McGeary J, et al: Relapse after cognitive behavior therapy of depression: potential implications for longer courses of treatment. Am J Psychiatry 149:1046–1052, 1992

Turkington D, Kingdon D, Rathod S, et al: Outcomes of an effectiveness trial of cognitive-behavioural intervention by mental health nurses in schizophrenia. Br J Psychiatry 189:36–40, 2006

Turkington D, Scott JL, Sensky T, et al: A randomized controlled trial of cognitive-behavior therapy for persistent symptoms in schizophrenia: a five-year follow-up. Schizophr Res 98:1–7, 2008

Appendix 1

Worksheets and Checklists

Contents

Cognitive-Behavior Therapy
Case Formulation Worksheet

Patient Name:		Date:
Diagnoses/Symptoms:		
Formative Influences:		
Situational Issues:		
Biological, Genetic, and Medical Factors:		
Strengths/Assets:		
Treatment Goals:		
Event 1	Event 2	Event 3
Automatic Thoughts	Automatic Thoughts	Automatic Thoughts
Emotions	Emotions	Emotions
Behaviors	Behaviors	Behaviors
Schemas:		
Working Hypothesis:		
Treatment Plan:		

Note. Available at: www.appi.org/pdf/62362.

Weekly Activity Schedule

Instructions: Write down your activities for each hour and then rate them on a scale of 0–10 for mastery (**m**) or degree of accomplishment and for pleasure (**p**) or amount of enjoyment you experienced. A rating of 0 would mean that you had no sense of mastery or pleasure. A rating of 10 would mean that you experienced maximum mastery or pleasure.

	Sunday	Monday	Tuesday	Wednesday	Thursday	Friday	Saturday
8:00 A.M.							
9:00 A.M.							
10:00 A.M.							
11:00 A.M.							
12:00 P.M.							
1:00 P.M.							
2:00 P.M.							
3:00 P.M.							
4:00 P.M.							
5:00 P.M.							
6:00 P.M.							
7:00 P.M.							
8:00 P.M.							
9:00 P.M.							

Note. Available at: www.appi.org/pdf/62362.

Thought Change Record

Situation	Automatic thought(s)	Emotion(s)	Rational response	Outcome
Describe a. Actual event leading to unpleasant emotion *or* b. Stream of thoughts leading to unpleasant emotion *or* c. Unpleasant physiological sensations.	a. *Write* automatic thought(s) that preceded emotion(s). b. *Rate* belief in automatic thought(s), 0%–100%.	a. *Specify* sad, anxious, angry, etc. b. *Rate* degree of emotion, 1%–100%.	a. *Identify* cognitive errors. b. *Write* rational response to automatic thought(s). c. *Rate* belief in rational response, 0%–100%.	a. *Specify and rate* subsequent emotion(s), 0%–100%. b. *Describe* changes in behavior.

Note.   Available at: www.appi.org/pdf/62362.

Definitions of Cognitive Errors

- **Ignoring the evidence**
  When you ignore the evidence, you make a judgment (usually about your shortcomings or about something you think you cannot do) without looking at all the information. This cognitive error has also been called the *mental filter* because you filter, or screen out, valuable information about topics such as 1) positive experiences from the past, 2) your strengths, and 3) support that others can give.
- **Jumping to conclusions**
  If you are depressed or anxious, you might jump to conclusions. You might immediately think of the worst possible interpretations of situations. Once these negative images come into your mind, you might become certain that bad things will happen.
- **Overgeneralizing**
  Sometimes you might let a single problem mean so much to you that it colors your view of everything in your life. You can give a small difficulty or flaw so much significance that it seems to define the entire picture. This type of cognitive error is called overgeneralizing.
- **Magnifying or minimizing**
  One of the most common cognitive errors is magnifying or minimizing the significance of things in your life. When you are depressed or anxious, you might magnify your faults and minimize your strengths. You also might magnify the risks of difficulties in situations and minimize the options or resources that you have to manage the problem.

  An extreme form of magnifying is sometimes called *catastrophizing*. When you catastrophize, you automatically think that the worst possible thing will happen. If you are having a panic attack, your mind races with thoughts such as these: "I'm going to have a heart attack or stroke" or "I'm going to totally lose control." Depressed persons may think they are bound to fail or that they are about to lose everything.
- **Personalizing**
  Personalizing is a classic feature of anxiety and depression in which you get caught up in taking personal blame for everything that seems to go wrong. When you personalize, you accept full responsibility for a troubling situation or problem even when there is no good evidence to back your conclusion. This type of cognitive error undermines your self-esteem and makes you more depressed.

  Of course, you need to accept responsibility when you have made mistakes. Owning up to problems can help you start to turn things around. However, if you can recognize the times that you are person-

Note. Available at: www.appi.org/pdf/62362.

alizing, you can avoid putting yourself down unnecessarily, and you can start to develop a healthier style of thinking.

- **All-or-none thinking**
One of the most damaging of the cognitive errors—all-or-none thinking—is demonstrated by the following types of thoughts: "Nothing ever goes my way"; "There's no way I could handle it"; "I always mess up"; "She's got it all"; "Everything is going wrong." When you let all-or-none thinking go unchecked, you see the world in absolute terms. Everything is all good or all bad. You believe that others are doing great and you are doing just the opposite.

    All-or-none thinking also can interfere with your working on tasks. Imagine what would happen if you thought that you had to achieve 100% success or you should not even try at all. It is usually better to set reasonable goals and to realize that people are rarely complete successes or total failures. Most things in life fall somewhere in between.

Note.   Available at: www.appi.org/pdf/62362.

Automatic Thoughts Checklist

Instructions: Place a check mark beside each negative automatic thought that you have had in the past 2 weeks.

_____ I should be doing better in life.

_____ He/she doesn't understand me.

_____ I've let him/her down.

_____ I just can't enjoy things anymore.

_____ Why am I so weak?

_____ I always keep messing things up.

_____ My life's going nowhere.

_____ I can't handle it.

_____ I'm failing.

_____ It's too much for me.

_____ I don't have much of a future.

_____ Things are out of control.

_____ I feel like giving up.

_____ Something bad is sure to happen.

_____ There must be something wrong with me.

Note.   Available at: www.appi.org/pdf/62362.

Brief Checklist of Adaptive Core Beliefs

Instructions: Place a check mark beside each core belief that you have.

____ I'm a solid person.

____ If I work hard at something, I can master it.

____ I'm a survivor.

____ Others trust me.

____ I care about other people.

____ People respect me.

____ If I prepare in advance, I usually do better.

____ I deserve to be respected.

____ I like to be challenged.

____ I'm intelligent.

____ I can figure things out.

____ I'm friendly.

____ I can handle stress.

____ I can learn from my mistakes and be a better person.

____ I'm a good spouse (and/or parent, child friend, lover).

Note. Available at: www.appi.org/pdf/62362.

Sleep Diary

	Monday	Tuesday	Wednesday	Thursday	Friday	Saturday	Sunday
Bedtime							
Time fell asleep							
Hours asleep							
Sleep breaks							
Wake-up time							
Naps?							
Quality of sleep							
Alcohol/ medications?							

Note. Available at: www.appi.org/pdf/62362.

List of 60 Coping Strategies for Hallucinations

Distraction
1. Hum
2. Talk to yourself
3. Listen to modern music
4. Listen to classical music
5. Prayer
6. Meditation
7. Use a mantra
8. Painting
9. Imagery
10. Walk in the fresh air
11. Phone a friend
12. Exercise
13. Use a relaxation tape
14. Yoga
15. Take a warm bath
16. Call your mental health professional
17. Attend the day center/drop in
18. Watch TV
19. Do a crossword or other puzzle
20. Play a computer game
21. Try a new hobby

Focusing
1. Correct the cognitive distortions in the voices
2. Respond rationally to voice content
3. Use subvocalization
4. Dismiss the voices
5. Remind yourself that no one else can hear the voice
6. Phone a voice buddy and tell him or her the voice is active
7. Remember to take antipsychotic medication
8. Demonstrate controllability by bringing the voices on
9. Give the voices a 10-minute slot at a specific time each day
10. Play a cognitive therapy tape discussing voice control
11. Use a normalizing explanation
12. Use rational responses to reduce anger
13. List the evidence in favor of the voice content
14. List the evidence against the voice content

Note.   Available at: www.appi.org/pdf/62362.

15. Use guided imagery to practice coping with the voices differently
16. Role-play for and against the voices
17. Remind yourself that voices are not actions and need not be viewed that way
18. Remind yourself that the voices don't seem to know much
19. Remind yourself that you don't need to obey the voices
20. Talk to someone you trust about the voice content
21. Use rational responses to reduce shame
22. Use rational responses to reduce anxiety
23. Use a diary to manage stress
24. Use a diary to manage your time
25. Plan your daily activities the night before
26. Use a voice diary in a scientific manner
27. Mindfulness
28. Try an earplug (right ear first if right-handed)

Meta-cognitive Methods

1. Use schema-focused techniques
2. Acceptance
3. Assertiveness
4. Use a biological model
5. Consider shamanistic views of voice hearing
6. Consider cultural aspects of voice hearing
7. Keep a list of daily behaviors to prove that you are not as bad as the voices say
8. Use a continuum relating your own worth to that of other people
9. List your positive experiences in life
10. List your achievements, friendships, etc.
11. Act against the voices (show them that you are better than they say)

Note. Available at: www.appi.org/pdf/62362.

List of Self-Report Symptom Rating Scales

- Beck Anxiety Inventory
  www.pearsonassessments.com/pai
    Beck AT, Epstein N, Brown G, et al: An inventory for measuring clinical anxiety: psychometric properties. J Consult Clin Psychol 56:893–897, 1988

- Beck Depression Inventory
  www.pearsonassessments.com/pai
    Beck AT, Ward CH, Mendelson M, et al: An inventory for measuring depression. Arch Gen Psychiatry 4:561–571, 1961

- Patient Health Questionnaire–9
  www.mapi-trust.org/test/129-phq
    Kroenke K, Spitzer RL, Williams JB: The PHQ-9: validity of a brief depression severity measure. J Gen Intern Med 16:606–613, 2001

- Penn State Worry Questionnaire
    Meyer TJ, Miller ML, Metzger RL, et al: Development and validation of the Penn State Worry Questionnaire. Behav Res Ther 28:487–495, 1990

- Psychotic Symptom Rating Scales
    Haddock G, McCarron J, Tarrier N, et al: Scales to measure dimensions of hallucinations and delusions: the Psychotic Symptom Rating Scales (PSYRATS). Psychol Med 29:879–889, 1999

- Quick Inventory of Depressive Symptomatology
  www.ids-qids.org
    Rush AJ, Trivedi MH, Ibrahim HM, et al: The 16-item Quick Inventory of Depressive Symptomatology (QIDS) Clinician Rating (QIDS-C) and Self-Report (QIDS-SR): a psychometric evaluation in patients with chronic major depression. Biol Psychiatry 54:573–583, 2003

Note.   Available at: www.appi.org/pdf/62362.

Appendix 2

CBT Resources for Patients and Families

Books

Managing Mood and Anxiety Disorders

Antony MM, Norton PJ: The Anti-Anxiety Workbook: Proven Strategies to Overcome Worry, Phobias, Panic, and Obsessions. New York, Guilford, 2009

Basco MR: Never Good Enough. New York, Free Press, 1999

Basco MR: The Bipolar Workbook. New York, Guilford, 2006

Burns DD: Feeling Good. New York, Morrow, 1999

Craske MG, Barlow DH: Mastery of Your Anxiety and Panic, 3rd Edition. San Antonio, TX, Psychological Corporation, 2000

Foa EB, Wilson R: Stop Obsessing! How to Overcome Your Obsessions and Compulsions. New York, Bantam Books, 1991

Greenberger D, Padesky CA: Mind Over Mood. New York, Guilford, 1995

Jamison KR: Touched With Fire: Manic-Depressive Illness and the Artistic Temperament. New York, Simon & Schuster, 1996

Kabat-Zinn J: Full Catastrophe Living: Using the Wisdom of Your Body to Face Stress, Pain, and Illness. New York, Hyperion, 1990

Last CG: When Someone You Love Is Bipolar: Help and Support for You and Your Partner. New York, Guilford, 2009

Miklowitz DJ: The Bipolar Survival Guide: What You and Your Family Need to Know. New York, Guilford, 2002

Williams M, Teasdale J, Segal Z, et al: The Mindful Way Through Depression. New York, Guilford, 2007

Wright JH, Basco MR: Getting Your Life Back: The Complete Guide to Recovery From Depression. New York, Touchstone, 2002

Note.   Appendix 2 is available at: www.appi.org/pdf/62362.

Personal Accounts of Mental Illness

Duke P: Brilliant Madness: Living With Manic Depressive Illness. New York, Bantam Books, 1992

Jamison KR: An Unquiet Mind. New York, Knopf, 1995

Nasar SA: A Beautiful Mind: The Life of Mathematical Genius and Nobel Laureate John Nash. New York, Touchstone, 1998

Shields B: Down Came the Rain. New York, Hyperion, 2005

Styron W: Darkness Visible: A Memoir of Madness. New York, Random House, 1990

Improving Sleep

Edinger J, Carney C: Overcoming Insomnia: A Cognitive Behavioral Approach—Therapist Guide. New York, Oxford University Press, 2008

Hauri P, Linde S: No More Sleepless Nights. Hoboken, NJ, Wiley, 1996

Jacobs G, Benson H: Say Good Night to Insomnia: The Six-Week, Drug-Free Program Developed at Harvard Medical School. New York, Owl Books, 1999

Morin CM: Relief From Insomnia: Getting the Sleep of Your Dreams. New York, Doubleday, 1996

Managing Psychosis

Freeman D, Freeman J, Garety P: Overcoming Paranoid and Suspicious Thoughts. London, Robinson, 2006

Mueser KT, Gingerich S: The Complete Family Guide to Schizophrenia. New York, Guilford, 2006

Romme M, Escher S: Understanding Voices: Coping with Auditory Hallucinations and Confusing Realities. London, Handsell, 1996

Turkington D, Kingdon D, Rathod S, et al: Back to Life, Back to Normality: Cognitive Therapy, Recovery and Psychosis. Cambridge, UK, Cambridge University Press, 2009

Web Sites

General Information on Psychiatric Treatment and/or CBT

- Academy of Cognitive Therapy
  www.academyofct.org

- Depression and Bipolar Support Alliance
  www.dbsalliance.org

- Depression and Related Affective Disorders Association
  www.drada.org

- Massachusetts General Hospital Mood and Anxiety Disorders Institute
www2.massgeneral.org/madiresourcecenter/index.asp
- National Alliance on Mental Illness
www.nami.org
- National Institute of Mental Health
www.nimh.nih.gov
- University of Louisville Depression Center
www.louisville.edu/depression
- University of Michigan Depression Center
www.depressioncenter.org

Psychoeducation for CBT

- MoodGYM Training Program
www.moodgym.anu.edu.au

Helping Persons With Psychosis

- Hearing Voices Network
www.hearing-voices.org
Provides practical advice for understanding voice hearing.
- Gloucestershire Hearing Voices & Recovery Groups
www.hearingvoices.org.uk/info_resources11.htm
Provides examples of coping skills for voice hearing.
- Paranoid Thoughts
www.paranoidthoughts.com
Gives helpful advice on coping with paranoia.

Improving Sleep

- www.cbtforinsomnia.com
Provides interactive CBT Web-based program.
- www.helpguide.org/life/insomnia_treatment.htm
Provides psychoeducation about insomnia, cognitive-behavior therapy and relaxation tips, sleep diary, and links to other sites.
- www.sleepfoundation.org
Has available podcasts, videos, print materials about different types of sleep disorders, and online sleep store.

Online Support Groups

- Depression and Bipolar Support Alliance
  www.dbsalliance.org
- Walkers in Darkness (for people with mood disorders)
  www.walkers.org

Computer-Assisted CBT Programs

- Beating the Blues
  www.beatingtheblues.co.uk
- FearFighter: Panic and Phobia Treatment
  www.fearfighter.com
- Good Days Ahead: The Multimedia Program for Cognitive Therapy
  www.mindstreet.com
- Virtual reality programs by Rothbaum and associates
  www.virtuallybetter.com

Resources for Relaxation Training and Practice

- Benson-Henry Institute for Mind Body Medicine (audio CD)
  www.massgeneral.org/bhi
- Letting Go of Stress: Four Effective Techniques for Relaxation and Stress Reduction (audio CD by Emmett Miller and Steven Halpern)
  Available from various music vendors
- Progressive Muscle Relaxation (audio CD by Frank Dattilio, Ph.D.)
  www.dattilio.com
- Time for Healing: Relaxation for Mind and Body (audio set by Catherine Regan, Ph.D.)
  Bull Publishing Company
  www.bullpub.com/healing.html

Appendix 3

CBT Educational Resources for Clinicians

Courses and Workshops

- Annual Meeting of the American Psychiatric Association
  www.psych.org
- Annual Meeting of the Association for Behavioral and Cognitive Therapies
  www.abct.org
- Annual Meeting of the American Psychological Association
  www.apa.org

Certification in CBT

- Academy of Cognitive Therapy
  www.academyofct.org

Extramural Fellowship

- Beck Institute for Cognitive Therapy and Research
  www.beckinstitute.org

Computer-Assisted CBT Training

- Praxis
  www.praxiscbtonline.co.uk

Recommended Reading List

Barlow DH, Cherney JA: Psychological Treatment of Panic. New York, Guilford, 1988

Basco MR, Rush AJ: Cognitive-Behavioral Therapy for Bipolar Disorder, 2nd Edition. New York, Guilford, 2005

Beck AT, Rush AJ, Shaw BF, et al: Cognitive Therapy of Depression. New York, Guilford, 1979

Beck AT, Emery GD, Greenberg RL: Anxiety Disorders and Phobias: A Cognitive Perspective. New York, Basic Books, 1985

Beck AT, Freeman A, Davis DD, et al: Cognitive Therapy of Personality Disorders, 2nd Edition. New York, Guilford, 2004

Beck J: Cognitive Therapy: Basics and Beyond. New York, Guilford, 1995

Chadwick P: Person Based Cognitive Therapy for Distressing Psychosis. Chichester, UK, Wiley, 2006

Clark DA, Beck AT, Alford BA: Scientific Foundations of Cognitive Theory and Therapy of Depression. New York, Wiley, 1999

Frank E: Treating Bipolar Disorder: A Clinician's Guide to Interpersonal and Social Rhythm Therapy. New York, Guilford, 2005

Frankl VE: Man's Search for Meaning: An Introduction to Logotherapy. Boston, MA, Beacon Press, 1992

Haddock G, Slade PD (eds): Cognitive Behavioral Interventions with Psychotic Disorders. London, Routledge, 1996

Kabat-Zinn J: Full Catastrophe Living: Using the Wisdom of Your Body to Fight Stress, Pain, and Illness. New York, Hyperion, 1990

Kingdon D, Turkington D: A Case Study Guide to Cognitive Therapy for Psychosis. Chichester, UK, Wiley, 2002

Kingdon DG, Turkington D: Cognitive Therapy of Schizophrenia. New York, Guilford, 2005

Romme M, Escher S: Making Sense of Voices: A Guide for Professionals Who Work With Voice Hearers. London, Mind, 2000

Safran J, Segal Z: Interpersonal Processes in Cognitive Therapy. New York, Basic Books, 1990

Segal Z, Williams JMG, Teasdale JD: Mindfulness-Based Cognitive Therapy for Depression: A New Approach to Preventing Relapse. New York, Guilford, 2002

Sudak D: Cognitive Behavioral Therapy for Clinicians. Philadelphia, PA, Lippincott Williams & Wilkins, 2006

Wright JH, Thase ME, Beck AT, et al (eds): Cognitive Therapy With Inpatients: Developing a Cognitive Milieu. New York, Guilford, 1992

Wright JH, Basco MR, Thase ME: Learning Cognitive-Behavior Therapy: An Illustrated Guide. Washington, DC, American Psychiatric Publishing, 2006

Wright JH, Turkington D, Kingdon DG, et al: Cognitive-Behavior Therapy for Severe Mental Illness: An Illustrated Guide. Washington, DC, American Psychiatric Publishing, 2009

Appendix 4

DVD Guide

Instructions

Place the DVD in a DVD player or a computer with a DVD drive. A title page will be displayed. Select **Next** to view the Menu screens with video titles listed. Select individual videos to view as desired.

If you are viewing the DVD on a personal computer, control options such as Menu, Pause, Play, or DVD Properties should be displayed. If they are not displayed, clicking on the right mouse button will often provide control options.

The "DVD Menu" or "Disc Menu" button on your DVD player remote control or on your computer control options (as described above) can be selected while you are viewing video illustrations to return to the Menu screens for the video titles. Alternatively, you can fast forward through each video to reach the end of the illustration and return to the Menu screens.

Video Illustrations

Number	Title	Time (minutes)
1	A Brief CBT Session: Dr. Wright and Barbara	12:05
2	Modifying Automatic Thoughts I: Dr. Sudak and Grace	10:40
3	CBT for Adherence I: Dr. Wright and Barbara	10:46
4	CBT for Adherence II: Dr. Turkington and Helen	9:13
5	Behavioral Methods for Depression: Dr. Thase and Darrell	10:48
6	Modifying Automatic Thoughts II: Dr. Sudak and Grace	7:28

Video Illustrations (*continued*)

Number	Title	Time (minutes)
7	Generating Hope: Dr. Thase and Darrell	11:00
8	Breathing Retraining: Dr. Wright and Gina[†]	7:08
9	Exposure Therapy I: Dr. Wright and Rick	10:52
10	Exposure Therapy II: Dr. Wright and Rick	7:30
11	CBT for Insomnia: Dr. Sudak and Grace	10:07
12	Working With Delusions I: Dr. Turkington and Helen	12:38
13	Working With Delusions II: Dr. Turkington and Helen	8:24
14	Coping With Hallucinations: Dr. Turkington and Helen	9:45
15	CBT for Substance Abuse I: Dr. Thase and Darrell	12:10
16	CBT for Substance Abuse II: Dr. Thase and Darrell	9:40
17	Breaking Through Procrastination: Dr. Sudak and Grace	8:11
18	Helping a Patient With a Medical Disorder I: Dr. Sudak and Allan	12:24
19	Helping a Patient With a Medical Disorder II: Dr. Sudak and Allan	5:16
	Total time	**186:05**

[†]Video Illustration 8 is used with permission from Wright JH, Basco MR, Thase ME: *Learning Cognitive-Behavior Therapy: An Illustrated Guide*. Washington, DC, American Psychiatric Publishing, 2006. Copyright © 2006 Jesse H. Wright, M.D., Ph.D.

Index

*Page numbers printed in **boldface** type refer to tables or figures.*
Those followed by "n" indicate footnotes.